COMPUTER-BASED INSTRUCTION IN MILITARY ENVIRONMENTS

DEFENSE RESEARCH SERIES

Volume 1 Computer-Based Instruction in Military Environments
Edited by Robert J. Seidel and Peter D. Weddle

Computer-Based Instruction in Military Environments

Edited by

ROBERT J. SEIDEL
U.S. Army Research Institute
Alexandria, Virginia

and

PETER D. WEDDLE
Hay Systems, Inc.
Washington, D.C.

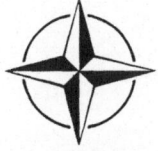

PLENUM PRESS • NEW YORK AND LONDON
Published in cooperation with NATO Defense Research Group

Library of Congress Cataloging in Publication Data

Computer-based instruction in military environments / edited by Robert J. Seidel and Peter D. Weddle.

    p. cm. — (Defense research series; v. 1)
  Based on the proceedings of a symposium held Apr. 15-17, 1985, in Brussels, Belgium.
    "Published in cooperation with NATO Defense Research Group."
    Bibliography: p.
    Includes index.
    ISBN-13:978-1-4612-8243-3   e-ISBN-13:978-1-4613-0915-4
    DOI: 10.1007/978-1-4613-0915-4

  1. Military education—Europe—Congresses. 2. Military education—North America—Congresses. 3. Computer-assisted instruction—Europe—Congresses. 4. Computer-assisted instruction—North America—Congresses. 5. North Atlantic Treaty Organization—Armed Forces—Congresses. I. Seidel, Robert J., date. II. Weddle, Peter D. III. NATO Defense Research Group. IV. Series.
  Q505.C66   1987
  355'.007—dc19   87-16610
                                                                                                                     CIP

Based on the proceedings of a symposium by NATO Defense Research Group Panel VIII on Computer-Based Instruction in Military Environments, held April 15-17, 1985, in Brussels, Belgium

© 1987 Plenum Press, New York
Softcover reprint of the hardcover 1st edition 1987

A Division of Plenum Publishing Corporation
233 Spring Street, New York, N.Y. 10013

All rights reserved

No part of this book may be reproduced, stored in a retrieval system, or transmitted in any form or by any means, electronic, mechanical, photocopying, microfilming, recording, or otherwise, without written permission from the Publisher

FOREWORD

This collection of papers is the result of a symposium sponsored by NATO's Defense Research Group Panel VIII in the Spring of 1985. The symposium came into being when it became obvious to the NATO countries that research, development and utilization of advanced technologies for training was the best means of increasing both training effectiveness and efficiency.

This symposium was the second in a series of three devoted to training. The series was structured to cover all aspects of training. The first series addressed the value of training, the second one dealt with the application of training technologies and the third and last of the series focused on academic issues concerned with the effect of prior learning on subsequent learning.

The fact that a major American publisher has determined that computer based instruction is the technology of greatest interest to the NATO community is not surprising. Advances in microprocessor technology have revolutionized both how and where we train. During this symposium there were a limited number of carefully chosen exhibits to demonstrate the various applications of computer based training techniques. In the following papers you will find both a practical and scientific basis for the way current and future training and training systems should be designed, applied and utilized.

We know that training must be done faster and more effectively. Computer based instruction can save up to 30 percent in time compared to conventional methods. When this savings is translated into financial and other resources it can be substantial. However, it was also realized during the symposium that depending on what and where we are training, this savings might have to be used for retraining. In other words, if the material learned is not retained adequately there is not going to be a real savings. This particular payoff should be viewed with some caution and greater effort should be expended on the many payoffs of computer based instructional techniques.

As you study these papers be aware that they are only part of the many research projects that currently support this burgeoning computer based training effort. During the symposium we were constantly reminded that computer based instruction is a rapidly growing industry. Its potential applications exceed what is now being considered by the user. The increased use of expert systems, voice recognition and synthesis, flat panel displays, high density memory devices, automated curriculum development, computer graphics and imagery video discs, and touch sensitive surfaces all provide the opportunities for using computers to provide better education and training. However it is obvious from these papers that there is still much to be done in the future to use what we have and will soon have available.

There were 35 papers submitted to this symposium. Unfortunately, only 24 could be accepted for presentation (23 of which appear in this volume, -ed.), supplemented by 2 invited addresses, due to time limitations. The fact that NATO sponsored such a symposium series emphasizes the importance of training. Expensive weapon systems are only of value to those paying the bill when they are operated and maintained correctly. To have this occur requires proper training and retention of that specialized skill. These papers demonstrate how far we have progressed in the area of training using microprocessor based capabilities. As the present and past chairmen of the NATO panel which sponsored this series we are appreciative of the scientific rigor displayed by the academic, industrial and military experts who are devoted to improved training.

                                              Capt. Paul Chatelier
                                                Office of the U.S. Secretary
                                                    of Defense

                                              Professor R. Bernotat
                                              Chairman of NATO Defense
                                              Research Group Panel VIII

PREFACE

The papers which follow demonstrate both the importance of training to the preparedness of the NATO Alliance and the truly international character of advances being made in human science research. Our intent in editing this volume is to extend the awareness of those two facts.

We would like to thank the authors of the papers for their cooperation and contribution to the development of this book. We have made every effort, including the use of their English translations, to preserve the exact word and essence of their presentations. Our thanks go, as well, to Patricia M. Ryan, Joanne Pomponio, Carol-Ruth Korch and Jessie McVean for their assistance in the preparation of the manuscript.

> Dr. Robert J. Seidel
> U.S. Army Research Institute for the
>   Behavioral and Social Sciences
>
> Mr. Peter D. Weddle
> HAY Systems, Incorporated

CONTENTS

An Overview of Computer-Based Instruction in Military Environments . . .   1
   C.L. Wiggs and R.J. Seidel

INTELLIGENT CAI

An Intelligent Computer Assisted Instruction System for Maintenance
     Training 11
   L.H. Nawrocki

The Conversion of an Expert System to an Intelligent CAI System 21
   S.J. Bevan and P.R. Wetherall

Self-Organised Learning within an Intelligent Teaching System 29
   R.R. Todd

Portable, Intelligent Simulation for ASW Training 41
   E.D. McWilliams and G.L. Ricard

DEVELOPMENT OF PROTOTYPES

CAITER: A Computer-Based Instruction Terminal 59
   A. Brebner, H.J. Hallworth and G. McKinnon

The Use of Computers in Training in the British Army 69
   D.K. Dana

Weapon Training and Simulation 89
   C. Saint-Raymond

CBI in the Royal Air Force: A Case Study of Two Part-Task Trainers . . . 95
   M.E. Court and D.A. Sharrock

Development of a Prototype Computer-Based Testing and Assessment
     System 105
   E.J. Anastasio and R. Serotkin-Getty

IMPLEMENTATION AND EVALUATION

Implementation of Computer-Based Training: A System Evaluation and
     Lessons Learned 145
   J.Y. Yasutake

Evaluating New Technology: Formative Evaluation of Intelligent
     Computer-Assisted Instruction 155
   E.L. Baker

AIDS TO RESOURCE USAGE, RESOURCE SHARING AND AUTHORING

Online Help: Design Issues for Authoring Systems 163
   T.M. Duffy and M.D. Langston

A User-Maintained Database for Trainers in Military Environments 179
   A. Meyers

Computer-Based Instruction in the Department of Defense: Enhancing
   Application of the Technology 197
   J.F. Funaro and N.E. Lane

Turning Educators into Authors: A Case Study in the Acquisition of
   Authoring Skills 203
   A.L. Droar and A. Kennedy

RESEARCH IN TRADITIONAL AND NON-TRADITIONAL ENVIRONMENTS

New Frontiers for Computer Aided Training 215
   G.P. Noja

The Development and Test of a Hand-Held Computerized Training Aid . . . 231
   R.A. Wisher

Consideration of Instruction and Training in Human Operator Models . . . 239
   J. Marguin

Computer-Assisted Programmed Cases: A Learning Method for Improving
   the Understanding of Persons 249
   L. Van den Brande

Electronic Delivery of Job Performance Aids 261
   W.E. Hartung

NEW THEORY

Video-Game Technology and Training Research 271
   C. Heaton

Experience-Consolidation Systems: A Sketch of a Theory of
   Computer-Based Instruction in Ill-Structured Domains 285
   R.J. Spiro

The Use of Intelligent Authoring Tools to Enhance CBI in Technical
   Training 293
   R.S. Perez and R.J. Seidel

INVITED ADDRESSES

Cognitive Science, Artificial Intelligence and Complex Training 313
   W. Feurzeig

Authoring Tools: Past, Present, and Future 331
   G. Kearsley

Index 341

AN OVERVIEW OF COMPUTER-BASED INSTRUCTION IN MILITARY ENVIRONMENTS[1]

C. L. Wiggs and R. J. Seidel

U.S. Army Research Institute
Alexandria, Virginia, U.S.A.

INTRODUCTION

This chapter is based on presentations made at the Computer Based Instruction symposium, however the presentations have been expanded upon, or amended, in order to become current. The chapter sketches the history of Computer Based Instruction (CBI) and provides a rationale and context for NATO interest in CBI in military training. Lastly, it focuses on highlights of issues to be covered in the subsequent chapters.

In general, the purpose of the symposium was to: 1) describe the current state-of-the-art in Computer Based Instruction in military environments, 2) identify implementation issues, 3) highlight high-gain areas, and 4) identify advanced technologies that will soon be available.

BACKGROUND

The history of Computer-Based Instruction can be traced back to the work of Pressey (1927) and Skinner (1958) on "teaching machines." Briefly, teaching machines were designed to provide response sensitive feedback to each student. Thus, the machines provided interactive, individualized learning experiences. Although the teaching machines were successful for teaching simple mathematics and spelling, when it came to learning, which required more complex and less straightforward responses, the machines had to be modified. A great deal of modification has taken place in the transformation from the rudimentary teaching machines to Computer-Based Instruction (CBI). Nevertheless, computers are just beginning to have a truly significant impact on public education and the training realm.

Kearsley, Hunter, and Seidel (1983) examined two decades of CBI projects, reviewing over 50 major CBI projects in terms of their theoretical and practical significance to the field of education and training. The review, which encompassed experiments, demonstrations,

---

[1]The opinions expressed in this chapter represent the opinion of the authors and in no way reflect any official position of the U.S. Army.

theory, innovation, and invention, provides ample evidence that computers can be used in educational ways compared to "traditional instruction" (i.e., classroom lectures, text, actual equipment). The problems inherent in a traditional classroom environment generally stem from the lack of interaction between the instructor and individual student. The pace is set for the imaginary "average" student; thus, the progression through the course is generally too fast or too slow for many of the students. The latter group of students may become bored and many not fulfill its potential. The former group, however, is of particular concern, in that it can never actually "catch up." As most courses are designed in a hierarchical fashion (Gagne, 1977), the slower students must understand the concepts presented earlier in the course before they can understand the more complex concepts presented later. Furthermore, individual questions cannot always be attended to by the instructor in the traditional classroom environment.

The introduction of CBI increases the opportunity for student-instructor interaction due to individualizing instruction. Each student has the equivalent of a private tutor attending to his particular learning progress on a dedicated basis. The major applications of computers to education and training have traditionally been in testing, student management (i.e. computer-managed instruction), drills/tutorials (i.e. computer-assisted instruction), simulations/games, and guidance (Kearsley & Seidel, 1985). The success of these CBI applications has been demonstrated across a wide range of limited instructional applications and types of learners in the domains of education and training.

One of those instructional domains which has revealed progress and provides promising prospects for CBI is military training. Since the early 1960s military services have supported research and development of CBI as a means for meeting "the training mission" (i.e. to provide a high quality product). Effectively managed training has been referred to as "the key to readiness and successful soldier and team performance" (United States Army Research Institute [USARI], FY 1987-1991), but accomplishing the training mission is neither a simple nor an inexpensive task. Training costs are increasing steadily and the modern military systems are becoming more complex. Yet higher levels of performance must be generated at a lower, or at least constant, cost.

Historically, the complex systems in the military have resided with the flight trainers (e.g., Cream, Eggemeier, & Klein, 1978; Smode, 1974) since about 1920. When the first flight trainers appeared, they were used for training military pilots. With the development of commercial aviation, flight simulators became more widely used. In the more recent years in the military, operation and maintenance of all kinds of equipment and systems has become increasingly common (e.g., Farrow, 1982). Now that computers are becoming more and more part of the work place in all of the military environments computer-based simulators are becoming increasingly relevant to the military training process.

The military training situation poses different instructional problems than those in public and private schools. One difference is that the methods of instruction that are cost effective for the military may not be cost effective for other learning environments (Orlansky & String, 1981). In the educational domain, students remain at school for required periods of time and are not paid while there. The schools, then, receive no direct benefits for instructional methods which result in faster student progress. The focus is on student achievement in a fixed time interval. The military, on the other hand, has emphasized the feasibility of saving student time while maintaining a high level of student achievement, for military personnel receive pay and allowances while they are in training school. Thus, any procedure that can reduce the time required for training, without significantly affecting the amount or quality of information acquired by the students, can reduce the cost of training. Furthermore, upon graduation from training schools, military personnel are assigned to operational commands where they receive on-the-job, team-and-unit, and field-exercise training. These types of training strongly influence military readiness. Thus, it is beneficial for personnel to increase the amount of time spent in operational assignments during their military careers.

Specific problems have been noted in the present U.S. military training which need to be addressed (USARI, FY 1987-1991). First, despite the availability of remedial programs, U.S. soldiers continue to have inadequate basic skills (reading, writing, math, and language). Furthermore, literacy problems are not restricted to entry level soldiers. Skill deficiencies also develop as soldiers advance to new jobs requiring higher levels of literacy. Considering the fact that current remedial programs for U.S. Military have been unsuccessful, either new approaches must be made in teaching basic skills, or instruction must be presented in an alternative medium (i.e. non-verbal). Secondly, training programs are also needed to improve essential combat skills. It has been noted that soldier skills in detection, recognition, identification, and acquisition of targets need improvement as well as the use of small arms systems (soldier and weapon).

The future poses new problems with the evolution of a future military environment. The impact of high-technology weapons and navigation instruments is crucial. However, the advanced performing capabilities built into new military systems will be realized only if military personnel are adequately trained to properly operate and maintain these complex systems. New training concepts and programs are needed, as are cost saving procedures for rapidly updating databases and materials for the user and maintenance communities.

In general, the military's training programs are strained by reductions in training time available, yet there is an increased need for highly skilled personnel to maintain, repair, and use complex, high-technology weapon systems. Furthermore, there is a greater emphasis on training to higher standards. However, training resources, such as instructors and ranges, fuel, and ammunition for field training, are becoming scarce. The challenge is to provide more effective training using fewer resources.

CBI has the potential to meet this challenge, particularly in noting the following trends which have occurred; there has been a dramatic increase in the level of computer availability and usage due to the prevalence of microcomputers and the commercial availability of educational software (i.e. courseware). This has lowered the costs of CBI to fit within the budget range of most training departments. The recent involvement of major U.S. publishers in the software industry is beginning to produce a wide selection of educational and training software. Furthermore, the improvement in the input and output capabilities of computers has increased the potential for all forms of instruction. Even inexpensive microcomputers are capable of color-graphics displays, touch input via joysticks, light pens, graphics tablets, or a mouse, sound and speech generators, and function keys. The most recent machines feature high-resolution displays for screen partitioning (windowing) and can display different type styles (Kearsley & Seidel, 1985).

Taking all of what has been stated into account, the feasibility is high that CBI holds the promise to offer a cost-effective training solution for the problems existing in the military environment. It is appropriate therefore to appraise the existing use of computers for military training and to make prognoses for the future. It was in this context that the NATO Symposium on CBI in the military took place.

THE SYMPOSIUM FOCUS

The NATO Symposium on CBI in military environments brought together experts in academic, industrial, and military environments from the participating countries. One hundred and twenty-five representatives participated in the symposium. Twenty-four papers were delivered (23 of which appear in this volume, -ed.), supplemented by two invited addresses.

The classification scheme ordering the presentation of the papers originated as a means of organizing Kearsley et al.'s (1983) review of research studies and programs conducted in the CBI domain. Six significant areas emerged relevant to NATO: 1) the development of prototypes, 2) major implementations and evaluations, 3) aids to resource usage, resource sharing and authoring, 4) intelligent computer assisted instruction (ICAI), 5) research in traditional and non-traditional environments and 6) new theory. These areas will be described below.

The Development of Prototypes

This category encompassed projects which have led to the development of hardware, software, and courseware of new CBI systems. Some of the early systems which served as models for successive CBI systems include the adaptive models in drill-and-practice programs (Suppes, Jerman, & Brian, 1968), an interactive problem-solving system that provides tutorial assistance (Barr, Beared, & Atkinson, 1975), a speech synthesis system (Sanders, Benbassat, & Smith, 1976), along with three major systems: PLATO, IBM 1500, and TICCIT. The research significance of most of the prototype systems was that they provided opportunities for a large number of individuals to gain practical experience with CBI, often in operational settings. In the NATO context, several projects exemplified the developments in international military training. For example, the use of computers as simulators in the field has been a successful new area. Specifically, Saint Raymond (Chapter 8, this volume) reported a prototype of computer-based weapon simulators installed directly on the weapon system for the French Army. Also, Court and Sharrock (Chapter 9, this volume) described combining simulation and instruction as part-task trainers in the Royal Air Force.

Prototypical technology with video capabilities (e.g. videodiscs and better computer graphics) and audio developments (e.g. voice input and output) have enhanced the trainee learning station. Brebner, Hallworth, and McKinnon (Chapter 6, this volume) described a prototype CBI terminal which incorporates these facilities in a multimedia form instead of relying on text.

Major Implementations and Evaluations

This category covered projects which have involved large-scale implementation of CBI and their corresponding evaluations. Generally, these implementations have taken place in regular classrooms and involved years of usage. A number of different types of CBI evaluations have been conducted ranging from qualitative to quantitative, formative to summative, and descriptive to comparative. In general, most CBI evaluations have been methodologically weak since they are done according to real world constraints. However, the general conclusions from implementation projects and their evaluations have been that CBI on a large scale was both effective and practical under the appropriate conditions. Baker (Chapter 12, this volume) substantiated this claim with an evaluation of CBI which encompassed three different training projects; each focused on different types of users (maintenance technicians, college freshmen, and elementary students) and different types of training tasks.

One of the major benefits demonstrated by CBI implementation projects is the reduction in student course time (Orlansky & String, 1981). Yasutake (Chapter 11, this volume) reported a significant time savings by comparing conventional and computer-based training for several technical training courses in the U.S. Air Force. The study covered a four-year demonstration period with 20,000 students. Along with the benefits of CBI, implementation and evaluation of CBI have also identified problems which arise and need to be attended to (these problems will be covered later).

Aids to Resource Usage, Resource Sharing, and Authoring

A great deal of attention has been devoted to the dissemination and sharing of information and ideas -- in the CBI field. Meyers (Chapter 14, this volume) described a system for disseminating information via nine different user-maintained data bases for trainers. The data base provides a clearinghouse for information on training. Besides the user of computer resources as a means for delivering information, this section also covers the dissemination of CBI information and materials.

The problems of NATO countries are to (a) know what instructional materials, software, and hardware systems exist in other countries, and (b) be able to benefit from these resources via networking, satellites, conferences, and publications. Major efforts have been made in the U.S. to document the available CBI Software and Courseware (e.g. the ENTELEK CAI/CMI catalog; Lekan (1968); and Wang (1976)) as well as to publish periodicals which evaluate the quality and effectiveness of CBI software/courseware (e.g. Journal of Courseware Review). Funaro and Lane (Chapter 15, this volume) addressed CBI resource sharing via networking in the U.S. Department of Defense. The network provides a central clearinghouse system for CBI information and courseware access. A mechanism for accomplishing this in NATO could be the expansion of bilateral data exchange agreements already begun. Incompatibility of different systems still represents a major obstacle to widespread sharing of courseware.

A major area of research unique to CBI has been the development of author languages and systems for creating interactive programs. Author languages and authoring systems were primarily designed to make the development of instructional lessons easier and to encourage the transportability, and thus, the sharing of courseware. Author languages provide a set of features especially suited to the kind of programming environment in which very little, if any, actual programming is needed. Instead, the author provides the subject matter and instructional logic via conversational interactions (i.e. prompting) or some type of menu/form driven approach. Most major CBI systems have their own author language or authoring systems, but a number of efforts has been made to develop system independent author languages (e.g. PILOT). Several presentations identified user resistance to CBI as a result of confusion due to the proliferation of languages, architectures, and authoring systems. The authoring issue was addressed by Droar and Kennedy (Chapter 16, this volume) in a computer-based education and training project at Chichester College of Technology. The project's results revealed that user friendliness was a key element in successful acquisition of authoring skills by educators. Duffy (Chapter 13, this volume) addressed the needs of the user in his design of a dynamic on-line help system embedded in the authoring system.

Avner (1979) suggested that authoring languages do increase the efficiency of CBI development. However, there is little evidence which supports the premise that author languages would improve courseware sharing. One drawback of author languages or authoring systems is that they have sometimes constrained the author to relatively narrow models of instructions.

Intelligent Computer-Assisted Instruction (ICAI)

ICAI departs from the other CBI systems in that ICAI programs derive from the study of computer science (specifically Artificial Intelligence) instead of instructional psychology. Thus, ICAI programs are fundamentally different in their structure and function. Specifically, ICAI programs involve knowledge networks which are acted upon by tutoring rules in order to generate student dialogs or problems. They are "mixed initiative" in nature; that is, either the student or the computer can take the initiative in proposing a question or idea. Foremost, the programs use sophisticated student models that allow them to understand what the student is/is not learning. It is this capability to understand what is being taught and why a student makes a mistake that makes ICAI programs "intelligent."

Several projects were presented concerning the development of ICAI systems, each suggesting a unique function. Nawrocki (Chapter 2, this volume) presented the merits of an ICAI system for maintaining training which serves as a diagnostic decision aid for the trainee. Bevan and Wetherall (Chapter 3, this volume) described the project of converting an expert system into an effective tutoring system. Todd (Chapter 4, this volume) has applied learner control of instruction in the context of a methodology called "Self-Organised Learning" within the existing framework of an Intelligent Teaching System. Finally, Ricard and McWilliams (Chapter 5, this volume) reported on a microcomputer in which a combination of simulation, computer-assisted instruction, and an embedded rule based expert system was developed as a portable aircrew trainer for the U.S. Navy.

ICAI demonstrates the kind of individualized instruction which computers are truly capable of providing, and is considered one of the most promising areas of current CBI research. The major obstacles which must be overcome in order to make a full impact in current training institutions include offering suitable ICAI systems with improved pedagogical models at affordable prices and a wider availability of ICAI expertise and knowledge.

Research in Traditional and Non-Traditional Environments

There has been a significant increase in research on improving training effectiveness as well as student learning styles. A current focus has been on creating novel learning environments for the student, often using graphics, simulations, and interconnected microcomputer networks. For example, Noja (Chapter 17, this volume) presented a computer aided training approach used by Gajon Systems which incorporated a terminal placed at the master desk for the instructor, connected with multiple lines to each student station-microcomputer.

Efforts to demonstrate that computers can be used as a tool of the student have developed alternatives to the original philosophy of CBI in which computers were a tool of the instructor used to deliver information.

CBI projects have also had access in non-traditional teaching environments (i.e. outside of the classroom). Microprocessor based portable systems developed for the U.S. Army were described by Wisher and Hartung as being advantageous in that they can deliver technical training to soldiers at flexible times in varied locations. Wisher (Chapter 18, this volume) described the portability of the hand-held tutor as useful, in that trainees may practice skills in situations when time is generally wasted (e.g. during transportation, waiting in line, etc.). Hartung (Chapter 21, this volume) presented a description of a prototype electronic job aid, called Personal Electronic Aid for Maintenance (PEAM), which has been effective in that useable technical information is delivered at the work site where maintenance is performed. Although there are only a few non-traditional places of CBI, they offer evidence of how CBI could fundamentally change the location of training and therefore our current military training institutions. The NATO countries could benefit greatly from synthesis of the research in both traditional and non-traditional environments.

New Theory

This category includes work in CBI which has directly or indirectly resulted in the generation of new instructional and cognitive theories. A number of new areas in instructional theory, such as adaptive testing Anastasio (Chapter 10, this volume) and the use of simulations and games in instruction Heaton (Chapter 22, this volume), have emerged because of CBI. New instructional models specifically developed for CBI have emerged which take into account the special capabilities of interactive instruction. In fact, Spiro (Chapter 23, this volume) suggests that the capabilities of CBI should be taken advantage of to prepare trainees for the novelty and complexity of the real world (i.e. ill-structured domains) rather than abstract, well-structured kinds of instruction.

GENERAL DISCUSSION

Whereas the technological advances in CBI are important, a general panel discussion concerning the future of CBI emphasized that work on how to use these advances is most important. There was little disagreement with the current assertion that CBI is not a "thing"; it is a tool. By itself it is inert; the use of the computer technology amplifies human teaching abilities and makes CBI a powerful instructional vehicle. Thus, the phrases commonly heard, such as "CBI has not truly fulfilled its potential" or "the promise of CBI has not been realized" are not so much a result of technological lag. Rather, the common ground among the panel members was that the major issues of the future were not technological (with the exception of ICAI), but instead the primary issues were identified as implementation, quality instruction, and the application of better cognitive science theories within the CBI context.

Implementation

Yasutake's experience at the U.S. Air Force Human Research Lab suggests that the promise of CBI has not been realized because of practical, organizational issues. Although CBI is demonstrated as a useful technique, there are few examples of large scale implementations. Thus, the issues of the future have to do with: 1) why this is so, 2) what can be done about it, and 3) what is necessary in order to make CBI more widely used within the military organizational community.

An implementation issue which surfaced in Yasutake's paper concerned users' reactions. Although students reacted favorably to CBI, the instructors reacted negatively. Thus, the resistance of individual instructors to CBI is an important implementation issue. Dana's presentation of the application of CBI at the Royal Signals Trade Training School revealed similar findings to those of Yasutake regarding instructor resistance to CBI: instructor attitudes had to be changed for successful use of the computer to occur. The potential value of computer use for cost-effective part-task simulation in operator training (as well as the potential gains in using embedded training on the operational computer and expert systems, or AI, for maintenance training) is indicated in Dana's paper given that these resistances can be overcome.

In general, the strong resistance to change is a problem that CBI has always faced. Overcoming this resistance is a challenge for widespread use of CBI. Seidel described one approach in the U.S. Army, called Training Technology Field Activities (TTFAs), to overcome this problem. TTFAs are new efforts designed as a partnership between the research, training-policy, and user communities. They hold promise as a model to bridge the gap between proof of the technologies and their use in U.S. Army schools.

Quality Instruction

Kearsley also discussed the problems concerning implementation; particularly the unsuccessful implementation of the individualized approach of CBI into the context of the current training structure, which is group based. A related issue, according to Kearsley, is how to retrain currently employed staff members to effectively and appropriately use computers in training. The nature of training educators has traditionally centered on content rather than on the use of computers as tools to teach effectively. The principal issue, Kearsley asserts, is how to motivate instructors to provide quality instruction. It is important to tackle the issue of what makes teaching programs good or bad, lest there be a danger of wasting a major technological investment. Feurzeig also emphasized the need for quality instruction within CBI and further specified that, although much of the current research emphasizes prescriptive or tutorial aspects, it is also important to have guided practice.

To summarize, CBI should be an effective tool for delivering quality, individualized instruction. Despite two decades of research in CBI, however, researchers know very little about how to individualize instruction, nor do they understand much about the effects of major instructional variables underlying CBI (Kearsley et al., 1983). Whereas most instructional theory has been developed from traditional instruction (most of which is presented via text), CBI offers completely different variables to examine and distinct powers of its own. CBI, combined with new video/computer graphic imagery techniques, has the potential to combine the qualities of instruction available in both pictorial and digital or verbal modes. Thus, there is a need for new instructional theories, new courseware development tools and techniques. An important step for the development of effective courseware is to use a teamwork process among subject matter experts, teachers, and designers of instruction, where each provides unique and complementary knowledge for the development of better instruction. Resource sharing and networking of updated information about CBI is important for the development of quality instruction and is beginning to be disseminated. Furthermore, quality courseware is becoming more accessible.

The development of instructional theories and courseware will continue to change in parallel to the advancement of evolving CBI systems. Automation of instructional development will play an important part in improving quality and efficiency in the instructional process. For example, Kearsley noted, while conducting research on this system, that each instructional activity has two parts: the first is the mechanical-clerical activity, which generally involves rearranging or tabulating data and is easy to automate. The second is a true cognitive activity, which is judgmental and experimental in nature. The latter is harder to automate, as well as being the activity we know the least about theoretically or from the instructional science point of view. It is this activity where artificial intelligence (or ICAI) has been required and investigated.

Cognitive Theories

Where Kearsley implied that cognitive and instructional theories may evolve as we continue to research CBI systems, Spiro suggested an opposite approach; i.e. work on cognitive and instructional science theories is needed to guide the development of future CBI. He asserted that, for better training to occur, we must have a clearer idea of the purpose and nature of the training, which should be guided by a cognitive model of how knowledge is structured in the individual. Although Spiro continues to narrow this discussion by putting forth "the apprentice model as an appropriate model of instruction," his original point suggests that there should be more than a one-way interaction between designers and users of CBI systems, re-emphasizing the gap which exists between research and implementation. Cognitive theorists, designers of instruction, and those who use (or implement) CBI systems must communicate, so that CBI will be nurtured to evolve within the "cybernetic" process.

Sociological Differences

The importance of communication is also evident in identifying cross-cultural differences between the various NATO countries. Discussion brought up the following sociological differences:

First, it was suggested that there may be more of an emphasis on individualizing instruction in the United States, whereas the United Kingdom expressed the importance of team training. Although spokespersons of the U.S. agreed that social interaction and group processes are important components of effective instruction, they agreed that there may be too strong an emphasis on individualizing instruction in the U.S.

Second, a spokesperson from the United Kingdom suggested that the military populations being taught may differ between countries. In the U.S. military, several CBI implementations have taken into account the fact that military personnel generally have low-literate skills (Spiro, Hartung). Training, then, has been adapted accordingly (such as decreasing the importance of the written word in training). A spokesperson from the United Kingdom brought to the attention of the Symposium that this is not an issue with the Royal Navy, as the entrance standards are very high in the military of the U.K. The work presented by Kennedy and Droar, however, demonstrated that low level literacy is an issue in the U.K. with (Chichester) Community college students. Although the populations within the U.K. are different (military students in Royal Navy/college students at Chichester), it does suggest low-level literacy is a factor that may need attention within different areas within each country.

The third sociological difference noted concerns the future results of advancing technologies. Spokespersons from the Royal Air Force and the Royal Navy of the U.K. and the Netherlands Air Force agreed that as the aircraft gets smarter, we need a lower lever technician to maintain them. Thus, there could be a reduction in training time. Spokespersons from the U.S., on the other hand, asserted that more complex technology in military systems will demand that maintenance requirements be addressed by more intelligent people at some level, perhaps in the system design stages. It will be the designer's responsibility to develop systems that allow the user to maintain applications without being exposed to the internal complexity of the system.

In short, the present selection of research is broad enough to render a good picture of the contemporary state of CBI in military environments. It is a dynamic state, given the technological advances which were covered. Nevertheless, it is apparent that the understanding and implementations of such systems are still in their infancy.

REFERENCES

Avner, R. A. (1979). Production of computer-based instructional materials. In H. F. O'Neil, Jr. (Ed.), "Issues in instructional systems development." New York: Academic Press.

Barr, A., Beard, M., & Atkinson, R.C. (1975). A rationale and description of a CAI program to teach the BASIC programming language. "Instructional Science," "4," 1-31.

Cream, B. W., Eggemeier, F. T., & Klein, G. A. (1978). A strategy for the development of training devices. "Human Factors," "20," 143-158.

Farrow, D. R. (1982, March). Reducing the risks of military aircrew training through simulation technology. "NSPI Journal," 13-18.

Gagne, R. M. (1977). "The conditions of learning" (3rd ed.). New York: Holt, Rinehart, & Winston.

Kearsley, G., Hunter, B., & Seidel, R. J. (1983, January). Two decades of computer-based instruction projects: What have we learned? Part 1. "THE Journal," "10(3)," 90-94.

Kearsley, G., Hunter, B., & Seidel, R. J. (1983, February). Two decades of computer-based instruction projects: What have we learned? Part 2. "THE Journal," "10(4)," 90-96.

Kearsley, G., & Seidel, R. J. (1985). Automation in training and education. "Human Factors," "27(1)," 61-74.

Lekan, H. (1968). "Index to computer-assisted instruction." Milwaukee: University of Wisconsin.

Orlansky, J., & String, J. (1981, Second quarter). Computer-based instruction for military training. "Defense Management Journal," 46-54.

Pressey, S. L. (1927). A machine for automatic teaching of drill material. "School and Society," "25," 1-14.

Sanders, W. R., Benbassat, G. V., & Smith, R. L. (1976). Speech synthesis for CAI: The MISS system and its applications. "ACME SIGCUE Bulletin," "8," 208-211.

Seidel, R. J., & Kearsley, G. (in press). The impact of computers on human learning. In J. Zeidner (Ed.), "Human Productivity Enhancement." New York: Praeger Press.

Skinner, B. F. (1958). Teaching machines. "Science," "128," 969-977.

Smode, A. F. (1974). Recent developments in instructor station design and utilization for flight simulators. "Human Factors," "16," 1-18.

Suppes, P., Jerman, M., & Brian, D. (1968). "Computer-assisted instruction: The 1965-66 Stanford arithmetic program." New York: Academic Press.

U.S. Army Research Institute. (FY 1987-1991). Science and technology plan. "Train the force" (Sections 3-3 to 3-48). Alexandria, VA: Author.

Wang, A. (1976). "Index to computer-based learning." Milwaukee: University of Wisconsin.

AN INTELLIGENT COMPUTER ASSISTED INSTRUCTION SYSTEM FOR MAINTENANCE TRAINING[1]

L. H. Nawrocki

Xerox Training Center
Leesburg, Virginia, U.S.A.

This chapter describes an ongoing, joint military and industrial project to develop and evaluate a prototype Intelligent Computer Assisted Instruction model (ICAI) for maintenance training. The project is directed toward determining the potential of ICAI as a means for ameliorating the increasingly adverse impact of economic, demographic and technology sophistication factors on the life cycle maintenance of complex systems. In addition, the project is anticipated to establish a foundation for the time and cost reduction of follow-on ICAI development efforts.

Maintenance Training Issues

As weapon systems become more complex, the capability to maintain these systems using traditional maintenance approaches has become concurrently more difficult and, typically, more costly. To alleviate this situation improvements have been made in engineering design techniques to increase the reliability of equipment and to provide built in diagnostic aids.

While engineering improvements have partially alleviated the maintenance problem, they have not eliminated the need for skilled maintenance personnel. Specialized skill training in the U.S. Army accounts for more than 50% of the annual training load and absorbs nearly $1.5 billion in delivery cost, with both load and cost expected to continue increasing (Military Manpower Training Report for FY 85, 1984). Ironically, the use of built-in diagnostics can often also increase the skill level required of maintenance technicians as the technician is left with the intermittent and interactive malfunctions beyond the scope of most diagnostic or job performance aids.

Improved accuracy in the selection of high ability individuals is another approach which can assist in reducing the training burden.

---

[1]The project discussed in this chapter was supported in part by the Army Research Institute for the Behavorial and Social Sciences under contract number MDA903-83-C-0189. The views and opinions expressed are those of the author and do not necessarily represent the policies of the Army Research Institute for the Behavorial and Social Sciences of the U.S. Government.

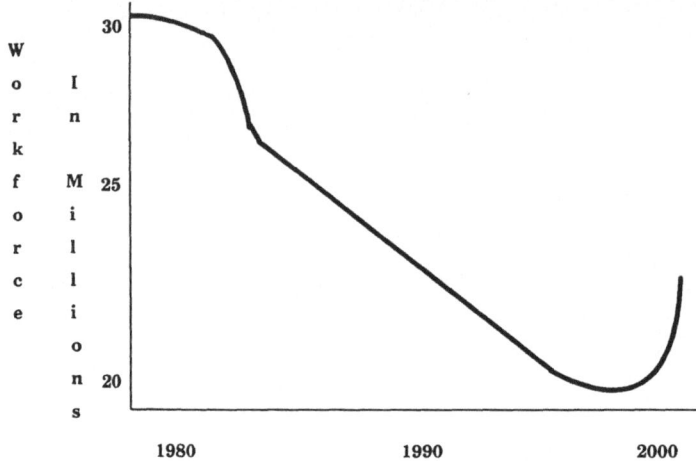

Figure 1. Available Workforce Projections

However, both this approach and the reliability engineering approaches are faced with a demographic counterforce. Figure 1 shows the downward trend in new workers available to enter the labor force (18-24 years of age) through the 1990's (Psotka, J.). Given this projection, it is unlikely that engineering or selection techniques alone can overcome the requirement for increased training.

The industrial experience in maintenance training has been analogous to that of the military. The cost of skilled labor has soared and the impact of a reduced labor force is beginning to exacerbate the problem. To remain competitive, both engineering improvements and increased use of diagnostic aids (both built-in and as adjuncts to the technicians "tool bag") have been initiated. The focus is on reducing unit manufacturing cost (hence profit or competitive price) while maintaining competitive levels of reliability. As in the military, these approaches may only partially address the problem.

Additional hardware components and software development costs for internal diagnostics may be more costly than obtaining and training technicians on a projected unit cost basis. On the other hand, the use of a higher proportion of lesser skilled technicians, supported by both internal and external job aids, may result in job dissatisfaction and hence a personnel turnover rate as costly as the savings in training reduction.

Thus, albeit with somewhat different measures of success, both the military and industrial environments are faced with demographic and cost variables negatively impacting on equipment maintainability. Engineering, selection and job aiding improvements do not necessarily eliminate the need for training. Finally, current training techniques do not adequately provide the level of expertise required at an acceptable cost.

ICAI Potential

One promising technology for more rapidly increasing individual knowledge and skill is that of Intelligent Computer Assisted Instruction (ICAI). An outgrowth of artificial intelligence research, particularly "expert systems", ICAI combines the delivery system advantages of computer instruction with the instructional advantages of a live, expert tutor. Expert, or "knowledgeable" computer based systems have reached the stage of

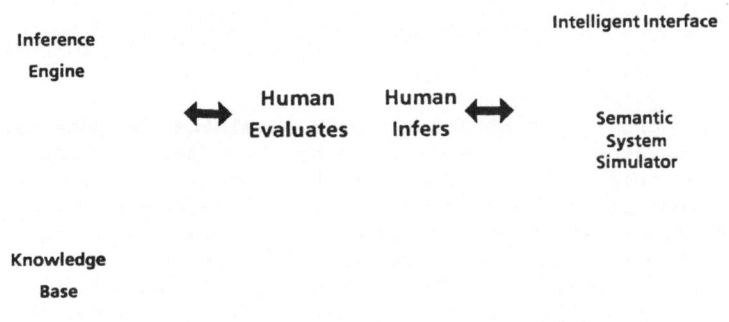

Figure 2. Alternative Expert System Approaches

cost effective application as decision aids, at least in limited domains (Winston, L.H. & Prendergast, K.A., 1984); D.'Ambrosio, B., 1985). The use of analogous technology as the basis for an instructional system has been demonstrated but, as yet, has not been rigorously evaluated as an effective application technique (Roberts, F.C. & Park, O., 1983).

In the somewhat oversimplified sense, traditional expert systems differ from ICAI systems as depicted in Figure 2. Expert systems per se, typically require the construction of a large set of rules (if...then) which serve as a knowledge base. The result of employing these rules is evaluated via a set of combinatorial algorithms, or inference engine. The result is a specification of a problem solution(s) with a probability of solution accuracy and a summary of the steps or rationale leading to that solution. The human user evaluates the solution and can introduce additional data to determine the influence of new data on probable solutions.

While an ICAI System can be similarly constructed, the differing role of the human suggests an alternative model. As the human assumes the role of making inference, the knowledge base link is via an intelligent interpreter or interface. The interface acts as an experienced tutor, responding to queries, providing guidance and "observing" behavior. Moreover, in the domain of diagnostic maintenance (troubleshooting) the knowledge base can be a semantic network of machine functions. That is, rather than a large set of rules, a machine can be described by a set of objects (components) and the parameters (values) associated with those objects as a function of their current state (operating status). A detailed discussion of expert system construction is provided in Hayes-Roth, Waterman and Lenat (1983).

Using the preceding model, the learner can experiment with the system, creating and testing hypotheses and developing an individualized strategy. The system acts as both a functional simulator and a mechanism for causal explanation. Thus, the system combines the advantages of simulation and an active learning environment. As the learner is able to compress discoveries normally experienced only by lengthy on-the-job exposures, it is possible for the learner to more rapidly develop skills associated with an expert.

The impact of compressed learning is that which underlies the rationale for the use of traditional training devices and simulators. The addition of an artificial intelligence capability should have even greater potential for decreasing the time to transition from novice to expert and increasing the probability of making this transition.

PROJECT DESCRIPTION

The current project is directed toward examining the potential of ICAI for improving maintenance training based on the model previously described. The project was initiated in December 1983 as a three phase effort. The goal is to evaluate both an ICAI development methodology and the training effectiveness of the system in an actual training environment. The task is focused on training sophisticated diagnostic skills for complex equipment. The first phase of the project addresses the content model of the ICAI simulation system. The second and third phases emphasize integration of the simulation with an instructional strategy and evaluating the training effectiveness, respectively.

Phase I: Content Model

The first phase was targeted toward selecting, analyzing and developing the core semantic simulation system. The Xerographic engine of the 1075/1090 copier was selected on the basis of being a complex electro-mechanical system requiring diagnostic logic representative of such systems in general; a significant, but manageable subsystem ; and a central part of the copier diagnostic training program. As a parallel effort during Phase I, a more traditional simulation was developed from a previous microcomputer based simulation project. Although this latter simulation represented a different copier, the similarities were sufficient to examine the feasibility of: developing a surface level diagnostic simulation and integrating this with the 1075/1090 deep simulation; and converting an existing fixed outcome simulation into a generic simulator using artificial intelligence techniques. Hardware for the development was the Xerox 1108, Workstation with a 1.5 MB, bit-mapped display system. Software was InterLisp, a version of Lisp which is embedded in a programming environment using windows, menus and powerful editing tools.

Technical Approach Following the determination and selection of the Xerographic engine as a testbed for the ICAI system, parallel efforts were initiated to analyze the physical engine properties and to explore training contexts appropriate for insertion of ICAI. Existing documents describing the Xerographic process were used to develop a preliminary description of the engine from both an engineering and troubleshooting standpoint. Experts (instructors) were then interviewed and later exposed to the preliminary simulation and asked to modify the design based on the causal (qualitative) determiners of how the machine functions and to describe the semantic rationale (explanation) of procedural diagnostic strategies. This process continued iteratively through Phase I.

To ascertain the appropriate training program applications, interviews were conducted with the technical training program managers, curriculum developers and instructors. Specific to the 1075, in addition, a member of the project team went through the existing training course as a student. This interview/participant information was analyzed in the context of course documentation. The outcome was a set of activities which could be matched against desirable features of the core simulation.

Results Figure 3 shows a somewhat schematic version of the current physical display. In actuality, the components are depicted more

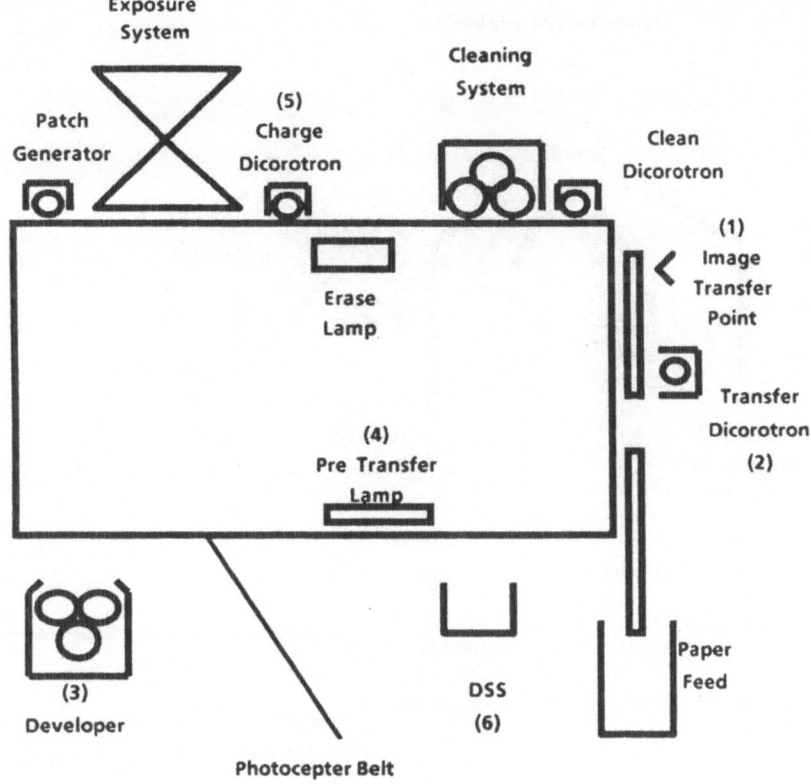

(N) = Components involved in "Paper Image Light" qualitative reasoning

Figure 3. Xerographic Model

realistically and the "belt" (the rectangular central box in Figure 3) moves around the components, changing electron charge and image pattern as appropriate. The troubleshooting model can be described as evidence, symptom, cause. In this model, physical evidence is interpreted in the light of formal knowledge or experience to specific symptoms; e.g., an inappropriate darkened area on the paper, or streak, is evidenced by such symptoms as constant width and being parallel to the paper travel direction. These symptoms can, in turn, be inferred as caused by the malfunction of one or more components (again through formal knowledge or experience). A cognitive prediction can be made that if component "x" is malfunctioning, it ought to produce an outcome leading to symptom "y". This prediction can be "tested" mentally, or by actually "fixing" the component. Although a bit more complicated than this description, the point is that a continuing observe, infer, hypothesize, test and evaluate loop can be implemented. Figure 4 shows one possible problem in the context of too light an image. The causal chain requires an inference about spatially related entities (solid line arrows) and logically related qualities (dotted line arrows). The numbers alongside the elements in Figure 4, show that the particular problem could involve any one of the components labeled correspondingly in Figure 3.

The overall system thus permits the student to: construct a "mental model" by exploring the simulation, thus forming symptom-cause maps; transfer previous knowledge by relating back to similar subsystems; develop

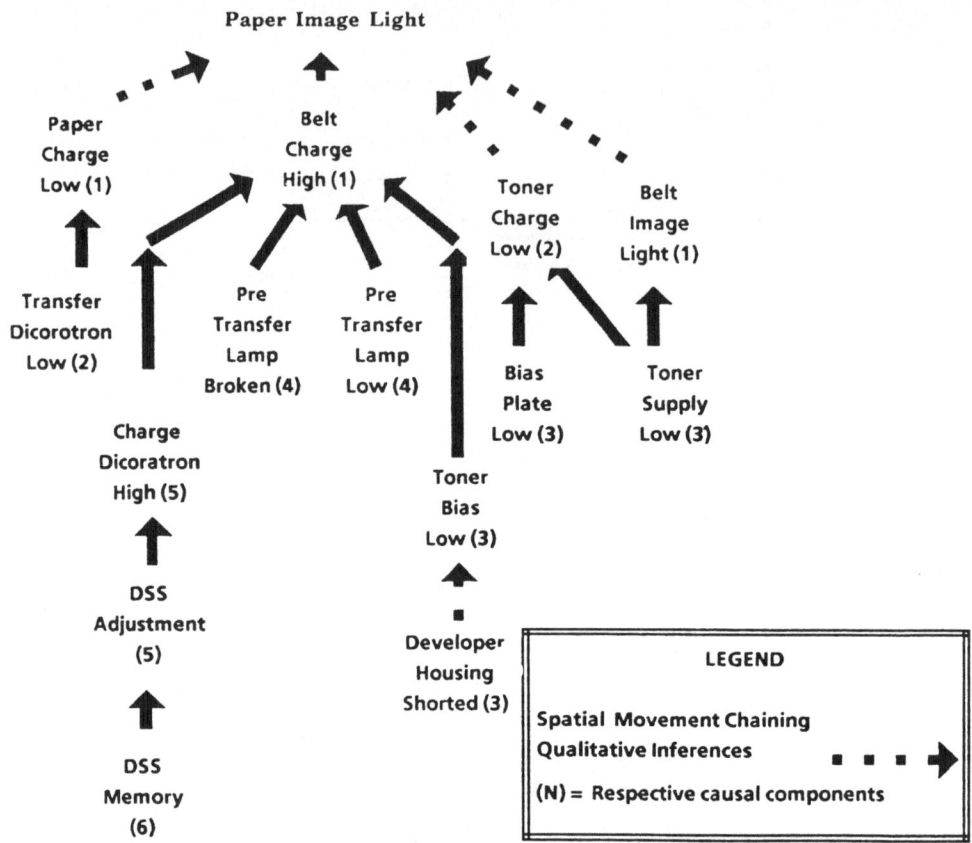

Figure 4. Causal Reasoning Chain for "Paper Image Light"

the general troubleshooting skills of recognizing symptoms via the collection of evidence, relate causes to predicted symptoms (backward chaining) and determine the information value of checks and tests. In other words, all those activities which form the set of cognitive knowledge and strategy known as expertise.

In the case of the surface model simulation, the emphasis was to develop a simulation of the "outside" of the entire copier to be used in conjunction with diagnostic job aids (referred to as Fault Isolation Procedures, or FIPS). In part, this development was suggested by a two part approach to troubleshooting strategy provided in the current service training program. The first strategy focuses on use of the FIP and emphasizes major module replacement for relatively noncomplex equipment. The second strategy combines FIP documents and an individual strategy based on generic knowledge and expertise. Given this distinction, the surface simulation was designed to reflect procedure following knowledge and the deep simulation oriented to problem solving skills. Linking these simulation levels would permit the notion of rapidly building expertise.

The training program situation turned out to be complicated by both timeliness and strategic planning factors. At the start of the project, major equipment and training were oriented to generic problem solving and conducted at a centralized training site - and this was the focus of the deep simulation development and evaluation plan. However, an increasing proportion of the training and equipment is now structured for FIP guided and machine specific maintenance and much of the training has been shifted to decentralized sites. In addition, while the development of curriculum remains at a central site, local variations are more likely to occur in training delivery. As a result, rather than develop an ICAI segment integrated with a particular machine, the project strategy was to rapidly install both simulation levels in a prototype version at test sites. Site users were asked to use the simulations as an addendum to existing training. The preliminary feedback suggested that there was a need to provide a more sophisticated version of output quality variations (print quality) and that a less complex deep simulation was required as an initial training entry point. This feedback was incorporated in Phase II.

Methodological Lessons   The issues arising and resolved during Phase I concerned primarily the distribution of labor in designing a core simulation and the dynamic nature of the classroom and field training programs. In part, the division of developmental labor was directed at determining the difficulty in using subject matter and instructional experts to develop ICAI simulations. This has turned out to be doable, but experience on this project suggests a 6-8 month learning curve before a reasonable ability to work in the hardware/software environment is attained. In addition, frequent interaction with "knowledge engineers" or cognitive psychologists is a necessity. Thus, our experience suggests that forming an ICAI applications team requires at least one experienced scientist and a 6 month minimum training period for dedicated instructional developers before initiating formal development.

The fluid training program environment has already been discussed in the Phase I Results section. Given the lengthy development time for a new ICAI system (processes learned in this project should permit reduction of this time, but a 12-18 month period appears reasonable), any such effort will require a more generic approach. An exception would be for training which is expected to be stable for 2-3 years, at least in terms of molar level objectives.

A final aspect of Phase I, less an issue than a challenge, has been to assist in the transfer of ICAI development to the U.S. Army technical personnel. Aside from project reviews and documents, this has been accomplished primarily by supplying a core Army technical team with both a comparable hardware/software environment and frequent on-site technical discussions. Suffice that the strategy is basically one of do it, show it, discuss it - i.e., a catalytic process.

Phase II: Instructional Model

Phase II was originally anticipated as development an overall instructional model for causal learning. As a result of Phase I user feedback, however, much of Phase II was directed at redesign of the conceptual simulations. Moreover, the maintenance community shift to more proceduralized skills required rethinking of the instructional goals. The focus for Phase II was turned toward developing a prototype training package which could be used to obtain information critical to final decisions for Phase III.

Technical Approach   To more rapidly prototype a field training package the xerographic simulation was revised to provide a more simplistic process simulation, but one which could be immediately integrated within the existing training program. The result was a basic xerography training module in which any one, or combination of, seven subsystems could be faulted to produce appropriate print output symptoms.

During this development, the effort required to embed the simulation with adjunct instructional supports (audiovisuals, instructor presented material and knowledge tests) made clear the need for on-line pedagogical tools. This led to the parallel development of a set of on-line developmental aids for creating, cross referencing and sequencing instructional materials. Concurrent with the xerographic simulation, the surface simulation was revised to include the use of an on-line analog multimeter simulation. At this point a natural divergence occurred. The xerographic process simulation evolved as a testbed to permit examination of alternative instructional strategies available through artificial intelligence cognitive models. The surface, FIP based, simulation became the testbed for evaluating software design structures for generic modeling of electronic circuits. Both simulations will permit the partial evaluation of instructional migration from procedural knowledge to problem solving skills.

Results The revised xerographic simulation was successfully piloted in two technical classes. In general, students were able to answer inference questions of the form described in the Phase I results. Students and instructors were very positive in their opinions on the utility of the simulation as a learning aid and the manner in which the simulation was integrated within the instructional context.

The surface simulation incorporating the multimeter and preliminary circuit generator were completed but the integrated capabilities remain to be tested.

The preliminary on-line instructional development aids are being balanced to include graphic and animation design tools and to permit computer-directed interface with peripheral training devices, to include videodisc. These tools are being packaged as an Instructional Development Environment (IDE) and will be used in Phase III development.

Methodological Lessons The most significant lesson during Phase II was the need for on-line develop tools. While not absolutely necessary, rapid prototyping for multiple ICAI simulations is unlikely without such tools. The ability to quickly design or redesign an ICAI module will enable the project team to iteratively examine and evaluate a variety of ICAI capabilities as opposed to focusing on a narrow, less generalized instructional domain.

Phase III: Evaluation

Phase III, not yet underway, is relatively simple to describe, but is the most difficult to structure and control. First, there is an interaction between that which is scientifically of interest and that which is possible in a real world training environment. This is true in either the military or industrial community and any new training technology is somewhat constrained by the operational need to get the job done. Below are five variables and the option for each, underlined options being those the project is focused upon and remaining options being those which may be examined should the resources and opportunity be present:

SITE:	Centralized	<u>Decentralized</u>
SKILL:	<u>Conceptual</u>	Procedural
TRAINEE:	Expert	<u>Novice</u>
CONDITION:	Controlled	<u>Field</u>
ICAI SYSTEMS:	<u>Integrated</u>	Independent

One potentially negative impact on the project is likely to become positive from the evaluation aspect. It is unlikely that the subsystems now being simulated will remain unchanged in the actual machines by the time formal evaluation is initiated. This is a typical real world situation though, and the test of the generalizable nature of the ICAI modeling approach is the degree to which the model can be rapidly updated. Our evidence to date is that this is a challenge which can be met, particularly as interface capabilities (e.g., IDE) are added to permit instructor modification of scenarios and internal system values without actual programming changes. One example is the feedback option. Learner feedback will make use of solution histories which are recorded as part of the interaction record. Based on the current state of this record, a number of semantic rationalizations, or dialogues, are candidates for evaluation in Phase III:

Task/Goal orientation:	"Since your goal is to accomplish XXX, you should next do YYY"
Conceptual Model orientation:	"XXX will effect YYY by accomplishing ZZZ, which in turn effects AAA and ..."
Human Cognition orientation:	"Now do XXX because you may otherwise forget/ misplace/ break/etc."
Contextual orientation	"You have insufficient parts/time/etc. to check XXX"

It is not clear at this stage of development how extensive feedback need be or will be. The tactics for developing this instructional interface will be largely dictated by field feedback on the prototype simulations. In addition, the ICAI systems are not proposed as stand-alone training systems, but are to be used in a context where basic knowledge has been provided by traditional means such that the learner is prepared for the discovery learning process. At this stage the most likely situation is instruction on surface simulations (FIP based) and transfer on a limited basis to the deep simulations. The major goal will be to permit a wider range of individualized experiences with new equipment than is currently possible using operational equipment.

Lastly, and most difficult, will be to extract meaningful measures of training transfer. Measures of performance relating to terminal training objectives are a given. What is being examined is the possibility of an additional set of longitudinal measures to evaluate impact, if any, on job performance. Currently, the primary job measure of interest is mean time to repair. Unfortunately, this measure is confounded in the field with numerous peripheral effects as a function of the particular site. We are now examining temporary measures which could be instituted in representative field locations with minimal disruption to operations.

SUMMARY

To date we have found that the major difference between implementing an ICAI approach, versus traditional instructional development, is that there is almost too much flexibility. In addition, the process is clearly more iterate and revise than what is recommended by existing instructional development models. As a result, the development of a simulation proceeds more rapidly than the corresponding instructional strategy. On the other hand, development of the simulation has proven to be more rapid than initially anticipated and permits the iterate/revise process in parallel with refinement of the training strategy.

REFERENCES

D'Ambrosio, B. (1985). Expert systems - myth or reality. "BYTE," 275-282.

Hayes-Roth, F., Waterman, D.A., and Lenat, D.B. (Eds.) (1983). "Building Expert Systems." Reading, MA: Addison-Wesley Publishing Company.

Psotka, J. "Personnel Communication," U.S. Army Research Institute for the Behavioral and Social Sciences.

Roberts, F.C. and Park, O. (1983). Intelligent Computer Assisted Instruction: An Explanation and Overview. "Educational Psychology," 7-11.

U.S. Department of Defense, (1984). "Military Manpower Training Report for FY 85."

Winston, P.H., & Prendergast, K.A. (Eds.) (1984). "The AI Business." Cambridge, MA: The MIT Press.

THE CONVERSION OF AN EXPERT SYSTEM TO AN INTELLIGENT CAI SYSTEM

S. J. Bevan and P. R. Wetherall

Royal Signals and Radar Establishment, MOD (PE)
Great Malvern, England

INTRODUCTION

   The process of building the knowledge base associated with an expert system is long and complex, and the information it contains very valuable. Most expert systems are designed to be used in a consultative manner by a non-expert in order to perform a task requiring expertise. The idea of using the same knowledge base in a tutoring role is very attractive.

   This approach has been adopted in the GUIDON system (Clancey, 1978) where the knowledge base from the MYCIN medical consultation system was used in a tutoring system. The implementation of GUIDON was difficult because the knowledge base needed to be augmented by rules that described the logical connections between rules in the knowledge base. The major drawback of the GUIDON was that its implementation was tied to the MYCIN knowledge base; in other words, there was little attempt to address the design of an intelligent tutoring system.

   An Intelligent Computer Aided Instruction (ICAI) system is one which uses knowledge based techniques in its implementation. Knowledge bases are used to represent the teaching domain and also to govern the operation of the instruction system. The advantages of this approach are twofold:

1. The use of a rule base to govern the operation of the instruction system enables the operational characteristics of the system to be easily modified.

2. Isolation of the domain dependent rules from the rules controlling the instruction system provides a generalised ICAI system which can be used for a variety of teaching domains.

   Such techniques have been used in the SOPHIE system (Brown, Burton, & Bell, 1977) and in the MENO-TUTOR system (Woolf & McDonald, 1984). The former is a single domain ICAI system for electronic troubleshooting; the latter is a generalised ICAI system which may be used for a variety of domains.

   As the Royal Signals and Radar Establishment (RSRE) has developed, and continues to develop, a variety of expert systems, an investigation into the problems of constructing a generalised ICAI system about an operational

---

© British Crown Copyright

expert system has been started. Not only is this seen as a way of capturing the knowledge base in the expert system for training purposes, but intelligent tutoring systems are also one way whereby operational staff can observe the performance of an expert system.

Originally the subject to be taught corresponded to a domain in which we already had an expert system shell and knowledge base. However, for operational reasons, a different domain, with similar characteristics, was chosen, and the knowledge base for the new domain prepared specifically to fit the expert system shell. Any conclusions we make about the conversion of an existing expert system should still be valid.

THE 'TUTOR' PROJECT

This generalised ICAI system is known as 'Tutor' (Davies, Dickens, & Ford, 1984) and is being implemented by LOGICA plc for RSRE. TUTOR is implemented in Prolog and runs on DEC VAX machines under the VMS operating system.

Initial development of the system was targeted at the rules which govern the driving actions to be taken at a set of traffic lights. This relatively simple domain was used to develop the TUTOR framework. The subject domain was then extended to cover certain aspects of motorway driving and rules for joining other roads taken from the United Kingdom's Highway Code. Examples in this paper will be taken from these domains as the subject matter is readily understood by most readers.

In parallel with the Highway Code implementation, RSRE has developed an expert system on the procedures used by Air Traffic Controllers when an aircraft is in an emergency. This expert system is now being integrated with the framework to produce a TUTOR system which teaches these emergency procedures. The performance of TUTOR in this domain will be assessed by educationalists later this year.

In the the section entitled "Tutor System Components," the main components of the ICAI framework are described. In the section entitled "Creating a New Tutoring Domain," we describe the work which needs to be done to create a new teaching domain for the TUTOR framework. The section entitled "Implementation" describes some of the implementation issues.

'TUTOR' SYSTEM COMPONENTS

General Structure

The overall design of the TUTOR framework derives from O'Shea's Five Ring Model (O'Shea, Bornat, Bouley, Eisenstadt, & Page 1981). In this, each interaction between TUTOR and student passes once round the cycle shown, in simplified form, in Figure 1. Based on the current assessment of the student's ability and knowledge, the teaching generator decides what kind of interaction to give the student next, e.g., exposition or problem to answer, and selects a particular topic to present. Directed by this strategy, it considers what has been presented in the past and provides the Administrator with all the detail needed to present a situation to the student, and if it is a problem, to the Domain Expert System (DES) for the correct solution. The Administrator interacts with the student through the Natural Language Interface (NLI), and can if necessary, pose subsidiary problems to the DES as a result of the student's own questioning. Finally each interaction with the student is recorded in the Student Model, so that the Teaching Generator can choose the next interaction.

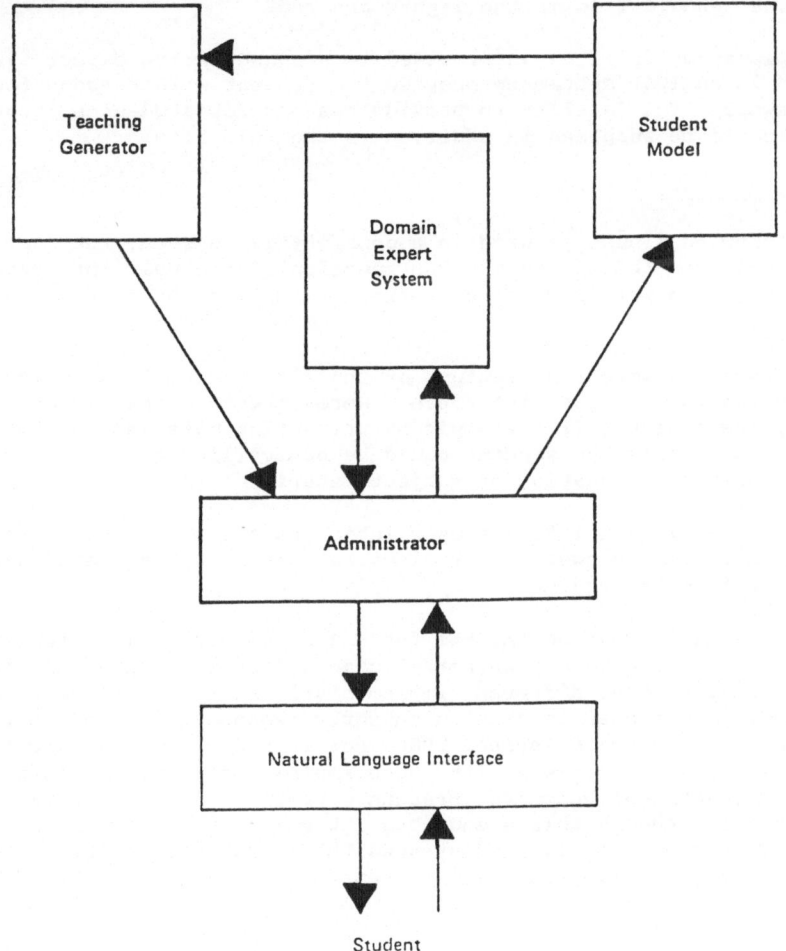

Figure 1. Overall Model of TUTOR

As well as the DES being a knowledge based component, the teaching generator, student model and NLI are being developed using knowledge based techniques. The TUTOR framework itself is thus an expert system in its own right, and should benefit from all the advantages claimed for the approach, in particular, relative ease of enhancing the rulebases of the individual components.

Domain dependency is limited to the DES itself, the knowledge base for the subject curriculum used by the Teaching Generator, and the vocabulary of the NLI. Student modelling, how to teach, and the structure of natural language, together with the Administrator, should all be domain independent and provide the generalised framework within which different subjects can be taught.

The Domain Expert System

This component of the ICAI system contains the domain specific rules as they would appear in a consultative expert system. Its function is to check that the student's answers can be used to answer queries that the student may pose to the system. For example, the student may ask supplementary questions about a scenario generated by the system:

'What should I do if the lights are red?'

The explanation facility as provided in a consultative expert system can be used in an ICAI system to provide the student with reasons for correct answers. The facility to provide reasons for student's incorrect answers needs to be supplied in addition to the rule base.

The Natural Language Interface

When a knowledge base is used in a consultative system, the user has little control over the dialogue. The function of the user interface in such a system is to get from the user the information the system needs to form a conclusion.

By contrast, an important feature of the ICAI system is what is known as a 'Mixed Initiative' user interface. Here, the teaching system could be controlling the dialogue (for example by presenting material and asking questions). Similarly the student could be controlling the dialogue by asking for further explanation of subject material.

To provide a mixed initiative user interface and also to give the user freedom in expressing answers to problems, a fairly sophisticated natural language interface is required.

One extra requirement on the NLI for a generalised ICAI system is to be able to modify the vocabulary when the subject domain is changed. At the time of writing, several different implementations of the NLI have been tried including augmented transition networks (Woods, 1970) and definite clause grammars (Pereira & Warren, 1980) but it has proved relatively difficult to change vocabulary with these implementations. It is thought that Lexical Functional Grammars (Bresnan & Kaplan, 1982) may provide a better solution although this avenue has not yet been explored. For the current TUTOR system, we have sidestepped the issue by simplifying the interface altogether, adopting menu driven techniques.

The Student Model

The function of the student model is to maintain a record of the student's knowledge of the subject domain. It can also be used to hold information about the student's preferred teaching strategies and level of expertise. In our ICAI system we currently recognize just three classes of student: complete novice, experienced, and competent but needing revision.

During observations of human tutors, it became apparent that the tutor taught 'clusters' of rules. For example a general principle would be presented and then the exceptions to the principle. In our student model we record the student's comprehension on two levels, concept belief and cluster belief. In the current implementation we simply record either success or failure at a given concept or cluster.

The Teaching Generator

The function of this component is to provide initial, corrective and revision teaching on individual topics in the syllabus, and also to generate problems for the student to solve which are consistent with the student model and the curriculum of material to be presented.

The curriculum for a given domain is represented by a 'Genetic Graph' (Goldstein, 1982). Concepts and rule clusters are represented as nodes in a network and directed arcs represent how the tutor is to progress between topics given the student's success or failure at earlier topics.

The teaching generator will determine the nature of a problem to present to the student and a number of constraints on the problem. The student will be asked questions on the unconstrained parts of the problem. For example in the traffic lights domain, the teaching generator may decide to test knowledge of driving actions when the road is wet and the car is near the lights. This leaves the state of the lights as an unconstrained part of the problem and the system is able to generate questions like:

'The lights are red, what would you do?'

CREATING A NEW TUTORING DOMAIN

Protocol Analysis

For each of the subject domains that we have implemented, we have made extensive studies of the dialogue between a human tutor teaching the subject material and the student. Analysis of these communication protocols between the tutor and the student provides much useful information for the domain dependent parts of the TUTOR system. This step seems equivalent to the Systems Analysis of conventional ADP.

Tailoring The NLI

Protocol analysis enables a domain specific vocabulary to be created. In addition, the forms of sentences used by a human tutor in teaching the subject can be found.

The Genetic Graph And Student Model

Protocol analysis also yields much of the information necessary to structure the genetic graph. First of all, the subject domain is broken down into the various components and the logical dependencies between the components can be found. This creates the syllabus for the teaching domain and also provides the structure of the student model. Finally, by observing how the human tutor moves through the domain, the structure of the genetic graph may be completed.

The Domain Expert System

For each subject domain, an expert system, complete with knowledge base, needs to be supplied. For the domains we have implemented to date, this knowledge base has been specially prepared. The domains have been in areas where the rule base is of a "legislative" nature and have shared a common expert system structure. The domains are also characterised by the need to perform a series of actions in the correct sequence, such as checking the mirror before indicating a turn.

If the domain rule base also provides an explanation facility, then this can be used by TUTOR to provide reasons for 'correct' answers to problems. Since conventional expert systems do not need explanations for 'incorrect' conclusions, we have found it necessary to provide a set of reasons to explain why a student's wrong answer to a given problem is incorrect.

General Knowledge Of The Domain

When the student is presented with a problem, the student may wish to query certain aspects of the problem. Some aspects will be directly related to the information that TUTOR is trying to get from the student; others may be added by TUTOR to create a more interesting problem. If the student should query any aspect, TUTOR needs to be able to provide some sort of answer.

For example: If TUTOR creates a problem where the road has become wet, the following dialogue may arise:

>STUDENT: 'I thought the road was dry.'
>TUTOR: 'There has been a shower.'

We have gone some way to providing general knowledge of the domain in the Traffic Lights and Highway Code prototypes. The more the TUTOR is to handle general queries, the more 'Human' it becomes.

However, this facility requires an adequate NLI as an available component. As discussed above, the Emergency Procedures domain has a driven input capability, so the provision of general knowledge in this domain has not been tackled.

In general, we would expect this part of the domain to come out of the protocol analysis which would identify likely aspects for the student to query. Appropriate knowledge could then be inserted into the knowledge base for explanations. The automatic generation of suitable responses ('there has been a shower') to queries and statements ('I thought the road was dry') about the general nature of the domain would require a capability in reasoning and justification which is not available 'off the shelf' and unlikely to be for many years yet.

IMPLEMENTATION

The structure of the DES is simplicity itself, and is based upon the concept of a sequence of actions to be followed in given circumstances for some particular objective, such as turning off a road – check mirror, give the turn signal, take up position for turn, give way to pedestrians, make the turn, etc. Each particular set of circumstances corresponds to a scene, and scenes are grouped together to describe an action sequence.

Two data structures are needed to implement this method:

1. A set of scene variables is associated with each action sequence together with the value of each variable defining a particular scene.

2. For each action, there is a rule which:

    - Identifies the particular scene(s) for which the action is valid

    - Checks that prerequisite actions have been executed

    - Changes the state of scene variables associated with the execution of the action

    - Changes the sequence if necessary

The ability to change the value of scene variables allows the system to run free within an action sequence without requiring external inputs. Extending this mechanism to permit changes of sequence enables a whole series of action sequences to be followed.

This formalism defines a particular kind of expert system which is capable of taking (recommending) a course of action according to a particular set of values for the external environment. There is nothing in the formalism which links the DES to the TUTOR system, although implementing TUTOR has caused it to diverge somewhat from the structure developed originally in RSRE.

Two particular extensions to the structure have been required to integrate the DES with TUTOR:

1. The rule defining each action is associated with the concepts that should have been grasped if the student is to identify the correct action given the particular scene.

2. A natural language interface to present scenes to the student, as well as the explanation system, has had to be provided.

Textual material for the presentation of scenes can be generated automatically for the majority of situations provided suitable names for actions, scene variables and their values, are chosen. We have not yet developed a satisfactory method of providing explanations automatically, as the DES does not necessarily include the underlying justification in its rule base, e.g., why it is necessary to look in the mirror before turning. Extension protocol analysis can also show up the errors made by students, so that particular explanations of why erroneous responses are wrong can be added to the knowledge base.

Thus the interface between DES and TUTOR consists of a definition of scene variables, the values of these which define individual scenes, the concepts associated with each action, and the textual material to present situations and justify actions.

CONCLUSIONS

The TUTOR system is still in its infancy and we have only just begun to tackle the problems of creating teaching systems for knowledge bases. Our work so far has shown that a sophisticated NLI is highly desirable for a 'human-like' TUTOR but its implementation is difficult.

There is scope for a better student modelling capability that records more than the student's success or failure at a given concept.

A long term goal of the TUTOR project is to be able to take knowledge bases which form part of advice giving systems and incorporate the rules into TUTOR and establish the links into the teaching material of TUTOR. With the present formalisms, it would be necessary to make the representation of the rule base conform to the one used by TUTOR.

A set of tools for creating the domain specific components of TUTOR could be envisaged in the future, but even the feasibility of this idea is open to debate. For some time to come, the creation of a teaching system from a rule base will be the task of an expert 'Teaching Engineer' in the same way that the creation of a rule base is the task of the 'Knowledge Engineer'.

ACKNOWLEDGEMENTS

Our thanks are due to Sue Middleton, also of RSRE, who developed the original expert system shell and who has continued to take an interest in its progress, and also the the Logica team - Nigel Davies, Simon Dickens,

Lindsey Ford and Rod Rivers – who have worked valiantly in all aspects of the implementation of TUTOR, as well as to all those who have assisted us in the knowledge engineering of the emergency procedures domain.

REFERENCES

Bresnan, J., & Kaplan, R. (1982). Lexical-functional grammar: A formal system for grammatical representation. "The mental representation of grammatical relations." Cambridge, MA: MIT Press.

Brown, J.S., Burton, R., & Bell, A. (1977). SOPHIE: A sophisticated instructional environment for teaching electronic troubleshooting. "International Journal of Man Machine Studies," "7."

Clancey, W. (1978). Tutoring rules for guiding a case method dialogue. "International Journal of Man Machine Studies," "11."

Davies, N.G., Dickens, S.L., & Ford, L. (1984). TUTOR: A prototype ICAI system. "Proceedings of Expert Systems 84." England: Warwick University.

Goldstein, I.P. (1982). The genetic graph: A representation for the evaluation of procedural knowledge. "Intelligent tutoring systems." Academic Press.

O'Shea, T., Bornat, R., Bouley, B. du, Eisenstadt, M., & Page, I. (1981). Tools for designing intelligent computer tutor. "Proceedings of 1981 NATO Conference on Human and Artificial Intelligence." North Holland.

Pereira, F., & Warren, D. (1980). Definite clause grammars for language analysis – A survey of the formalisms and their comparison with augmented transition networks. "Artificial Intelligence," "13(3)."

Woods, W. (1970). Transition network grammars for natural language analysis. "CACM," "13(10)."

Woolf, B., & McDonald, D.D. (1984, September). Building a computer tutor. "IEEE Computer."

SELF-ORGANISED LEARNING WITHIN AN INTELLIGENT TEACHING SYSTEM

R. R. Todd

Admiralty Research Establishment
Teddington, Middlesex, U.K.

INTRODUCTION

Ideally computer-based instruction should combine the flexibility of a gifted personal tutor with the consistency of a machine. The gifted teacher brings qualities of perceptiveness and responsiveness to the tutorial interaction which make it possible for instruction to be tailored to the personal and changing needs of the learner. This is a major aim of Intelligent Teaching Systems (Sleeman & Brown, 1982), which are being developed at the Admiralty Research Establishment, Applied Psychology Unit (APU). This paper reports research on the application of the theory and methodology of Self-Organised Learning (Thomas & Harri-Augstein, 1985) to the development of an Intelligent Teaching System. The domain, submarine command tactics, is simulated in a war game HUNKS, an abbreviation of HUNter Killer Simulation.

AN INTELLIGENT TEACHING SYSTEM

The skeleton framework of the Intelligent Teaching System (ITS) is shown in Figure 1 (Sheppard, 1981). The learner is able to engage in HUNKS play via the Interface; this interface also serves for the communication of instructional guidance and support from the Support Generator to the learner. The system is able to make its support intelligible to the learner, by virtue of its knowledge of him/her as a HUNKS player. This knowledge is acquired by the Modeller by direct interrogation of the learner during game play through the interface, which is simultaneously observed by the Modeller. The interrogation results in the construction of a Model of the learner as a HUNKS player. The system also includes a Referent model with which the Learner model may be compared in the Model Comparator. This Referent Model may represent an expert player of HUNKS. If this Expert has an authoritative status within the instructional programme, it can provide a goal for the instruction. In this case, the learner's skill as a HUNKS player is evaluated against the Expert model, and the Support Generator operates to reduce or eliminate the difference between the Learner model and the Expert model. It is worth noting that the domain expertise, represented in the Expert model, is functionally distinct from the instructional expertise, supplied by the Support Generator.

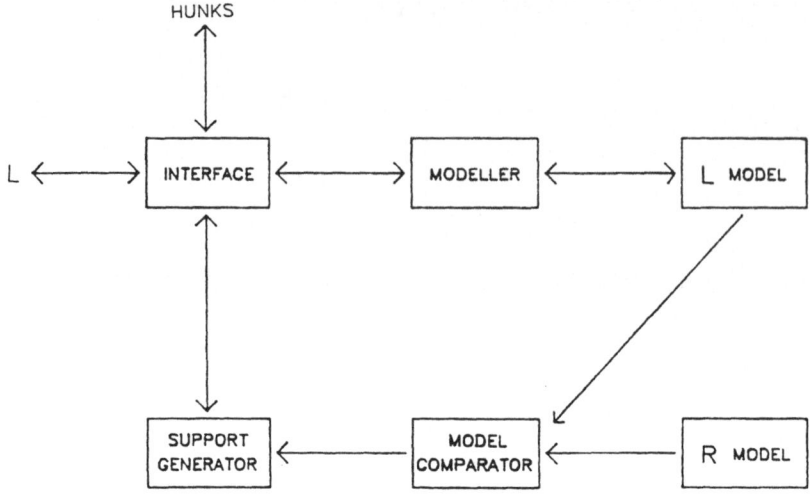

Figure 1. An Intelligent Teaching System

An ITS may be seen as a development from current computer-based instruction systems. Many CBI systems incorporate automatic assessment of the learner's level of knowledge or skill; this feature provides the system with some perceptiveness of the learner's needs. However, assessment is usually a very much abbreviated sampling of the learner's knowledge or skill, based on a few summary measures of performance or a test score assumed to be representative of his capability in the domain (or subdomain). A CBI system may also show some degree of responsiveness to the individual by selecting for him an appropriate pathway through the instructional material, but this is usually restricted to a simple branching lesson structure. Alternative pathways represent its capacity for response variation, and together with self-pacing are the chief means by which the system accommodates individual needs. In contrast, the capability of an ITS to construct an elaborated model of the learner as game player provides it with a perceptiveness of the learner's current state which is not normally achieved in CBI. The comparison with an Expert model enables the system to locate precisely the lacunae in the learner model and thus to identify the current personal needs of the learner. The learner model also provides for support to be couched in terms which the learner is known to understand. The capacity of an ITS to respond appropriately to the learner's needs depends on the degree of elaboration of the Support Generator. In these ways an ITS is able to adapt to the individual learner to a degree not achieved by most CBI systems.

This description of an ITS framework allows many interpretations. Different styles of teaching may be associated with dissimilar instructional goals and dissimilar methods. These will be reflected in differing contents for the Support Generator, possibly also in special purpose modellers, and in distinct mechanisms for the control of the instructional process. In part, the choice between alternative realisations of an ITS may depend on the nature of the task to be learned. The view of HUNKS play adopted here has led to the choice of Self-Organised Learning as a compatible approach to be realised within an ITS.

DOMAIN

The game of HUNKS, in spite of its formal simplicity, elegantly captures many of the features of the submarine command decision-making environment. Previous work at APU (Todd, 1982) has shown that submarine tactics requires, among others, skills which are inventive and adaptive. Given almost any tactical problem, no two submariners are likely to agree on its solution: to some extent, it is a question of individual style. Tactics need to be inventive, to cope with the unexpected event or one which has never been encountered before. Finally, the domain is an evolving one: changes in sensors, weaponry or vessel capabilities on either side can present new tactical problems or offer new solutions. In these aspects, the domain of submarine command decision-making does not lend itself to training based on an Expert model. Tactics which replicate those of an Expert would lead to stereotyped behaviour, ultimately predictable to an opponent, and lacking in adaptability. For the present day context, training based on an Expert model is undesirable; for tactics of the future, the relevant Expert does not exist. Training which does not rely on an authoritative "expert" version of task competence presents a challenging problem for the training designer, in particular within CBI.

The whole relationship between the learner, the domain and the instructor changes when there is no domain expert to call upon and refer to. A new basis for defining a training objective has to be found, together with alternative criteria for assessing the learner's progress and determining his needs. If the Expert-based training environment is regarded as one in which the learner, via the instructor, interrogates the expert about the domain, and is informed by him under the direction of the instructor, the Expert-less training environment by contrast appears as one in which there is no known answer to the learner's questions. The learner's position resembles that of a researcher.

SELF-ORGANIZED LEARNING

An approach to learning which is particularly well suited to this problem is Self-Organised Learning. The theory and methodology were originated and developed over twenty years by L. Thomas and E. Harri-Augstein (1983a) at the Centre for the Study of Human Learning (CSHL), Brunel University, and have been shown to be applicable to many skill areas or domains. Because their approach is strongly centred on the individual learner, and does not rely on an authoritative domain Expert, it appeared to offer an attractive solution to the problem of HUNKS learning within an ITS. The current collaboration between CSHL and APU is directed towards the implementation of their theory and its associated methodology within an ITS.

A basic premise in Self-Organised Learning theory is that most people fail to realise their potential as learners, because their experiences of education and training environments have required them simply to submit to being taught. As a result, they have never learned how to learn. When students engage in Self-Organised Learning rather than dependent learning, studies have repeatedly shown (Thomas & Harri-Augstein, 1976) that learning is accelerated and the resulting achievement is much superior.

The Self-Organised learner acts as a researcher or "personal scientist" within the domain (Thomas & Harri-Augstein, 1983a; Kelly, 1955). His or her learning is conducted as a personal exploration of the domain; an investigation of the cause and effect relationships that hold within it, by carefully planned probes and detailed appraisal of the results. He takes the same deliberately questioning approach to his own learning processes, regarding them as equally open to experimentation. Three attributes in particular distinguish the Self-Organised from the dependent learner:

- The Self-Organised learner is self-aware: he is conscious of his own experience and behaviour in the domain and in learning, and understands his own processes. This is in contrast to the dependent learner who relies on the Teacher to monitor such aspects of the learner's activities as are relevant in the Teacher's view.

- The Self-Organised learner is self-directing: he is able to function purposefully towards goals he has defined himself. The dependent learner on the other hand responds passively under the Teacher's definition of purposes.

- The Self-Organised learner is self-critical: he can construct his own evaluative criteria and assess his achievement and progress himself. He can observe the behaviour of others within his own evaluation scheme, and make productive use of comparisons with himself. He differs here from the dependent learner, who is reliant on the Teacher's assessment against criteria which are often covert.

These different roles or perspectives within the individual are in communication and can act on each other; the learner can sustain a dialogue with himself.

The purpose of the Self-Organised Learning methodology is to enable the learner to become Self-Organised. Most learners are initially unable to generate and maintain these communicating perspectives, and the dialogue needs to be articulated and supported through a Learning Manager (Thomas & Harri-Augstein, 1983b). A substantial body of techniques, collectively termed the Intelligent Learning System, has been developed by Thomas and Harri-Augstein to provide this conversational support, and to encourage a learner to become Self-Organised. His new learning skills are gained and practised within a particular domain, so that he is simultaneously engaged in learning the domain and in learning how to learn. The aim of the current work is a machine implementation of these techniques for the HUNKS domain, i.e. to produce a computerised "manager". The next section outlines these techniques, with their theoretical foundations, in an Idealised Version of an Intelligent Teaching System for Self-Organised Learning (ITSSOL).

The learning environment for promoting Self-Organised Learning is a radical departure from conventional CBI and also from other interpretations of an ITS. In particular, the role of the "Instructor" in CBI is completely reformulated in the "Learning Manager" in Self-Organised Learning. While the "Instructor" acts to impart the "Expert's" knowledge to the learner, and assesses his progress against the Expert, the "Learning Manager" acts to enhance the effectiveness of the learner's exploratory interactions with the domain, and to promote his autonomy as a learner. The "Learning Manager" has no need of a domain Expert as referent. There is a second important difference. In most teaching systems, learning is coterminous with teaching, and is discontinued when instructional support is withdrawn. In an ITS designed to promote Self-Organised Learning, the learner becomes progressively more able to direct and control his own learning, and the support provided by the Learning Manager becomes no longer needed. The function of the Learning Manager is designed to be obsolescent, and is gradually withdrawn as the learner becomes able to take over its function himself, and to continue learning autonomously.

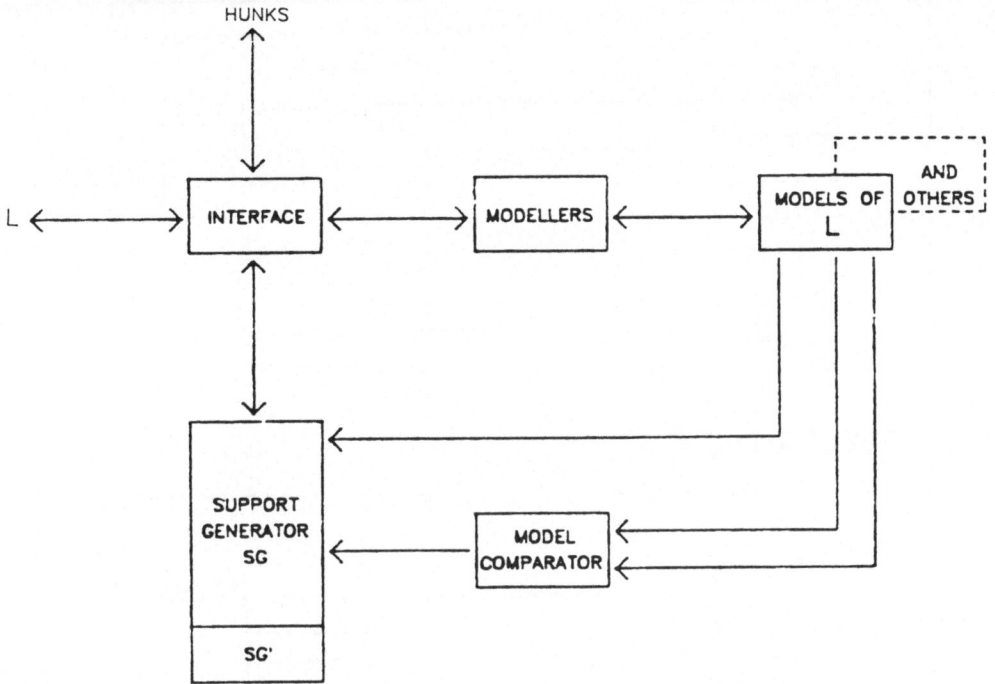

Figure 2. ITSSOL: Idealised Version

ITSSOL: AN IDEALISED VERSION

The idealised system towards which we are working is an integration of certain components of an ITS being developed at APU with components of an Intelligent Learning System developed over many years by Thomas and Harri-Augstein and more recently in collaboration with APU (1983b).

Figure 2 shows the idealised system in a representation parallel to the ITS framework of Figure 1. The single modeller in the ITS skeleton is replaced by multiple modellers in Figure 2. The use of multiple models is an integral part of Self-Organised Learning theory; they enable the learner to explore different facets of his experience and behaviour, to observe himself from different perspectives, and they encourage him to generate multiple internal representations of his experience and behaviour. The intention is not to restrict the learner in his construction of internal models, but to promote the possibility of alternatives through the parallel and comparative use of those provided. In comparison with Figure 1, the idealised version shows the reduced emphasis on machine comparison of models, and the flexible rather than mandatory use of Referent models, which reflect the underlying theoretical principles. These Referent models no longer have the status of an authoritative Expert. They include models of colearners, non-authoritative experts and possibly earlier versions of the learner himself, and are available for the learner's use, to encourage flexibility and to enhance his development as a critical observer.

Most of the operations of the Learning Manager are represented within the Support Generator, which can act to provide guidance and support which is sensitive to the individual learner. His needs are known to the Support Generator from the learner models. Other aspects of the Learning Manager's function are represented elsewhere in the system, in the modellers themselves. The sequence of an elicitation procedure in a modeller, for

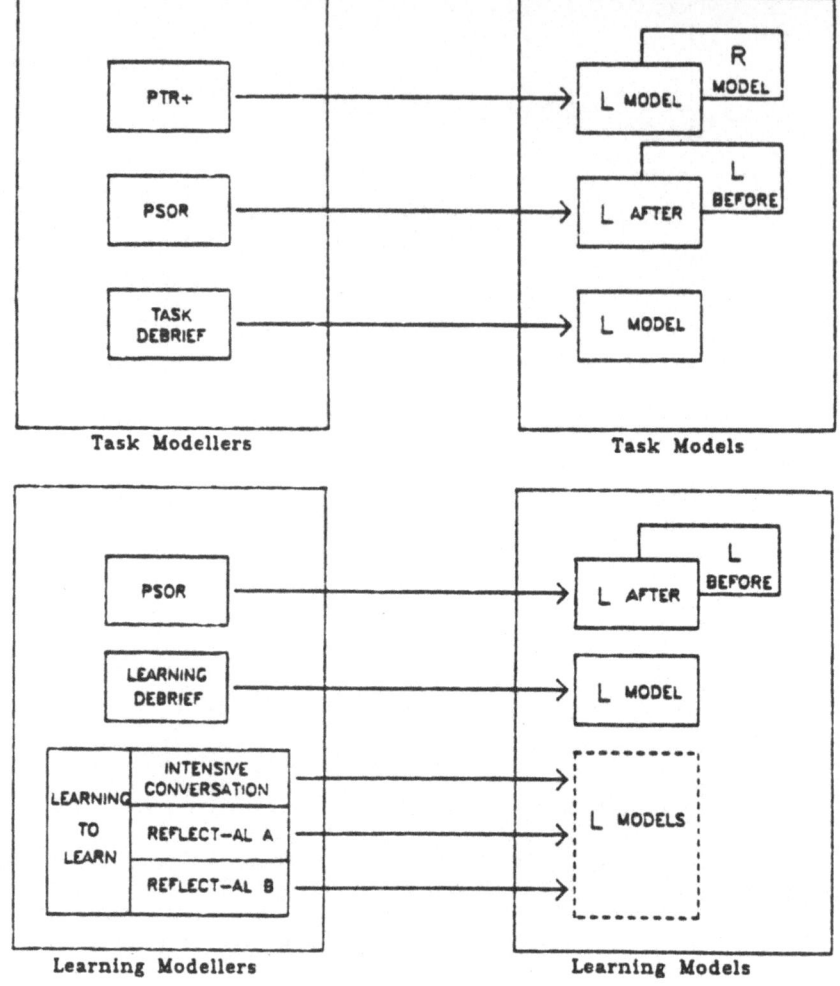

Figure 3. Modelling in ITSSOL: Idealised Version

example, exerts a directive influence on the responding learner. This kind of guidance is not adaptive to the individual but is invariant across learners. The interventions of the Learning Manager can be more or less heavily directive. An activity which imposes a fixed sequence on the learner corresponds to a high degree of directiveness, whereas an activity which offers the learner many or repeated choices is much less strongly directive.

Since the system works to promote Self-Organised Learning, the functions of the Learning Manager are gradually taken over by the learner himself. This includes the control exercised by the Support Generator SG. The withdrawal of this control probably also depends indirectly on the contents or use of the various models, and is mediated by a secondary control function SG .

Figure 3 is an expansion of the modelling component in Figure 2, the Idealised version of ITSSOL. It shows the modellers in two groups: one concerned with modelling the learner's activity in the domain, his task; the second concerned with the modelling of learning itself.

The three task modellers capture different aspects of the learner's experience and behaviour in the HUNKS game, and serve different purposes. The modeller based on PTR (Personalised Task Representation) is being constructed at APU. The PTR modeller (Gregory, 1979, 1981) captures the learner's HUNKS play, and its causal and teleological bases through direct interrogation of the learner. The resultant model of the learner is intended to be operable, i.e. when sufficiently complete, it can substitute for the learner and play as he would himself. Similarly it is open to interrogation by means of the PTR questions, and will respond as the learner would. Models of other players are available for inspection and use as machine players by the learner. Since they have been constructed by the PTR modeller, they can also describe and explain their own play in response to PTR questions, although naturally their accounts will be in the terms of their originators. It is our expectation that PTR modelling will have the effect of focussing the learner's attention on the rational basis of his play as structured by the PTR questions. The principal value of PTR modelling within the system however is in terms of its product, the PTR model, which can be deployed by the learner or by the Support Generator in various ways to promote learning. A bespoke version of the PTR modeller is expected to be needed for integration with the components of the Intelligent Learning System.

The function of the second modeller is in complete contrast to this. The PSOR modeller provides the learner with the facility to formulate and execute contracts relating to the task. A contract is both a plan for the next episode of HUNKS activity and a commitment which the learner makes with himself. Its fixed components (abbreviated as P, S, O, and R) are:

- Purpose: the learner defines his own intentions.

- Strategy: the learner specifies the means by which he will achieve his purpose.

- Outcome: the learner generates criteria by which he will assess the quality of the outcome of his strategy.

- Review: a retrospective appraisal of his purpose-definition, choice of strategy, and outcome criteria.

When the learner is provisionally satisfied with his purpose, strategy, and outcome, he executes his PSOR contract. His ensuing activity will frequently engage him in HUNKS play. Finally, the learner reviews his performance in the light of his contract, and re-examines his contract. Occasions where the contract has not been successfully executed are regarded as particularly significant learning opportunities: they confront the learner with inconsistencies or inadequacies in his internal model of the task. The comparison between before- and after-task versions of his contract is used by the Support Generator to identify the direction of development, and by the learner in the formulation of the next contract. Like the PSOR contract itself, the comparison is a means to an end; its purpose is to encourage the learner to think positively and constructively. In the course of learning, a sequence of contracts will have different foci, different scopes and differing time scales. Unlike the PTR modeller, PSOR modelling is more closely concerned with the process of formulating and executing the contract than with the contents of the contract. The elicitation and execution of the "model" are themselves aspects of the Learning Manager's support.

The Task Debrief is an activity which is normally interpolated between the learner's HUNKS play and his contract review. It is a modeller in the sense that it leads the learner to represent aspects of his performance in

a particular structure. As with PSOR, its primary purpose is to engage the
learner in a process rather than to extract a product. He is asked to
recall his game play episode, and to reconstruct it and analyse it with the
help of a replay of the episode. The exercise helps the learner to
integrate his remembered experience with the objective record of his
behaviour, which allows him to test and develop his perceptions and
expectations within the game of HUNKS against observed event sequences.
These activities enhance the learner's awareness of himself as a HUNKS
player, and enable him to be a more effective "personal scientist" in the
domain. The Debrief stimulates the learner to reorganise his experience,
which in turn generates content for his subsequent contract review.

Both PSOR and the Debrief procedure can be applied to the modelling of
learning as well as to the modelling of the task. The structure of the
activity remains exactly the same; the only difference is in the content.
At early stages, learners frequently find it difficult to think and speak
about their learning; they lack awareness of themselves as learners. The
support of the Learning Manager encourages this transition, and enables the
learner to act as "personal scientist" with respect to his own learning. A
further group of activities, the Learning-to-Learn procedures, serve both
to widen the learner's perspective and to sharpen his focus on his own
learning. The Idealised version of ITSSOL includes three such procedures
among the learning modellers. The Intensive Conversation can be regarded
as a remedial activity for the learner whose PSOR contracts fail because
they are poorly formulated. It leads him into a detailed examination of
each of the contract components, so that he becomes better able to produce
well-differentiated and significant contents for his PSOR contracts.
Because the Intensive Conversation increases the learner's capability to
use PSOR contracts productively, it increases his ability to learn. The
Reflect-and-Learn procedures shift the learner's attention to a broader
perspective on his own learning, by directing him to survey either a group
of his contracts (Reflect-Al B) or his experiences of games learning in
general (Reflect-Al A). These Learning-to-Learn procedures incorporate
Repertory Grid technology.

ITSSOL: CURRENT VERSION

The current version of the system (developed by Thomas and
Harri-Augstein, 1976, at CSHL) is implemented on an Apple II microcomputer
in Applesoft Basic. The components which are already available as software
are shown in Figure 4. The HUNKS game is also implemented on an Apple,
together with a computer player which can provide an opponent for the
learner in game play.

The system comprises a suite of programs which explain themselves to
the learner, offer him choices of activity, and lead him through the
elicitation procedures of model building. The learner can choose to be
addressed as a "Novice", when he will receive full explanatory annotations
to the procedures, or as an "Expert", when the explanations are withheld.
The learner is free to traverse the elicitation and associated procedures
in almost any order he chooses, although some routes are suggested as more
sensible than others. The dialogue conducted via the VDU and the keyboard
is augmented by hard copy printouts of the learner's models which may be
accompanied by non-evaluative comments which draw the learner's attention
to omissions in the model or suggestions for the learner to reflect on.
The system cannot comment on the meaning of any of the contents of the
learner models, because it has no language understanding mechanism.

There are essentially three activities available to the learner,
corresponding to the three modellers in Figure 4:   PSOR contracts, the

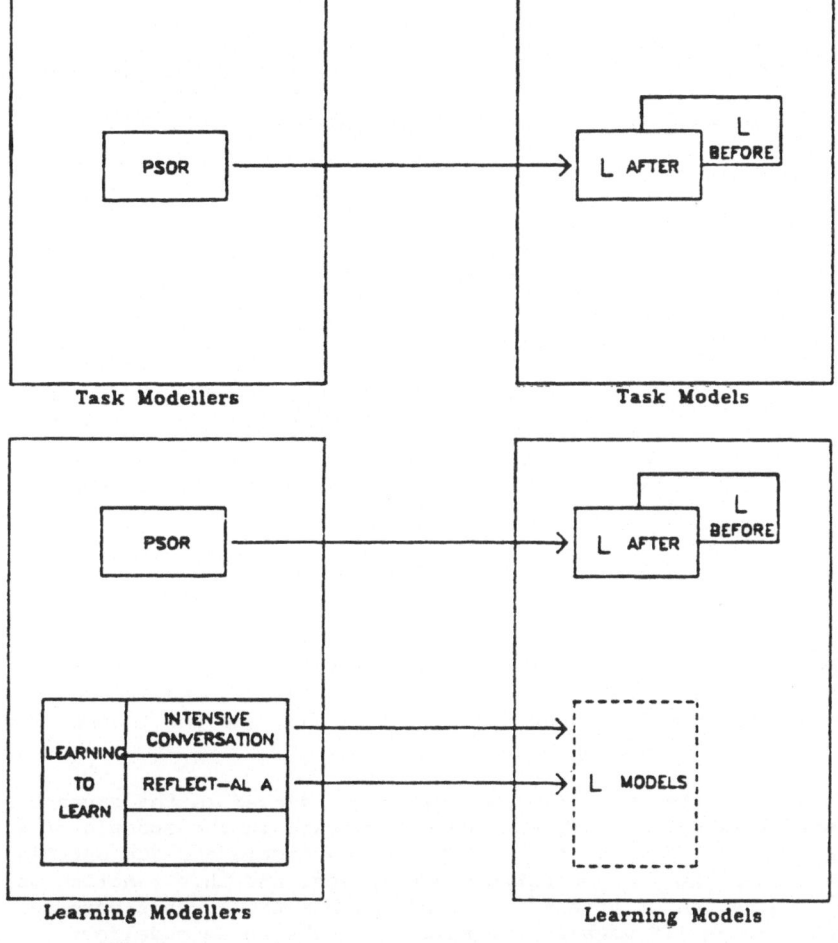

Figure 4. Modelling in ITSSOL: Current Version

Intensive Conversation, and Reflect-al A, concerned with the learner's experience of games. PSOR contracts may address either the HUNKS task itself or HUNKS learning; the system provides no constraints on the contents of the learner's contracts.

The PSOR modeller leads the learner through the elicitation of his contract, prompting him always to formulate his contract with the utmost care and to revise its contents, repeatedly if necessary. This emphasis reflects the importance attached to the process of contract-making as one which itself induces change in the learner. Together with the definition of the contract topic, its purpose, strategy, outcome and outcome criteria, the learner is asked to specify the resources he will need or draw upon to execute his contract. An expansion of the contract follows, although here as elsewhere the learner can opt out of the suggested sequence. The learner is asked to specify both a superordinate context and a set of subordinate elements for each of the components of his contract, so that he is constructing a three level hierarchy. Again he has the opportunity to revise his contract. When he is at least provisionally satisfied, he attempts to execute it in game play. The suggested sequel to game play is the contract review procedure, in which the learner reconstructs all the

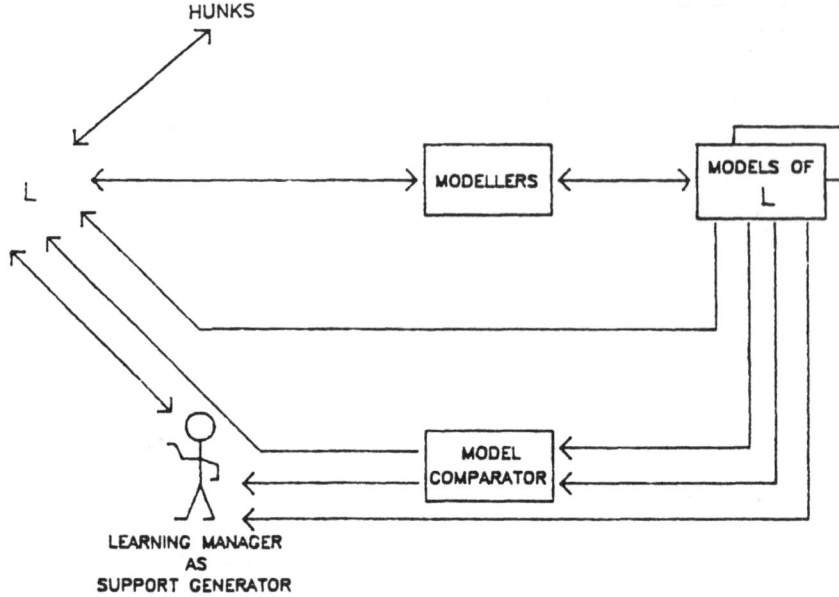

Figure 5. Current Version as an ITS

components of his contract and his resource list in the light of his experience in game play. A comparison of his Before- and After-task versions of a contract is provided as a printout, and the learner invited to reflect on the differences.

Each of the three modelling activities conducted in the current version of the system is self-contained, and can operate in the absence of a human Learning Manager. However the system does not include a Support Generator which can steer the learner between activities, and this function has to be performed in person at present. Figure 5 shows the current version represented as an ITS parallel to Figure 1. The three modellers can be supplemented by a pencil-and-paper version of the Debrief, which is most appropriately used after HUNKS play and before contract review. The pencil-and-paper version of a procedure can be seen as an intermediate stage in the implementation of a procedure which initially exists only in the head of the skilled Learning Manager. This process of externalising and articulating the art of the Learning Manager is the first step towards a machine implementation, and is served by a research strategy based on empirical study.

THE RESEARCH STRATEGY

The development of the current version of an ITS based on Self-Organised Learning towards the idealised version is expected to be an incremental process. At each stage, further aspects of the Learning Manager's function will be incorporated within the system. Each intermediate version will be tested in operation, and the empirical trials will serve in the identification of the next series of additions and modifications to the system.

Figure 6 illustrates this strategy (Thomas, 1976). It shows a learner in interaction with an intermediate version of the system. The human Learning Manager acts as a critical observer to his interaction, in order

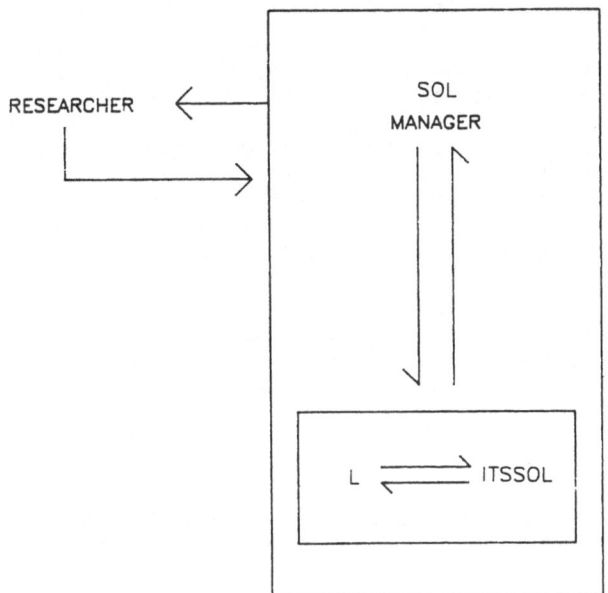

Figure 6

to identify shortcomings in the system. He also acts as a participant in the interaction, supplementing and structuring the Self-Organised Learning support provided to the learner. In this role, he or she is observed by a Researcher, who analyses the interventions of the Learning Manager. This analysis is continued subsequently, with the Learning Manager contributing his experience and retrospectively sharing in the Researcher's role. The result of this analysis is a specification for the changes and extensions to the system which will produce a closer approximation to the idealised version. Once this specification has been implemented, the new version is itself the subject of empirical trials in a repetition of the development cycle.

The current version of the system, shown in Figures 4 and 5, has been the subject of empirical study in line with this strategy. The expected benefits of the study were three-fold:

1. Feedback for the researchers on the usability and comprehensibility of the current system, at the level of the lucidity of explanations provided by the system, the transparency of its structure, the suitability of input and printout facilities, and the style of the dialogue the system conducts with the learner.

2. Articulation of the manager's role. The management of the learning conversation is a highly skilled activity, and difficult for its practitioners to articulate, depending as it does on tacit knowledge and sensitive response to the learner's needs. Video records of trial sessions were able to show exactly what interventions the manager made, to steer the learner towards productive use of the system, to supplement its existing procedures, and to introduce techniques as yet not present in the system.

3. Demonstration in a publicly communicable manner of the principles of self-organised learning technology.

SUMMARY

A particular problem arises in training when it is impossible or inappropriate to make reference to an authoritative expert in the task. It is suggested that in some respects submarine command tactics presents a training problem of this kind. This paper describes the structure and evolution of an Intelligent Teaching System designed to address this problem, using the war game HUNKS to simulate the command task environment. The work makes use of the well-developed theoretical principles of Self-Organised Learning and its associated research strategy in the progressive implementation of ITSSOL. This approach appears particularly well suited to individual training, in tasks which are primarily cognitive in content, and as a possible solution to the problem of training in the absence of an expert, ITSSOL potentially offers a valuable contribution to the development of advanced CBI systems.

ACKNOWLEDGEMENTS

The author wishes to acknowledge the collaboration with L. F. Thomas and E. S. Harri-Augstein under ARE/APU Contract No. 2066/034.

REFERENCES

Gregory, R. (1979). "Personalised task representation" (AMTE(E) TM 79103).
Gregory, R. (1981). "Personalised task representation" (AMTE(E) TM 81104).
Kelly, G. (1955). "The psychology of personal contracts" (Vols. 1 & 2). New York: Norton.
Sheppard, C. (1981). "Rationale and work programme 1981-83." Teddington, Middx. UK: Admiralty Research Establishment, Applied Psychology Unit, Man-Computer Studies Section.
Sleeman, D. H., & Brown, J. S. (1982). "Intelligent tutoring systems." New York: Academic Press.
Thomas, L. F (1976). "Nothing more theoretical than good practice" (SSRC Report). Brunel University, Centre for the Study of Human Learning.
Thomas L. F., & Harri-Augstein, E. S. (1976). "The self-organised-learner and the printed word" (Final Progress Report SSRC). Brunel University, Centre for the Study of Human Learning.
lhomas L. F., & Harri-Augstein, E. S. (1983a). The personal scientist as self-organised learner: A conversational technology for reflecting on behaviour and experience. In J. Adams Webber (Ed.), "Applications of personal construct psychology." Academic Press.
Thomas L. F., & Harri-Augstein, E. S. (1983b). "The self-organised learner and computer-aided learning systems" (Final Report, ARE/APU Contract No. 2066/020). Teddington, Middx. UK: Admiralty Research Establishment, Applied Psychology Unit.
Thomas L. F., & Harri-Augstein, E. S. (1985). "Self-organised learning." London: Routledge and Kegan Paul.
Todd, R. R. (1982). "Initial report on submarine command tactics training" (E1/P2.10/13/82).

PORTABLE, INTELLIGENT SIMULATION FOR ASW TRAINING

E. D. McWilliams* and G. L. Ricard**

*The CRT Corporation
Rockville, Maryland, U.S.A.

**Naval Training Equipment Center
Orlando, Florida, U.S.A.

INTRODUCTION

The purpose of this paper is twofold: first, we would like to discuss some Navy-sponsored research and development work in Computer-based Instruction (CBI) where the aim is to add "intelligence" to the CBI, and second, to describe one such system. The military services have to train large numbers of people to perform a wide variety of somewhat specialized jobs, and to this process, they devote considerable resources and personnel. It is little wonder that technical developments that offer to make instruction better or more efficient have generated a great deal of interest.

And so it has been with computers. Because of their ability to store alphanumeric material and present it along with graphical representations, computers were quickly adopted by educators as machines that could support instruction. By the addition of the capability to ask questions of students and then to branch to different sections of material to be learned, the computing machinery seemed to have been given some of the characteristics of human instructors, and the education community was quick to see the potential of this new technology and to apply it. Several large projects were started for the development and presentation of CBI (see for instance Meyers, 1984 or Wilson, 1984) and many courses were developed specifically for CBI, for programs of both military training and civilian education.

By and large, CBI programs have been successful. Since the same material was, for the most part, presented in the same manner as a conventional instructor would do it, CBI did not produce substantially more or better learning on the parts of students, but it did produce faster learning, probably because students had control of the pace of their instruction and could skip over material they knew or could quickly master and then dwell on material which was more difficult. CBI thus seems more efficient than conventional teaching in that similar levels of mastery are produced about 30 percent faster, and this has been found true for secondary and college education (see Kulik, Bangert, and Williams, 1983; and Kulik, Kulik and Cohen, 1980) as well as for military training programs (Orlansky and String, 1980). Twenty years of work on CBI has produced substantial literature and one might see Kearsley (1983) or Kearsley, Hunter, and Seidel (1983) for a summarization. While the development of CBI material is laborious and advancement of the technology will probably be slow (Montague and Wulfeck, 1984), it is clear that CBI is appropriate for many training programs (Montague, 1984) and that the application of computing techniques to problems of education will continue.

Within the training research and development activities of the military, there is interest in capitalizing on one of the inherent strengths of the computer - that is, the ability to make comparisons and decisions quickly - to extend the range of applications of CBI. Much of the technology for this development comes from developments in the field of artificial intelligence (AI), particularly from the area of expert systems. Expert systems are more properly, systems for representing expertise in computer software in a manner upon which the machine can act. There are a variety of techniques for simulating such expertise - one is to represent knowledge about a domain as a set of rules (called "production rules") defining what the "expert" will conclude if specified conditions are met; another is to place related information into file-like structures ("frames") which, when accessed, make available a great deal of stereotypical information or knowledge that frequently applies under certain circumstances.

Regardless of the means chosen to represent expertise, several large AI demonstration projects have shown that the techniques work well enough for them to be seriously considered for a variety of applied problems. The movement of expert systems from the laboratory to industrial and military operations has begun, and the U.S. Navy is near the forefront of this movement. There are several projects in the Navy to develop expert systems for operational use. For the most part, these systems are to act as information handlers or decision aids. Although the objectives vary somewhat, the aim is often to reduce the workload of the human decision-maker by enabling a computer to do part of the thinking and decision-making, particularly in situations where the decision must be made under constraints of time or requires the consideration of large volumes of data. The requirement to process information and make decisions is common to many jobs, of course, including that of an instructor in a military training program. If "conventional" CBI is already useful for military training, it appears possible to make it even more useful by adding "intelligence" to it so that the CBI system itself can be more responsive to student performance. It also appears possible that the knowledge about a task or the performance of a task can be incorporated into an expert CBI system so as to provide assistance in a variety of activities that are required of the instructors in training programs.

And the job of military instructor has a lot of variety. For instance, instructors must plan for and present lectures, select simulations or other special exercises, brief students, demonstrate desired performance, appraise, score, and correct trainee performance, provide constructive feedback and debriefings, and possibly enter scores into a record-keeping system. Furthermore, over the long run, instructors have to assess the training that they are providing and, if necessary, take steps to improve it.

Over the past 15 years, the Human Factors Division of the Naval Training Equipment Center has sponsored many projects to develop capabilities for computers to support instructors in Navy training programs. Projects that have been supported have attempted to develop computer-based capabilities for one or more of the tasks outlined above. Systems to measure performance, maintain records, generate training materials, control training, and provide numerous other services, have been the object of considerable research and development. With this interest in AI, particularly expert systems, is a continuation of this interest in applying computers to the problems of military training.

As in the programs to apply the techniques of expert systems to operational jobs, the justification for using them in CBI applications is workload reduction, for either instructors or students. The development of powerful microcomputers has stimulated interest in training where adequate simulations of a task may be encoded into a microcomputer and the techniques of expert systems can be used to incorporate information for making instructional decisions. The goal is to create portable, stand-alone training devices that require a minimum of assistance from instructors (who are often too busy to be burdened by additional duties). The information that can be included in an expert system can be about the task being trained, about instruction, or about the trainee, and from the work over the past decade, it is clear that the knowledge can be used to add a variety of automated functions to a CBI system. Expert systems can, for instance, provide data base management functions such as the scanning of records for the purpose of quality control or personnel assignment. Or, closer to the learning process itself, expert systems could be developed to create learning scenarios and provide trainees with briefings on them.

Because of the importance of knowledge of results to the process of learning, current work has often emphasized the instructor's role of providing diagnostic feedback and advice, either during or after a student's performance of the task. The domain knowledge, then, is used to characterize what the student did and to assign meaning to the student's actions. The aim of focusing upon providing feedback and advice is to free students from their dependence upon the availability of instructors. Because the costs associated with military training are great, the appeal of a stand-alone trainer is high, particularly if the feedback from such a device not only reduced training time but also improved the trainee's performance.

The use of expert system techniques to increase the intelligence of CBI systems is important, but not critical, since these techniques represent merely the latest development in software technology. More critical is the process by which the CBI system is developed. We believe strongly in a continuous, integrated cycle of research and development, with frequent and intensive trial use of the system by operational fleet personnel. This process is one of experimentation, testing, and successive refinement, rather than attempting to define all requirements in advance. The CBI system evolves over time, with the system itself being used as a research instrument to provide behaviors and comments with each trial use. These behaviors are analyzed and the system is refined before it is used in the next field trial. This process of successive refinement is at variance with many CBI development projects, in which the requirements (down to the number of "hours" of courseware) are laid down at the outset and development proceeds in a relatively sequential fashion.

RECENT DEVELOPMENTS

Several developments within the past few years have brought such a trainer much more within reach. The first of these developments is a better understanding of the features of flight simulators that are most essential for the effective transfer of training to the aircraft. These features, described by Caro (1973) and Adams (1979), are: operational fidelity (the degree to which trainees can practice behaviors that are important to the task), knowledge of results (essentially error information), perceptual learning (to extract information), stimulus response learning, and motivation. Two other recent developments are equally pertinent to producing low-cost, effective training systems. The first of these is the microminiaturization of powerful computing systems. The second is the emergence of techniques for modelling expert performance in complex domains using computer programs. Each of these latter two developments will be reviewed in turn.

The inherent advantages of microcomputer systems for many demanding applications, particularly those requiring rapid updating of complex displays, instantaneous response, and continuous processing power, have been reported in the literature (Tenczar, 1981). One can now have up to 16 million bytes (MB) of Random-Access Memory (RAM) on many microcomputers, and several hundred MB of disk storage. Tenczar also pointed out the advantages in cost and reliability that microcomputers enjoy over large time-sharing systems. He described a microcomputer system specifically designed for demanding applications, including unusually powerful system software tools to facilitate the development of graphic, interactive programs.

The existence of such systems could be of fundamental importance for the development of high-performance, low-cost, real-time simulators that require graphical displays. They make possible, for the first time, inexpensive, portable simulators with high operational fidelity. This includes the ability to compute and display each important simulated interaction at the time that it would occur in the real world. As explained above, however, one would like to have a trainer that provides not only simulation, but specific diagnostic feedback and advice as well. This requires more than portable, low-cost hardware. It requires a relatively detailed model of both expert and trainee performance plus knowledge of when and how to provide advice. Fortunately, progress has been made recently in this area as well.

For instance, computer programs have been produced that can provide doctors, scientists, and engineers with useful advice on real, complex problems. Outstanding performance has been reported. DENDRAL (Buchanan and Mitchell, 1978), a program for determining the structure of a complex molecule is said to surpass even expert chemists in speed and accuracy, and its results have appeared in many published papers. A program for internal medicine (Pople, Myers, and Miller, 1975) has demonstrated the capability to correctly diagnose disease cases that are described in medical journals as being particularly difficult.

Some attempts to provide expert advice using computer programs were only performance based. That is, there was little attempt to constrain the system to reason like a human expert or to provide explanations in those terms. One such system, SOPHIE I (Brown and Burton, 1975), simulated and analyzed electronic circuits. It could judge a student's answer, but was unable to provide a very satisfying explanation of its reasoning. Such systems are referred to as "black box" or inarticulate systems, for obvious reasons.

In other projects, attempts have been made to provide computer programs that reason more like human experts, with correspondingly greater ability to explain performance in more comprehensible terms. Systems of this kind are sometimes called "glass box" or articulate systems. The NEOMYCIN system for training medical students to diagnose infectious diseases (Clancey, 1981), and the system by Burton and Brown (1979) for facilitating the acquisition of arithmetic skills through the use of an interactive computer-based game exemplify this approach. In this computer-based arithmetic game, the computer monitors a child's move, computes a set of relatively "expert" moves for the same situation, and maintains a record of both. When asked, it provides advice for improving the student's score by employing an arithmetic skill that had been ignored by the student but was employed in one of the expert moves. Burton and Brown call this a "Differential Diagnostic Model of Coaching", since it is based upon the difference between expert and student performance and is more akin to coaching than teaching. (Sleeman and Brown, 1982, contains many interesting papers about computer-based training.)

A number of useful heuristic principles have been derived from many studies of expert problem-solving and from attempts to model expertise for computer-based aiding or instruction. (See Feigenbaum, 1977; Davis, 1982.) The following principles involve the nature of expertise itself:

- Problem-solving performance appears to rely primarily upon extensive and well organized stores of knowledge about the specific task, rather than a set of domain independent methods.

- Problem-solving knowledge is often inexact, incomplete, and ill-specified, so that it is frequently necessary to help the expert to explicate and classify what he knows and how it is used.

- Expertise appears to be acquired incrementally.

Other principles have been derived from guiding the development of computer-based expert systems. The following are the most important for consideration here:

- Make the system flexible and transparent (a "glass box") to facilitate its evolution over a period of several years and many improvement cycles.

- Separate the knowledge base from the simulation programs, and separate both from the strategies for learning or instruction that will be attempted.

The recent literature contains several reports of attempts to provide computer-based, graphical simulations and expertise for a complex system, following the principles noted above. In the STEAMER project (Williams, Hollan, and Stevens, 1981) a dedicated, stand-alone computer has been programmed to simulate many aspects of a steam-generation plant, for ship propulsion. The operation of the plant can be displayed graphically as animated color diagrams, and can be controlled using a graphics interface. These and other features permit the trainee to manipulate or replace simulated components such as values, switches, and pumps, and observe the efforts upon parameters such as pressure, temperature, and rates of flow. Plans include a real-time tutor that can monitor and critique trainee performance, and can provide instruction and explanations at a conceptual, rather than procedural level.

In a trainer for plotting ship positions on a maneuvering board, Hutchins and McCandless (1982) and Hutchins, McCandless, Woodworth, and Dutton (1984) have combined a graphical representation of the plotboard with information to teach the concepts of relative motion. This system was specifically designed with the students' ease-of-use in mind. An analysis was made of their purposes in using various functions and then the functions were designed to serve those purposes.

The problems of flight training are not the same as those in medicine, chemistry, or steam generation. There are however, reasons for believing that techniques developed for solving problems in one domain can be applied to another. One of the problems of flight training is the constraint on time created by the high rates of speed of modern aircraft. Although the computers used in simulations are getting faster, the gain is often more than offset by the need to process additional information. Expert systems often require a large number of comparisons in order to reach a decision and, for flight training, it was not clear what functions an expert system could provide in real-time for a man-in-the-loop simulation.

A Trainer for Radar Intercept Operation (TRIO) is being developed to examine training functions that an expert system can provide for fast-paced air intercept training, where the closing rate of the interceptor and target can easily exceed 1000 knots. Feurzeig, Ash, and Ricard (1984) describe the TRIO system and the rule-based training capabilities developed to date. TRIO's expert system can examine events in the intercept and then alert the trainee to critical errors using a text-to-speech capability. After a more extensive analysis TRIO can debrief the intercept run, and (since TRIO's rules describe desired performance) TRIO can demonstrate expert performance to students. Because air intercepts occur so quickly, the CBI functions developed for TRIO tend to be those that instructors do either before or after intercept runs.

This need not always be the case however. The project that will be described in the remainder of this paper attempts to provide a portable, low-cost, real-time, intelligent trainer with high operational fidelity for every essential system and procedure used at one crew position in airborne Anti-Submarine Warfare (ASW). Many microcomputer capabilities are employed, as well as many of the techniques and principles from work on expert systems and training system design. Furthermore, the system provides advice in real-time, as the scenario is unfolding, as well as post-performance evaluation.

The system being developed, called the Portable Aircrew Trainer (PAT), is designed for research, practice, training, and instruction on strategies, tactics, and procedures for airborne ASW. The PAT will monitor and critique performance and be able to provide relatively expert advice and demonstration. It will operate singly for individual training or in a local network of PATs for instructor-monitoring or integrated crew training. The desk-top computer system for the prototypes PAT, with voice output, is presently available at a cost of about $30,000. The features of the PAT are described in greater detail later in this paper, following an explanation of the domain (airborne ASW) for which it has been developed.

THE TASK

An airborne ASW mission normally proceeds in sequential stages: search, localization, track, and attack. During the search phase, specific crew members monitor signals from floating sonobuoys or from the RADAR, forward-looking infrared detector (FLIR), or from the magnetic-anomaly detector (MAD), for indications of the presence of hostile submarines. Search often proceeds slowly, over large areas of the ocean, and with limited information.

If contact is gained through one of the sensory devices or by a visual sighting or other report, the mission enters the localization phase. During localization, additional sonobuoys and the other instruments are deployed methodically so as to gradually reduce the area of ocean containing the target to the point where the target's position can be fixed and contained with some degree of certainty. At this time, the mission shifts to the tracking phase, in which the target's course and speed are known and it can be followed with some confidence as it moves through an area of interest. It is frequently necessary to keep expanding the field of sonobuoys ahead of the target, or make other adjustments to avoid losing contact as the target changes depth, course, speed, or other aspects. Attack can be commenced when certain classified criteria are met.

Accuracy of navigation of the aircraft relative to the submarine is obviously of paramount importance. A special tactical navigational system (TACNAV) is provided for tactical situations such as this, to permit navigation with respect to floating sonobuoys or other objects. This system provides a continuous estimate of the velocity and position of the aircraft relative to a reference sonobuoy. The accuracy of the position of the aircraft can be checked and corrected by flying over a reference sonobuoy and executing a series of procedures (Romano, 1978). The aircraft normally finds such a sonobuoy by flying to it on the radio beacon by which the sonobuoy reports what it is detecting.

During at least the search and localization phases, "passive" sonobuoys are used, since they do not reveal their presence to the submarine. Passive sonobuoys put no additional sound into the water: they merely listen and transmit what they hear to the aircraft. During the track or attack phases, or if the submarine has been able to detect the presence of the aircraft, the crew may elect to use "active" sonobuoys that "ping" and listen for echoes reflected from the submarine. Actives are generally more accurate than passives, but this advantage is gained by sacrificing secrecy. The submarine can detect an active sonobuoy at long range.

The ability to gain and maintain contact with a submerged submarine is strongly influenced by environmental factors such as the change of ocean temperature with depth, the average ocean depth, winds and currents, ambient noise, and weather conditions. Performance characteristics of the aircraft and submarine are also important, as are those of the sonobuoys, MAD, RADAR and FLIR, each of which is sensitive only within a certain range and is subject to noise and inaccuracies. An aircraft can carry only a limited number of sonobuoys, and the navigational system for ASW is not perfectly accurate, causing navigational error or "drift" to accumulate.

In the U.S. Navy, the responsibility for the placement of sonobuoys and the deployment of the aircraft so as to maintain contact with and neutralize hostile targets, rests upon the Naval Flight Officer known as the Tactical Coordinator or TACCO. The TACCO is the mission co-commander in the Navy's P-3 or S-3 ASW aircraft. He monitors pertinent information provided to him by other crew members, by his own instruments, or by other participating naval units, and is responsible for the deployment of additional buoys and other resources to complete the mission successfully.

The TACCO is assisted in his tasks by a computer system in the aircraft that continually updates his position and makes possible the estimate of the relative positions of sonobuoys, fixes, and other objects of interest. This system provides many functions, including those for: estimating a submarine's velocity or predicting its future position based upon two or more previous fixes; correcting the aircraft's position when it is in error due to navigational draft; computing a correction to the aircraft's velocity; and correcting the positions of sonobuoys and fixes. The computer also permits the TACCO to build a priority queue of autopilot tasks to automatically steer the aircraft to a designated sonobuoy (for checking navigational drift), to one or more designated "fly-to-points" for dropping (or "expending") a sonobuoy, to a point where a weapon is to be dropped, to some other point of interest, or along a designated heading.

An ASW mission is complex and dynamic, with incomplete or conflicting information that requires considerable judgement and initiative from the TACCO, under time constraints. This makes it an interesting example of real-time problem-solving, and it has been studied from that viewpoint. The theoretical perspective, methodology, and preliminary findings are described elsewhere (McWilliams, 1981). The basic idea of the study was to document the behaviors of individual TACCOs by observing what information was requested, what inferences were made, and what actions were taken as each prosecuted a simulated ASW scenario. Individuals at different levels of experience were studied and contrasted in order to construct a model of expertise at the TACCO position.

The conduct of such a study required access to the TACCO position and control of the scenarios, neither of which was possible in the aircraft or high-fidelity simulators. The PAT simulator was initially conceived as a research instrument required for the study. In the five-year period of this project, the PAT has evolved through several versions of hardware and software. The features of the operational prototype, as of February, 1985, are described in the following section.

THE PAT

The general requirements for the simulator needed to study TACCOs were that it be portable; capable of simulating relatively complex ASW scenarios as they might be seen at the TACCO station in the P-3 or S-3

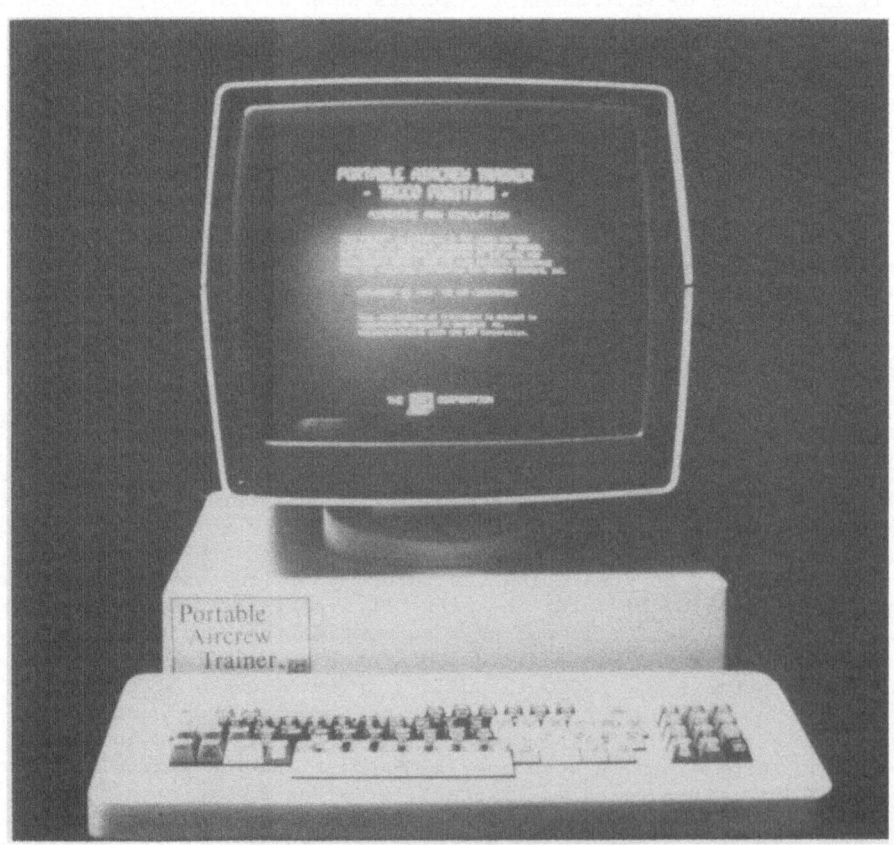

Figure 1. The PAT System
(Without Disk Storage and Voice Output Device)

problem-solving behaviors; and able to provide sufficient data storage and
control to permit the analysis of a TACCO's performance later by replaying
the scenario exactly as he played it. In addition, the system had to be
sufficiently powerful to use for development, and reliable enough to
operate in hot and humid conditions after being transported long distances
in the trunk of the investigator's car. The portable, low-cost,
high-performance microcomputer system developed by Regency Systems, Inc.,
and initially described by Tenczar (1981) was selected and employed. That
system, the RC-1, has been superseded by a later model, the R2-C, upon
which the PAT is presently based.

This (R2-C) system offers a number of features not commonly found on
small inexpensive equipment. The most important of these features for the
PAT project are: a high-resolution, color screen capable of detecting a
touch to within one-eighth of an inch; separate microprocessors for program
code, floating point operations, and touch input; 320 KB of RAM and 40 MB
of fast disk memory; audio output and networking capability; a keyset with
the ability to use each of the 80 keys for a different, programmer-defined
function; and many system software features that facilitate development.
The PAT display and keyset are shown in Figure 1.

To simulate airborne ASW, computer programs mathematically model the
most important characteristics and interactions of the various objects and
instruments, such as the aircraft, the ocean, submarines, sonobuoys, and
the RADAR and MAD. The aircraft can be "flown" using either an automatic
pilot (to points touched on the screen) or "manually", using the pad of
keys separated from the others on the keyboard. Surprisingly, the system
has enough processing capacity to permit the recomputation of all necessary
interactions about once each second, close to "real-time".

The Regency CRT and its touch-input device were used to simulate the
TACCO's display screen and "trackball", a device similar to a joy stick by
which the TACCO positions a cursor on the display. Most of the subsystems
required at the TACCO position, including instrumentation and other
avionics, have been modelled mathematically and are displayed graphically
as they would appear in the aircraft. Figure 2 is a printout of the CRT at
one instant in a simulated scenario. It shows the "tactical plot" of the
aircraft (◊), sonobuoys (◊) and (✗), fixes (⊕), and other objects, plus
alphanumeric information in separate "windows" around the border. At the
moment depicted, the aircraft is flying northeast at an altitude of 800
feet, there are two passive (DIFAR) buoys, tuned to radio channels 5 and 6,
and there is an active (DICASS) buoys tuned to channel 7. All of the buoys
are in contact with the target, and the range circle indicates that the
target is about 2060 yards from the active buoy.

The TACPLOT therefore provides a geographical representation, as viewed
from above. The other "windows" of the PAT display screen provides textual
information. Like the TACPLOT, each of these windows is updated
individually, in real time. The window just above the TACPLOT is used to
display the various alerts provided by software in the P-3 aircraft. The
window at the upper left displays the time, the scale of the TACPLOT, and
the queue of tasks for autopilot steering (shown enroute to buoy #7). The
window at the left of the TACPLOT is "time-shared". Currently, it shows
the status of the tactical navigation system, the dynamics of the aircraft,
and status of the MAD system. At the press of a key, this window is
reconfigured to display the types and numbers of buoys that are available,
the assignment of radio frequencies to buoys, and other status information.

The two windows at the lower left provide information unique to the
PAT, usually in response to operator requests. The lower window presently
indicates that the PAT is "paused". To the right of these is a "cue and

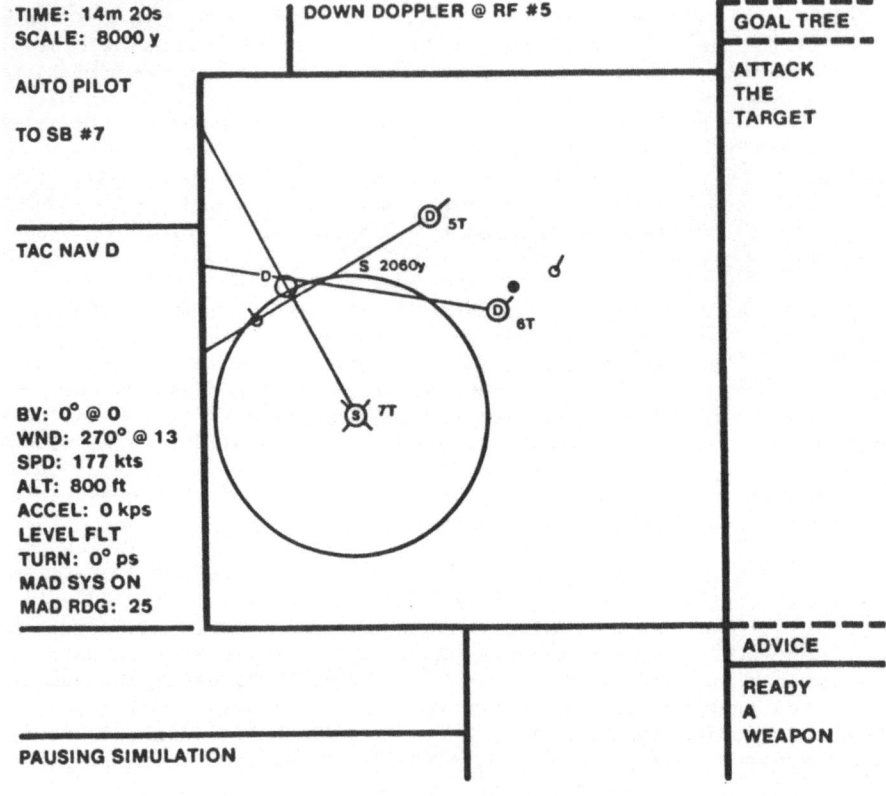

Figure 2. The PAT Simulated TACCO Display During the Prosecution of a Scenario

response" window where the P-3 software in the aircraft requests information from the operator and displays the operator's response. The PAT simulates these interactions as is done in the aircraft. Finally, the window to the right of the TACPLOT is time-shared, to display advice (if a trainee requests it) or special status information (if an instructor requests it). At present it displays the system's current advice and the goals that were used to derive the advice. In the case shown, the goal is to attack the target and the advice is to get a weapon ready, since the rule-based advisory system has concluded that the criteria for attacking the target have been met.

Communication between the operator and the simulation is greatly facilitated by the touch input panel attached to the CRT. The operator simply touches the point of the tactical plot to which he wants the simulator to attend, and then confirms his intensions by pressing a function key on the keyboard reserved for that purpose. The simulator accepts this position and saves its coordinates for whatever action the TACCO may take subsequently. The PAT's response to a touch of the CRT or a depression of a key is usually immediate and does not slow the simulation unless a disk access is required.

Voice output is provided using an analog device consisting of a 15-inch floppy disk containing approximately 30 minutes of pre-recorded, audio messages. Each message can be as short as a half second or as long as 30 minutes, and each is accessible in approximately a half second. Recording, editing, and playing messages is relatively easy; the sound is of high

quality, and the playing of audio messages does not slow the simulation.
(The audio device is available from Education Information Systems,
Incorporated, of Champaign, Illinois.)

The keyboard provides access to simulations of standard TACCO functions
for displaying and monitoring sensors; tracking targets; defining
Fly-To-Points and controlling the autopilot; deploying weapons; monitoring
and controlling the navigational error; and controlling the display by
recentering, rescaling, or changing the level of detail. Other keys were
programmed to permit the TACCO to exercise the "special" features of the
PAT, such as pausing or controlling the speed of the simulation;
controlling the audio device; invoking the advisor for assistance;
providing any of several dozen pertinent pieces of information that would
normally be available to him from crew members or other sources; and
controlling the flight of the aircraft. The TACCO can take actions and
obtain information when the system is either paused or running: the
keyboard is "live" at all times.

Once provided with a set of initial values for the environment,
aircraft, submarine, sonobuoys, and other factors, the simulation runs in
real time, responding to the operator's directives to climb, turn, release
or "ping" a sonobuoy, etc.; fulfilling operator requests for information;
and updating and displaying all interactions and changes each second. Play
continues until some pre-determined objective has been met or until the
player runs out of time. The system automatically saves all important
performance data on disk, to permit replay and evaluative data reporting.

The study of ASW and TACCO behavior is proceeding in parallel with the
development of the PAT. The investigator uses the PAT to study individual
TACCOs. Each TACCO is given some pertinent background information
concerning the scenario, and is asked to prosecute it as he would in the
aircraft. He is free to request information and take actions that are
normally available to him, using the PAT system as described earlier. Each
TACCO's performance and comments are analyzed, and the model of expert
performance and the PAT are improved and used to study other TACCOs.

This approach has yielded a research instrument of considerable power
and flexibility for studying the performance of TACCOs in airborne ASW. It
can provide a wide range of relatively realistic scenarios, with familiar
cues, symbology, avionics, interactions, and audio reports. The challenge
of a scenario can be specifically controlled, to permit observations of
TACCO performance on specific subproblems that complicate airborne ASW.

For example, the range of sensitivity of sonobuoys, MAD and other
sensors can be varied, along with the number of sonobuoys and weapons. The
simulated MAD is perturbed by aircraft maneuvers, as it is in the air, and
sonobuoys may fail to operate when dropped at high speed, high altitude, or
at other unpredictable times. Furthermore, the simulator can be
initialized to generate a false MAD signal at some point in the scenario.
The program does so at a point when a MAD contact is not completely
unreasonable but is highly unlikely based upon other information available
to the TACCO.

The study of TACCOs using the PAT is sill underway. Experience in the
use of various versions of it to study approximately a dozen individuals
indicates (McWilliams, 1981) that an individual TACCO behaves relatively
consistently, and that few of them take advantage of the chance to pause
the scenario for information or assistance. Furthermore, more experienced
TACCOs appear to engage in more planning early in the scenario to obtain
and save information that is frequently useful later. This appears to be
similar to the "posting" of information by experts, reported by Lesgold,

Feltovich, Glaser, and Wang (1981). Experience does not however, result in error-free performance. For example, experts as well as novices are sometimes susceptible to spurious MAD signals.

The results are considered quite tentative, since they were derived from relatively few TACCOs, using preliminary versions of the simulator that lacked passive sonobuoys and RADAR. The most recent version of the PAT, described below, has higher fidelity, including passive sonobuoys and RADAR, plus several special features designed specifically for training that will now be discussed.

SPECIAL FEATURES

It seems likely that most of the features of the simulator that are useful for research will be useful for training as well. This includes the ability to readily generate scenarios with specific challenges and the ability to replay scenarios. Other features have been added specifically for practice and training. Each of these features is dynamic, that is each can be invoked while a scenario is being played. These include abilities to control the speed and "place" of the scenario, to monitor and influence the performance of a trainee, and to obtain expert advice. Each of these features will be discussed briefly.

Scenario Control

It is envisioned that the PAT may be used for evaluation or qualifying tests, in which a scenario must be prosecuted in real time, without pausing or backing up. For more general practice, however, a scenario can be initialized to permit these actions. A trainee can, therefore "freeze" the scenario, and obtain information from the PAT while in the frozen state. This feature enables the trainee to "catch up" if the scenario is unfolding faster than he can prosecute it. The PAT can also be "backed up" by the operator, to return the simulator to a previously played point. This provides opportunities for the trainee to repeatedly prosecute a troublesome or difficult portion of a scenario, perhaps trying different tactics.

Furthermore, during replay of a scenario, the trainee can skip forward, checkpoint-by-checkpoint, to reach quickly any point of special interest. It is also possible to switch from replay to the "retry" mode, permitting either the trainee or the instructor to retry a scenario, from any point. This feature enables a trainee or his instructor to try (or demonstrate) alternative approaches, with all of the consequences that subsequently ensue.

Instructor Monitoring and Control

Two PATs can be connected in a local network, in which one PAT can simulate the pilot station from which the aircraft can be "flown" using the PAT flight control keys. The TACCO is thereby freed from the task of flight control and can concentrate completely, at his PAT, upon his special responsibilities. This networking feature also permits the instructor unobtrusively to monitor the TACCO's performance and the true state of the scenario and vary the challenge dynamically, as it unfolds. For example, if the TACCO is getting hopelessly behind on the problem, the instructor can reduce the submarine's speed or depth and drive it back within range of distant sonobuoys or other sensory instruments. The converse is also possible, of course: the sonobuoys or the MAD can be made less sensitive or fail altogether. Such control permits the instructor to salvage a training session that would otherwise be a waste of time.

The operator also has the ability to generate (initialize) new scenarios or change existing ones readily, using the touch input, display control, and all other features of the system. The scenario is then available immediately for play or testing. This feature will certainly be used by instructors, but it may also prove useful to let a trainee use it. He could set some of the variables himself, such as the ocean temperature profile or submarine evasion tactics, then play the scenario and observe the results. If properly structured and constrained by the instructor or the PAT itself, such an approach might be a relatively effective CBI technique.

```
*
if      not(A-WEAPON-IS-READY)
then    READY-A-WEAPON
to      HAVE-A-WEAPON-SET-FOR-BEST-DEPTH-AND-ARMED-FOR-RELEASE
do      ADVISE
else
actv    REDUCE-MPD-DRIFT
*
if      not(IMMEDIATE-ATTACK-IS-CALLED-FOR)
and     (THE-A/C-IS-DRIFTING-WRT-MOTSB
or      not(MPD-DRIFT-WAS-RECENTLY-CHECKED))
then    REDUCE-MPD-DRIFT
to      IMPROVE-NAVIGATIONAL-ACCURACY-JUST-BEFORE-WEAPON-DROP
do      ADVISE
actv    CORRECT-THE-TACPLOT
else
actv    GET.A-GOOD-WPN.POINT
*
if      not(THERE-IS-A-WEAPON-POINT)
or      not(THE-WEAPON-POINT-IS-GOOD)
then    GET.A-GOOD-WPN.POINT
to      PROVIDE-A-GOOD-FTP-FOR-A/C-STEERING-AND-WEAPON-DROP
do      ADVISE-GET-WFTP-POINTER
else
actv    REDUCE-ALTITUDE-FOR.ATTACK
*
if      THE-A/C-IS-TOO-HIGH-FOR-ATTACK
then    REDUCE-ALTITUDE-FOR.ATTACK
to      INCREASE-THE-RANGE-OF-THE-MAGNETIC-ANOMOLY-DETECTOR
do      ADVISE
else
actv    DECREASE-SPEED-TO.FTP
*
if      THE-SPEED-TO-THE-FTP-IS-HIGH
then    DECREASE-SPEED-TO.FTP
to      ARRIVE-AT-FTP-AT-LOW-SPEED-TO-INCREASE-DWELL-TIME-THERE
do      ADVISE
else
actv    INCREASE-SPEED-TO.FTP
*
if      THE-SPEED-TO-THE-FTP-IS-LOW
then    INCREASE-SPEED-TO.FTP
to      REACH-THE-TARGET-MORE-QUICKLY
do      ADVISE
else
actv    ATTACK-THE.TARGET-DOWNTRACK
*
if      not(THE-APPRCH-TO-THE-WFTP-IS-GOOD)
then    ATTACK-THE.TARGET-DOWNTRACK
to      OPTIMIZE-THE-EFFECTIVENESS-OF-THE-WEAPON-AND-THE-MAD
do      ADVISE
else
actv    REDUCE-NOISE-IN.MAD
*
```

Table 1. A Fragment of the PAT-RTAS Rulebase

Automatic Monitoring and Advice

One subsystem of the trainer, presently only partially implemented, dynamically monitors and analyzes the state of the scenario and the trainee's actions. A fragment of the present basis for such monitoring is the set of ASW subgoals in Table 1. This is a subset of the rules that are considered for advice during the track and attack phase. Approximately 100 state variables are presently being monitored. Some of these are simply binary conditions (Yes/No, Absent/Present, On/Off). Many state variables have times of occurrence associated with them. This subsystem is called the Real-Time Advisory System (RTAS).

The RTAS permits the PAT to provide immediate diagnostic feedback. At present, two levels of advice are provided. The first level, when requested, simply searches the rule-base of expertise and the set of state/condition flags and provides a single, brief piece of advice concerning what it considers to be the most significant operator action for the most significant subproblem (or complication) present in the scenario. Play is not interrupted, and the operator is free to ignore the feedback. If the trainee wishes to see the basis for the advice, the PAT displays the hierarchy of goals immediately above the advice (See Figure 2). If the trainee wishes additional detail, the PAT can display a graphical, full-color display of the goal tree and evidence states, and dynamically trace how the advice was derived.

The second level of feedback, based upon the rule-base, is presented more forcefully. It is intended for use when the operator is having serious difficulty in one of the phases of ASW described earlier. When requested, the RTAS looks through a priority list of "critical incidents" that occurred earlier in the scenario (and were duly recorded by the RTAS). The RTAS chooses the incident of highest priority and returns the scenario to the place where the critical incident occurred. The simulation then enters the paused state, in which the trainee can request information or take actions that should permit him to avoid the consequences of the incident. The trainee cannot yet resume playing the scenario, however. The RTAS provides the information or takes the action requested by the trainee. If the request is pertinent to the critical incident, the RTAS commends the trainee for making it. If the trainee does not know what else to do, he can request advice, which the RTAS will provide, one piece at a time. In any case, the scenario will not be resumed until the trainee takes every pertinent action and requests every pertinent item of information. When he has done so, the RTAS releases the simulation from the paused state and the trainee can play the scenario again from that point. This second level of PAT assistance is called "direction", to reflect the degree of control that the PAT assumes when this level of assistance is requested.

The set of subproblems, with associated states and critical incidents is based upon the study of ASW and TACCOs begun by McWilliams (1981). Ultimately, the RTAS and related structures will embody the most appropriate behaviors observed or inferred from studying many experienced TACCOs, for all phases of ASW. Plans for the RTAS include the ability not only to advise the trainee, but to demonstrate appropriate performance as well. The RTAS will also be able to provide embedded explanations and instruction upon request, by using the simulator to produce and display important interactions and consequences. This feature resembles somewhat the "mini-labs" that Williams, Hollan, and Stevens (1981) have proposed to employ with STEAMER. The goal, of course, is to make the PAT more articulate, that is, more like a "glass box" (Goldstein and Papert, 1977) than a "black box".

CONCLUDING REMARKS

We have argued that adding information about a task or its performance can increase the instructional power of CBI systems and we have mentioned several such systems and described one - the PAT. Although the PAT started as a research device, it is currently being developed as an intelligent, microcomputer-based trainer for ASW. We feel that the development is sufficiently far along that it demonstrates the feasibility of the following important aspects of the project:

- Portable, low-cost microcomputer systems possess the computing power, graphic capabilities and other features necessary to simulate complex and dynamic systems, and can provide integrated and realistic practice and training on the procedures, tactics, and strategies required.

- The use of such a device as a research instrument in a domain such as ASW helps in understanding what constitutes and underlies expert behavior, and also facilitates system development.

- It is possible, within the same machine, to dynamically monitor individual trainee performance and provide pertinent advice and training.

- It is possible to develop all aspects of such a trainer using only the hardware and software provided with a microcomputer system.

It appears, therefore, that a good start has been made toward the long-term goal of developing a portable, low-cost, intelligent PAT. To conclude that something is feasible, however, does not imply that it is completed or that doing so will be easy. A good deal of work remains before a complete PAT system, with all of its instructional features, can be released for routine use. Let us consider some of the present limitations.

The PAT monitor/advisor subsystem is in preliminary form, with an incomplete and relatively untested model of the ASW goals and performance of the expert and the trainee. The present PAT cannot yet demonstrate expertise, adequately explain its advice, or provide true instruction. Furthermore, it is presently up to the trainee to select the level and time of the assistance. Except for the work of Burton and Brown (1979 and 1982), and Clancey (1981), there have been few studies about when and how to advise. It will undoubtedly require considerable experience with various versions of the advisor and various trainees before completely satisfactory strategies and structures emerge.

It is also not clear how to adequately monitor and temporarily order the multitude of states that can occur when a scenario is played. One cannot preserve everything, even with the considerable memory and processing power that is available. We have found little in the literature to guide us concerning this matter.

Even with the problems noted here, however, it seems likely that the PAT would already be useful for training in airborne ASW. As of this writing (February, 1985) one PAT system is installed and operating in one ASW Wing of the U.S. Navy, where fleet personnel are using it and are evaluating its utility. No decision has been made concerning wider use, but the results thus far seem encouraging.

Work is continuing toward the goal of a fully implemented PAT, in accord with the principles of simulation, training, and expert system development referenced in this paper. When that goal is reached, some interesting opportunities will arise. A fully operational PAT will be sufficiently inexpensive and portable enough to be carried along on deployment or on an aircraft carrier, and could be installed in every ASW squadron. Since the PAT simulator programs are generalized, one could extend the software to simulate the avionics and procedures for other ASW positions, such as the sensory operators (SENSOs). Two PATs in a squadroom could then provide individual practice and training for either TACCOs or SENSOs, or integrated crew training for a TACCO-SENSO team, prosecuting a common scenario. Such capability could contribute to significant changes in the acquisition and use of high-fidelity simulators. It could also deepen the understanding and appreciation of the importance of closely coupling empirical research and engineering development in the production of training systems.

REFERENCES

Adams, J.A. (1979). On the evaluation of training devices. "Human Factors," "21," 711-720.

Brown, J.S. & Burton, R.R. (1975). Multiple representations of knowledge for tutorial reasoning. In Bobrow, D. & Collins, A. (Eds.), "Representation and understanding: Studies in cognitive science" (pp. 311-349). New York: Academic Press.

Buchanan, B.G. & Mitchell, T.M. (1978). Model-directed learning of production rules. In Waterman, D. & Hayes-Roth, F. (Eds.) "Pattern directed inference systems" (pp. 297-312). New York: Academic Press.

Burton, R.R. & Brown, J.S. (1979). An investigation of computer coaching for informal learning activities. "International Journal of Man-Machine Studies," "11," 5-24.

Burton, R.R. & Brown, J.S. (1982). An investigation of computer coaching for informal learning activities. In Sleeman, D. & Brown, J.S. (Eds.), "Intelligent tutoring systems" (pp. 79-98). New York: Academic Press.

Caro, P.W. (1973). Aircraft simulators and pilot training. "Human Factors," "15," 502-509.

Clancey, W.J. (1981). "Methodology for building an intelligent tutoring system" (Tech. Rep. STAN-CS-81-894). Stanford, CA: Stanford University, Department of Computer Science.

Davis, R. (1982). Expert systems: where are we? And where do we go from here? "The AI Magazine" (pp. 3-22).

Feigenbaum, E.A. (1977). The art of artificial intelligence: I. Themes and case studies of knowledge engineering. "Proceedings of the Fifth International Joint Conference on Artificial Intelligence" (pp. 1014-1029). Pittsburgh, PA: Carnegie-Mellon University, Department of Computer Science.

Feurzeig, W., Ash, W., & Ricard, G.L. (1984). TRIO, an expert system for air intercept training. "In Proceedings of the Sixth Interservice/Industry Training Equipment Conference and Exhibition" (pp. 45-48). Orlando, Fl.: Naval Training Equipment Center.

Goldstein, I. & Papert, S. (1977). Artificial intelligence, language, and the study of knowledge. "Cognitive Science," "1," 1-21.

Hutchins, E. & McCandless, T. (1982). "MANBOARD: A graphic display program for training relative motion concepts" (Tech. Rep. NPRDC TR 82-10). San Diego: Naval Personnel Research and Development Center.

Hutchins, E., McCandless, T., Woodworth, G., & Dutton, B. (1984). "Maneuvering board training system: Analysis and redesign" (Tech. Rep. NPRDC TR 84-19). San Diego: Naval Personnel Research and Development Center.

Kearsley, G. (1983). "Computer-based training." Reading, MA: Addison-Wesley.

Kearsley, G., Hunter, B., & Seidel, R.J. (1983 January). Two decades of computer-based instruction projects: What have we learned? Part 1. "T.H.E. Journal," "10(3)," 90-94.

Kearsley, G., Hunter, B., & Seidel, R.J. (1983, February). Two decades of computer-based instruction projects: What have we learned? Part 2. "T.H.E. Journal," "10(4)," 90-96.

Kulik, J.A., Bangert, R.L., & Williams, G.W. (1983). Effects of computer-based teaching on secondary school students. "Journal of Educational Psychology," "75," 19-26.

Kulik, J.A., Kulik, C.C., & Cohen, P.A. (1980). Effectiveness of computer-based college teaching: A meta-analysis of findings. "Review of Educational Research," "50," 525-544.

Lesgold, A.M., Feltovich, P.J., Glaser, R., & Wang, Y. (1981). "The acquisition of perceptual diagnostic skill in radiology" (Tech. Rep. PDS-1). Pittsburgh: Learning Research and Development Center, University of Pittsburgh.

McWilliams, E.D. (1981). "A study of airborn tactical navigation." Unpublished doctoral dissertation, University of Maryland, College Park.

Meyers, R. (1984). Plato: Historical roots, current applications, and future prospects. "Training Technology Journal," "1(2)," 26-32.

Montague, W.E. (1984). "Computer-based systems for Navy classroom training" (Tech. Rep. NPRDC TR 85-11). San Diego: Naval Personnel Research and Development Center.

Montague, W.E. & Wulfeck, W.H., II (1984). Computer-based instruction: Will it improve instructional quality? "Training Technology Journal," "1(2)," 4-19.

Orlansky, J. & String, J. (1980). "Cost effectiveness of computer-based instruction in military training" (IDA paper P1375). Arlington, VA.: Institute of Defense Analysis.

Pople, H.E., Myers, J.D., and Miller, R.A. (1975). DIALOG, a model of diagnostic logic for internal medicine. "Proceedings of the Fourth International Joint Conference on Artificial Intelligence" (pp. 848-855). Los Altos, CA: William Kaufmann.

Romano, S.A. (1978). "Tactical navigation and plot stabilization" (Technical Memo from the S-3A software change review board coordinator). Rockville, MD: Tracor Sciences and Systems.

Sleeman, D. & Brown, J.S. (Eds.) (1982). "Intelligent tutoring system." New York: Academic Press.

Tenczar, P. (1981). CAI evolution: Mainframe to micro. In Zimmer, R.P. (Ed.), "Proceedings of the International Conference on Cybernetics and Society" (pp. 443-448). New York: Institute of Electrical and Electronic Engineers.

Williams, M., Hollan, J., & Stevens, A. (1981). An overview of STEAMER: An advanced computer-assisted instruction system for propulsion engineering. "Behavior Research Methods and Instrumentation," "13," 85-90.

Wilson, L. S. (1984). Presenting TICCIT: State-of-the-art computer-based instruction. "Training Technology Journal," "1(2)," 26-32.

CAITER: A COMPUTER BASED INSTRUCTION TERMINAL

A. Brebner*, H. J. Hallworth* and G. McKinnon**

*University of Calgary
 Calgary, Alberta, Canada

**Pedicom Electronic Teaching Systems, Ltd.
  Calgary, Alberta, Canada

A CBI TERMINAL SYSTEM

   The paper describes a terminal system, incorporating multi-media facilities, for the authoring and delivery of computer based instruction.

   For a period of 16 years the Faculty of Education Computer Applications Unit at the University of Calgary has been active in the development of terminal systems and special purpose languages for computer based instruction, and in the development and empirical evaluation of courseware for a variety of subject areas (Hallworth & Brebner, 1980). Several terminal systems have been designed in conjunction with the computer based education project in the Electrical Engineering Division of the National Research Council in Ottawa, and have been developed in prototype form by the NRC for experimental use in the Unit (Brahan & Hallworth, 1971). In 1977 a multi-media terminal system, based upon an early microcomputer, was produced in the Unit (Brebner & Hallworth, 1980; Hallworth & Brebner, 1979). Fifteen such terminals are only now being phased out of use.

   Based upon this background of experience in research, development, and evaluation of hardware, software, and courseware for computer based instruction, a new microcomputer based terminal system has now been produced (McKinnon, 1984).

   Provisionally named CAITER, this will provide an integrated system of hardware and software which is inexpensive, portable, stands alone and, if required, multilingual.

FUNCTIONS REQUIRED IN A CBI TERMINAL

   CAITER has been designed so that it will meet the significant requirements of a computer based instruction terminal system. It was considered that such a system must be adaptive to the needs of learners, that it must provide good support for courseware authors, that it must be adaptable to a variety of computing environments and that, in order to be accepted for widespread use, it must be low in cost with respect to both hardware on the one hand, and software and courseware on the other.

Adaptation to the Learner: Output Facilities

Computer based instruction systems are intended to facilitate student learning. Above all, therefore, they should be designed to allow the presentation of courseware so that it capitalizes upon the learner's needs and capabilities.

__Multi-Media Output__   It is unfortunate that so much courseware has been, and still is, text bound. At a time when only hard copy terminals were available, computer based instruction was, necessarily, almost entirely text. There is cause to believe it is largely for this reason that computer based instruction has not yet begun to produce the gains and achievements that will ultimately be possible.

Following the widespread acceptance of Piaget's description of human cognitive development, there would probably be general agreement that we begin our early learning in terms of schemata related to sensori- motor habits. These in turn develop through the "concrete" stage to the level of formal thinking using symbols. Our formal use of words, numbers, and other symbols comes last, and is based upon thinking centered around habits, concrete objects, and images of such objects. Many of us do not reach the stage of formal thinking; more of us reach it in only some limited parts of our cognitive operations; and all of us, when learning something new, proceed much more effectively if we are able to make use of concrete objects, or images of such objects.

When human thinking is considered in this light, it is clear that a CBI system should be multi-media. In most learning contexts, courseware should make use of graphics and images, either as an addition to or a replacement for words and numbers. Sound is also useful, particularly speech, in that it is an integral element in so much early learning and can be used to supplement visual information.

Further, all information should appear as rapidly as the student needs it. A fast response time is essential. This is particularly important in the case of graphics and images, which are typically slow to appear on CBI displays.

It is also essential that the system allow precise and reliable timing of audio output in relation to any display on the screen. This is now possible, but its importance should be noted, in that poor and unreliable timing have led to disastrous results in earlier CBI experiments.

Some of the better known projects such as PLATO and TICCIT have demonstrated the value of images, graphics, and audio. However, the technology they employed was not sufficiently flexible for the extensive use of computer based instruction that is now possible.

__Symbolic Output__   When learning material presented to the student is symbolic in form, that is, when it consists of words, numbers, or other symbolic characters, then the symbols used should be exactly those that are conventionally accepted and that the student is expected to learn.

Mathematical, statistical, and scientific symbols should appear as they normally do in typeset text; and second language characters should appear in their regular form. Further, all symbols should be appropriate size and should be positioned in the conventional manner: for example, axes and lines on graphs should be labelled as in a typeset text, and superscripts and subscripts should be placed in the correct positions:

- To make use of non-standard symbols, or to position symbols in a non-conventional manner, is simply to present extra difficulties to the student and to inhibit learning.
- It is also apparent that images should be detailed and sharp; and that lines or graphs, with any angle or curvature, should be at least as good as the student normally sees on a typeset text. In many cases, colour assists clarity and is certainly motivational.

Adaptation to the Learner: Input Facilities

The standard input device of CBI systems has been a keyboard similar to that used originally on a typewriter. For many learners this is probably the most appropriate device for general use, assuming that it provides the keys for any special characters that are required by the program.

In many learning situations it is an advantage to use a supplementary keyboard containing the symbols needed by a specific piece of courseware. Learners progress more rapidly when they choose from a restricted number of keys, particularly if the symbols are new to them. Bubble pad keyboard, for example, may be tailored to size and may be marked with any required symbols. If appropriate, these may be restricted to a binary choice. Further, such keyboards can be marked with pictures or icons, or the keys may be covered by real objects such as bills or coins. A CBI system designed to meet the needs of the learner must be able to interface such input devices with minimal difficulty and cost.

However, a keyboard generally requires that the learner has achieved a certain familiarity and competence with the symbols that are used. Again, a lower level of cognition may be reached by simply requiring that the learner recognize a picture, a drawing, or an icon, and position a cursor to select or move it. This is possible when the system includes an analogue to digital converter with appropriate input device such as a joystick, when the display has adequate resolution for the necessary images, and when software is available to enable an author to make use of this input mode.

Such "positional" input may also be used to simplify the response of a learner engaged in a high level cognitive task, such as marking points or tracks on a graph or map.

Provision of Author Support

The input and output of a CBI system are unlikely to be used to advantage, however, unless the system also provides adequate author support.

The large scale systems of the 1960s and 1970s excelled in this respect. The PLATO system had its own language, TUTOR, which continued to grow by accretion as new support for authors was required. Similarly, the TICCIT system supplied authors with easily used commands which would create frames for displaying questions or answers, develop graphics, or incorporate images into the programs. Both systems, like the Canadian National Research Council language NATAL, or the WICAT courseware development system, provide very easily used facilities for the recording of both student and program data.

There is still no widely used language that provides similar facilities on a microcomputer, and for a very good reason: such languages require a very large amount of memory and considerable processing power. TUTOR may be difficult to learn because of its large instruction set, but microcomputer versions of PLATO have so far been restrictive to the author because they provide too limited a subset of instructions. The TICCIT system was sometimes considered to impose too rigid a framework upon authors. NATAL, which originated on a PDP-10, has carried too great an overhead in its microcomputer implementation to date, although it might well be possible to divide it into a larger authoring system and a smaller delivery system.

Obviously, the provision of adequate author support on a low cost CBI system is a difficult problem.

Adaptability to Computing Environments

Similarly, none of the equipment available at present offers a solution to the problem of adapting a CBI system to a variety of computing environments.

Most computer based instruction in the 1960s and 1970s was developed on time sharing mainframes and minicomputers, using dumb terminals which were first hard copy and later display type. At a time when Grosch's law was still applicable, this made efficient use of the central processor. However, it did so at a price: telecommunications costs were high, particularly for remote terminals; and transmission speeds were low, resulting in slow graphic displays. The PLATO project has suffered in both respects.

More recently, the development of stand alone microcomputers has made possible much more widespread use of computer based instruction, of much lower quality. Graphics have been comparatively poor, image projection has been almost nonexistent, and record keeping facilities for a group of learners have either been ignored or have entailed severe logistical problems. Computer based instruction as provided by present microcomputers is to be commended, but at the same time regarded as quite inadequate.

Clearly, there is a need for a CBI system that is adaptive to a variety of computing environments: stand alone microcomputers; multiple user microcomputers; time shared minicomputers and mainframes; and distributed processing systems, possibly using local and long distance networks. At the present time there is no adequate CBI terminal system that can be used in all these environments.

Low Cost

Any CBI terminal system designed to fit into such a variety of computing environments should be not only effective and reliable, but also inexpensive, otherwise it will never be used on a wide scale.

The hardware should have a low manufacturing cost, based upon the use of custom chips. Further, this should be achieved while still retaining the facilities already indicated as necessary for an adequate CBI system.

The software should also be designed to maintain economy of operation. When it is acknowledged that the cost of software and courseware is growing so fast that it will soon outstrip the cost of hardware, several implications may be recognized. Courseware is not only expensive to develop, it is also difficult and therefore expensive to port to machines other than the one for which it was originally designed.

One reasonable solution would be to implement courseware in a widely used base language, for example C. However, since few CBI authors are able to program in a base language, it would then be necessary to develop macros which could be made available to authors as templates or mini-authoring systems. It is perhaps doubtful whether another fully fledged authoring system should be developed at the present time. Further, if one is desired, it is possible that NATAL will soon be available for a variety of machines.

A CBI terminal system adapted to a variety of computing environments would make portability a reality. Such a system, able to make use of a commonly used base language, but also to accept ASCII code generated by any language, would significantly reduce the cost of computer based instruction.

THE CAITER SYSTEM

CAITER has been designed to provide at low cost the functions required for effective computer based instruction in that it supports multi-media output, with a display that provides symbols adequate for all anticipated requirements, high resolution colour graphics, and synthetic speech to meet most CBI needs. It also offers versatile input facilities and author support, and is adaptable to a variety of computer environments.

Multi-Media Features

Symbols   The system supports either a monochrome or a colour monitor, with 512 X 480 pixels; and an eight level grey scale, or eight basic colours and 64 composite colours.

Considerable flexibility is offered in the display of both symbolic and graphic information.

The standard characters may be displayed in 30 lines of 64 characters, using a font of 8 X 16 pixels. There is also a resident set of Greek and mathematical symbols which use the same size font.

However, courseware authors may define and use any other symbols, using author support programs for the design of alternate characters. Again, such characters use a font size of 8 X 16 pixels. Composite characters may be built up by an optional overprinting facility. Larger characters requiring more than one block of pixels may be created by displaying their parts in adjacent blocks. These features are particularly useful in mathematics and science programs, also for second language instruction. Further, any character may be magnified up to 15 times, and may be rotated and placed in any position on the screen. It is therefore a simple matter to use superscripts and subscripts, to display the correct mathematical and scientific formulae using the appropriate symbols in their correct position, or to insert vertical labels on maps, graphs, and diagrams.

Using a colour monitor, CAITER allows control of both background and foreground colours when displaying symbols. With a monochrome monitor, this control is used to produce variable intensity of both characters and backgrounds.

In effect, the flexibility of CAITER's symbol display system approaches that of a person writing on a blackboard with coloured chalk. It is possible for the author to present to the student precisely those symbols that are required by the courseware, with the appropriate sizes and colours, in exactly the positions on the screen where they are needed. In this sense, the hardware and software system are designed to maximize learning from material presented in text format.

Graphics   CAITER also has extensive facilities for the display of graphical information. The resolution is equal to that of a PLATO terminal. Using a standard 525 line monitor, this is the maximum resolution that is practicable. However, CAITER has the added advantage of a range of colours or grey scale, as already indicated.

Lines may be from 1 to 15 pixels in width, in one of the eight basic colours. They may be drawn by an author for the creation of maps and diagrams by manipulation of a joystick, or by input from a graphics tablet. Again, author support programs make this a simple task. These simplify the drawing, for example, of straight lines, polygons, ellipses, or quadrants of circles. Screen areas may be filled by any of the eight solid colours or 64 composite colours; or with a monochrome monitor, any of the eight shades of grey. This assists student learning in a variety of lessons, for example where use is made of maps, or diagrammatic representations of equipment.

Other programs support the generation of graphical displays at run time, using either student input or randomly chosen data. This is useful in the drawing of graphs of mathematical functions, for example, where the parameters are input or randomly produced.

It is important to note that symbolic and graphical information may be freely mixed on any part of the screen.

The speed at which displays appear, even if they are complex graphs in colour, is much superior to that of other CBI systems available, even at considerably higher cost. In order to take full advantage of this feature, it is necessary to have a communications line operating at 9600 baud. In cases where such a baud rate is not possible, CAITER will still produce graphics of equal resolution but at a slower speed. In such circumstances it may be preferable to use a stand alone version of the system. Given the low cost and flexibility of CAITER, this will generally be possible.

   <u>Audio Output</u>   CAITER has a built-in synthetic speech system and a sound generator.

In deciding upon the type of speech output system to use, three considerations appeared important. First, the speech must be of high quality; second, it must not be confined to one language or one speaker, but must be available for a variety of languages and speakers; and third, it must be possible to produce not merely a few words and sentences, but a considerable amount of speech for various learning programs. Therefore text-to-speech systems were not considered as they do not provide sufficiently high quality output; phonetic systems were rejected as being confined, in general, to one natural language only; and fully digitized speech was not used because it requires too much memory, even when the code is compressed.

The chosen technology was linear predictive coding. This limits the system to output of pre-stored speech, in the form of code stored on ROM chips resident in CAITER, or on a disk in a host computer, or on a disk in a stand alone system. However, the linear predictive decoding chips are quite inexpensive, the speech is of good quality, and both the storage requirements and the transmission rate of 1800 baud are quite low. Further, considerable vocabularies are already available in ROM chips; and the technology is available, at comparatively low cost, to produce more code as necessary.

Each CAITER system is fitted with a linear predictive decoder chip, and with a basic single-word vocabulary in ROM. Other speech, consisting of single words, full sentences, or paragraphs, is produced from recorded utterances, using the particular type of voice required. The recording is processed to produce the necessary code, which is stored on disk.

It is considered that the system will make possible the development of courseware, using speech output, that is both effective and inexpensive.

CAITER's music and sound generator outputs a mixed sound from four sources. Three of these are pitch tunable, while the fourth produces periodic or non-periodic noise. The amplitudes of all four sources are controllable.

Sound generator outputs is useful for enhancing scientific courseware with realistic sound effects and providing melodies for music teaching.

CAITER has a built in speaker, also a jack for headphones.

<u>Image Projection</u>   Technology for image projection is currently being built into CAITER.

Numerous problems have arisen in connection with image projection techniques used by CBI projects in the past. Microfiche projection, as used in the University of Illinois PLATO project, has been notably unsuccessful and has not been adopted for the CDC version of PLATO.

The University of Calgary Faculty of Education Computer Applications unit has used random access slide projections under computer control since 1969. Several computer interfaces have been developed within the Unit, and have worked successfully for fifteen years, giving excellent image projection on a rear view screen. However, this apparatus is far too cumbersome for general use, and experience has indicated the importance of using a single display, namely the monitor.

The TICCIT system, using colour television sets, is in many respects excellent; but this system of audio output and image projection makes adaptation to other computing environments difficult, and also does not give a fast response time for single frames.

Video tape systems are unreliable due to the stretching of the tape. Video disks hold greater promise, but are still expensive for widespread use; and both the costs and logistics associated with authoring a disk are considerable.

It was therefore decided to use fully digitized images. One difficulty is that the technology to produce such images, using microcomputers such as the IBM PC, is only now becoming available commercially. However, several such systems have been announced recently. Further, although detailed images still require a large amount of storage, this requirement will become less significant as vertical head recording becomes common on disk systems.

This is therefore a feature of CAITER which will be added when justified by the economics of the technology.

<u>Student Interface: Input</u>

A regular keyboard is used to input the standard set of characters. The extended sets available may be accessed using the same keyboard, covered with a template.

However, a second 8-bit parallel input port is available so that a special purpose keyboard may also be attached. This may be a regular keyboard having certain keys marked with special characters as, for example, the characters needed in statistics, electronics, or second languages. Alternatively, as already indicated, such a keyboard may have keys marked by icons, pictures, or small objects such as transistors.

Further, CAITER has a built in joystick that may be used for positional input. Six additional analogue input channels are also available for attaching other joysticks, panpots, or variable switches.

In effect, this provides an extremely flexible input system that may be adapted to assist the student in interacting with a wide range of courseware.

When symbolic input is required, as in second language learning, mathematics, and the sciences, the student may learn to use the correct symbols: it is no longer necessary to demand that (s)he constantly translate to and from other symbols which are required by the limitations of the system, and which in fact inhibit learning.

Further, any positional input device may be used that best meets the needs of the student and the program. The student may draw graphs, input drawings, track a line, move a picture or part of a picture, or use the positional input to identify part of a text, graphic, or picture displayed on the screen.

The objective is to ensure that courseware may be adapted to student learning needs and, insofar as input is concerned, CAITER is able to achieve this more effectively than has previously been possible.

Author Support

CAITER is designed to accept ASCII code, which may originate from any computer language able to produce such code.

Author support programs are available for the interactive production and editing of alternate character sets, for automatic graphic generation, for use of the joystick to produce graphic displays, and for the development and editing of display files and speech output. Routines are also available to perform operations frequently required in CBI programs, for example, to evaluate mathematical expressions.

However, as indicated earlier, a large and increasing proportion of the cost of computer based instruction relates to the courseware. Instructional programs are expensive to produce, and become still more expensive if they must be retranslated for every computer system on which they are used. It is therefore essential to have effective tools for computer courseware authors, in order to reduce the time, insofar as possible, programmed in a widely acceptable base language.

Some earlier programs for CAITER were developed in BASIC, and the system can readily make use of code generated by this language.

However, author support routines have now been developed in the C language, which is widely available in microcomputers, minicomputers, and mainframes. The intent is to develop a library of such routines, from which units may be assembled to form a variety of template systems for use by authors in the generation of learning programs. This will allow authors who have experience in designing instruction, but no knowledge of computer programming, to generate specific types of programs in minimum time. All courseware will include record keeping facilities, and there will be no difficulty in developing new templates as required.

Adaptability to Computing Environments

To ensure flexibility of use, a CBI terminal system requires not only easily useable software developed in a widely available base language: it must also possess a capability to operate in a variety of computer hardware environments.

CAITER is therefore designed to be attached via a 9600 baud serial interface directly to a host computer, which may be a microcomputer, a minicomputer, or a mainframe, possibly operating in timesharing mode; to be part of a distributed processing system; or to be a stand alone machine with its own disk memory.

In timesharing environments in which there is some spare capacity, CAITER may most economically be used as a terminal attached to a host computer. In this case, courseware programs execute on the host and send high level commands encoded in ASCII to CAITER. A continuously running firmware program, stored in CAITER's ROM, interprets and implements these commands. Because the terminal input and output are interrupt driven, CAITER simultaneously receives and executes commands.

Courseware may be written in any host language that produces ASCII code, but in view of the author support routines available in C, this is the most appropriate language.

This is probably the least expensive way of achieving a multi-user installation, but performance is dependent upon availability of a host capable of providing data at 9600 baud.

In a distributed processing system, CAITER may be attached to a fileserver to accept courseware programs downloaded from a host over a local or long distance network. When a program has been run on CAITER, student and program performance data may be uploaded to the fileserver. In this type of environment the basic terminal requires, additionally, a single board computer.

CAITER may also be configured as a stand alone system. This configuration is particularly useful for situations where only a single learning station is required, or where transportability is desirable. To upgrade a basic terminal to a single user system, a single board computer and a 3.5 inch floppy disk drive must be added.

A CAITER, with its program and data, may be transferred from one computing environment to another. Since the terminal system does not change, the CBI system remains identical from the standpoint of the user: from his/her point of view, the environment remains constant.

CONTINUED DEVELOPMENT

An important feature of CAITER is that the hardware costs are low, and that such costs are becoming progressively lower while computing power and memory are increasing. This means that the system is affordable, and in this sense could be used on a large scale.

However, the most significant feature of CAITER is that, from a computer based instruction standpoint, it is a multi-media system tailored to the needs of the user. It is designed to make learning easy and effective because, instead of requiring that the learner adapt to the system, CAITER is adapted to the learner.

Moreover, the learner does not have to move out of his/her normal working environment in order to receive computer based instruction. CAITER is portable, and can be taken to the learner. It may be used effectively in most existing computing environments or as a stand alone. It uses software systems that are as portable as they can be, given the present state of the art. Further, the circuitry of the first production model of CAITER, using a custom chip and including a single board computer and disk drive if required, will be installed beneath a standard keyboard.

Since CAITER is designed to be flexible and to permit continued development as the technology becomes available, it can continue to grow and incorporate new facilities such as the display of digitized images and the use of more powerful microprocessors with larger memory.

The potential for continued development is based upon the fact that CAITER is in no way constrained by present hardware and software: its value resides in the concepts around which it has been developed, and in the custom chip circuitry which realizes these concepts.

REFERENCES

Alderman, D. L. (1978), "Evaluation of the TICCIT computer-assisted instructional system in the community college." Princeton, New Jersey: Educational Testing Service.
Avner, R. A. & Tenczar, P. (1979). CERL report X-4. Urbana, IL: University of Illinois.
Brahan, J. H., & Hallworth, H. J. (1971, March). "Computer-aided learning a cooperative research project." Paper presented to 18th International Scientific Congress on Electronics, Rome.
Brahan, J. W., Henneker, W. H. & Hlady, A. M.(1980). Natal-74 - concept to reality. "Proceedings of the Third Canadian Symposium on Instructional Technology," (pp. 233-240). Ottawa: National Research Council.
Brebner, A., & Hallworth, H. J. (1980). A multi-media CAI terminal based upon a microprocessor with applications for the handicapped. "Proceedings of the 18th Annual Convention of the Association for Educational Data Systems," (pp. 18-20). Washington, D.C.
Hallworth, H. J., & Brebner, A. (1979). "The microprocessor-based terminal: User's manual." Internal report, University of Calgary, Faculty of Education Computer Applications Unit, Alberta, Canada.
Hallworth, H. J., & Brebner, A. (1980). "Computer assisted instruction in schools," (p. 91). Edmonton, Alberta, Canada: Alberta Education.
McKinnon, G. (1984). "CAITER programming manual." Calgary, Alberta, Canada: Pedicom Electronic Teaching Systems Ltd.
Piaget, J. (1952). "The origin of intelligence in children." New York: International Universities Press.
Ralston, A. & Meek, C.L. (Eds.) (1976). "Encyclopedia of Computer Science," (p. 599). New York: Petrocelli/Charter.
"WISE" (1983). Provo, UT: WICAT Systems.

THE USE OF COMPUTERS IN TRAINING IN THE BRITISH ARMY

D. K. Dana

Army School of Training Support
Wilton Park, Bucks, U.K.

INTRODUCTION

The British Army adopted a formal systematic approach to training in the late 1960s (Annex A) and it soon became obvious that in order to monitor the efficiency and effectiveness of training courses, large amounts of data had to be analysed. As administrative computer systems became more readily available at a reasonable cost it was natural that trainers should turn to computers as a possible solution to the problems of producing accurate training data rapidly.

Computer controlled simulations have been in use for some time but it is only recently that a systematic analysis has been undertaken to link the level of fidelity required to master the skills required. Commercial pressures have in the past tended to persuade training establishments to buy high cost, high fidelity trainers.

MANAGEMENT OF TRAINING

Our first experiment in computer managed learning was a joint project involving International Computers Limited (ICL) and two universities. The Computer Assisted Management of Learning (CAMOL) system was introduced into the Royal Signals Trade Training School in 1976. This establishment handles upwards of 1,000 students on 80 courses with the annual throughput of 4,000 students.

The computer software was to be used to deal with test marking and analysis of test results and sorting, summarizing, recording and cross referencing data. The program had been developed for civilian educational establishments by ICL to help in student continuous assessment systems and was to be modified to suit the particular requirements of the Trade Training School. The project started with the analysis of the particular requirements of the military establishment and the types of data to be dealt with were:

    a. Test marks (objective and subjective)
    b. Numerical performance measures
    c. Binary pass/fail of training objectives and courses
    d. Scaling (5 points or less)

The requirements of the course managers and quality control cell were identified and reports designed to meet these needs. The system failed for a number of reasons. The causes were attributed to the method of software development and staff attitudes. The software was adapted from a continuous student assessment system of a university to the rigid pass/fail criteria referencing of an objective training system and this meant customising the software. This was achieved after 12 months. Appropriate reports that met the managements' stated requirements were able to be generated. Because of system software complexity the ability to change the system after the end of the development period to reflect any organizational changes was beyond the capabilities of the user and was therefore expensive.

Changes in the management structure of the organization and personalities took place soon after project completion and so the information contained in the reports sent to training managers was often inappropriate. Changes of staff at the managerial level at the time of system implementation meant that the committment to the system which had developed in the original staff because of their involvement in the project was no longer present to the same degree. This change in emphasis was seen by the remainder of the training staff who also saw in the system a method of monitoring their own performance as instructors. In addition it was found that by the time student information had been registered on the system and disseminated short courses were almost complete. The feedback in these cases was therefore of limited use to instructors who were still required to mark practical tests and subjective tests. In summary the failure of this first project could be attributed to three factors:

a. Inability of the software to meet organizational change

b. Loss of management committment because of staff changes

c. Lack of instructor support because no strategy was developed to manage change in the organization

STUDENT PERFORMANCE AND EVALUATION BY COMPUTER (SPEC)

The second project in use only one year later in a different training establishment developed in a different way and at a much slower pace. The system installed in 1977 was based on a system which started to be developed in 1971. At that stage it was merely a calculator but it provided invaluable experience to management and provided useful output to the Evaluation and Quality Control Cell. From these early beginnings developed the student monitoring facility designed to identify group and individual training weaknesses as early as possible in the training cycle. The operation of the system is best described by Figure 1.

Loop 1 is instructor feedback and gives simple analysis of test results, order of merit, and areas of weakness of both individuals and groups. By providing an analysis of each question, weaknesses of students can be identified which might otherwise be masked within overall test scores. Feedback to instructors was available within 20 minutes of completion of test. Loop 2 provides a range of reports designed to monitor and improve the quality of question bank items by analysing the reliability and validity of the test items. Loop 3 is the main student monitoring facility and provides standardized score profiles. These profiles are presented graphically and identify at a glance those students "at risk" thus allowing appropriate management action. (Annex B).

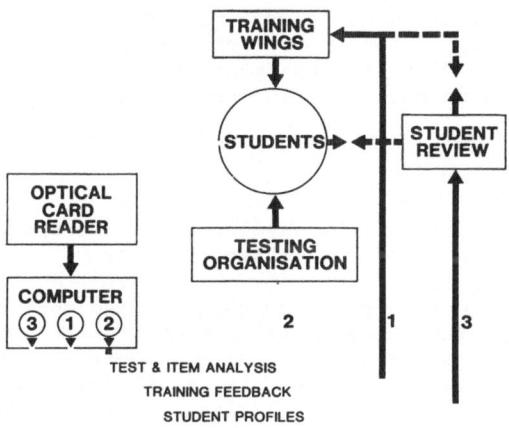

Figure 1. Computer-Aided Training Management System

SPEC was designed to meet the needs of an objective criteria referenced training system. The system requirement was formalized over a period of 2 years and interfaced with the organization and structure of the existing training system.

Staff attitudes towards the computer varied considerably. On the whole the system was well received by supervisory and management staff but with mixed feelings by instructors. Much of the reaction against the system was found to relate to the underlying instructional technology features of the system. Traditionally, achievement testing had tended to be neglected in Education and Training because of the sheer size of the computational task involved. The introduction of the computer suddenly focused instructors' minds on something that had merely been an interesting theory and forced them to make their own judgements on the subject. The hostile reaction was greatly reduced by holding a series of internal seminars and, where possible, by sending staff on in-service courses about testing techniques. In general the climate changed from one of fear of "big brother" to one in which there were frequent requests for the computer to be programmed to undertake more tasks. SPEC succeeded because:

a. It evolved as the evaluation and quality control system developed and thus interfaced successfully with the organization.

b. Management and supervisors were able to see the benefits of the monitoring process which allowed them to use the system generated reports with almost no explanation.

c. The effort was made to identify the fears of the instructors and develop a strategy to overcome them.

As the result of an evaluation in 1979, the main benefits of the system were found to be:

a. The necessity of relegation of students by one term was reduced from 40% to 10%. This represented annual savings of £90K.

b. Reallocation of technician apprentices to less academically focused trades because of a lack of ability was taking place one term earlier than previously expected. Because of the improvement in student performance, monitoring savings here amounted to £60K annually.

These savings of £150K annually were made for initial outlay of £36K for hardware and software. Upgrade systems are now to be found in 4 major training establishments with two additional bids under consideration. An extract of the evaluation report is included in Annex C.

COLLECTIVE TRAINING

The next area that began to be developed was the application of computers in direct support of collective training.

Technological advances in computer hardware and software at the end of the 1970s greatly improved the ability to simulate the complex information systems on which commanders depend to control warfare. The ability to generate data in real time introduced the capability to exercise both the individuals and the group in decision making in situations which approximate to the stressful conditions of war. A Battle Group Trainer (BGT) was developed to provide battalion and regimental commanders and their staffs with the opportunity to train collectively for their role. The BGT design included a high degree of environmental realism and is very much like a theatrical set. It uses actual vehicle bodies and realistic mock-ups to portray the situation of a battle group headquarters which has taken up temporary residence in an old farm and outbuildings. Light levels are varied and battle noises are heard in the background. Information flows into the headquarters through simulated radio networks from the control room. It was not designed as replacement for existing methods of training the headquarters but merely an adjunct to them. The Commanding Officer (CO) begins the training exercise by making his plan based on a scenario which is given to him. He issues his orders and coordinates compliance with his plans. Realism is again emphasised as this activity takes place near the trainer over live ground which the CO has been able to reconnoiter.

The next phase of the training is to "fight" the battle using the computer to support the simulation in the control room. The main tool used is a large scale master map showing features down to individual hedgegrows and ditches, own and enemy's men, individual vehicles and major equipments. Around this map sit the commanders of the subunits involved in the battle. These people fight the battle in respect to their own troops and report back to the Battle Group Headquarters staffs via the simulated communications systems. The play of the battle is free to the extent that it depends on the plans of the Commanding Officer and the action of his subordinate commanders. The computer subsystem is essential to generate the combat information by assessing such things as the likelihood of sightings, and of detection and the outcome of engagements between opposing units. Engagements are assessed using a database of hit and kill values which take into account the range, circumstances of opponents and weapons type. The computer subsystem also accounts for ammunition, records battle casualties and assesses the effects of artillery, mortar, helarm, fighters ground attack and air defense weapons systems. All the information generated is only available to the Battle Group HQ through the simulated communications net thus to some extent the "fog of war" can be simulated by controlling this information flow.

Those taking part in these exercises all considered then to be "very valuable" but no exercise had ever been undertaken to measure if the individual and collective tasks of the HQ actually correlated closely with those expected in action. It was decided to evaluate the Battle Group Trainer from three perspectives:

a. The Operational Perspective. How closely do the tasks undertaken by the HQ staff relate to both the build up to events and the subsequent functions? This information was gathered initially by interview and subsequently the task list circulated as a questionnaire.

b. The Commanding Officer's Perspective. Does the information received, decisions made and information transmitted coincide with the CO's perspective of how a Battle Group HQ operates?

c. The Training Perspective. Does the trainer add to the individual appointments within the Battle Group HQ over the previous training system?

The evaluation showed that the trainer was an effective simulator for staffs although some shortcomings were observed:

a. The tactical training aspects were limited but the trainer was extremely effective in practicing drills and procedures.

b. The use of real ground was considered a vital asset in itself which also enhanced the subsequent simulation.

c. The trainer has a particular value for COs as they often provide the first means of collective training for their staffs.

d. The trainer is versatile and flexible and can cater to and meet a number of needs for both Regular and Territorial Army Units.

e. Debriefing was inadequate.

f. There was a mismatch between the expectations of players and the simulated outcome of engagements. A more realistic graduation of the casualty assessment is required.

Most of the criticisms above have been rectified together with a number of additional minor enhancements.

Perhaps the most important part of the evaluation was to convert the training value into costs and savings. The basis of the measure was to attempt to calculate the increased value to be obtained from the salaries paid to personnel during subsequent field exercises. This was calculated by reducing the value of the improved collective training during field exercises by the cost of running the trainer including the salary of those attending the trainer. The net positive gain, assuming that those using the trainer improved in effectiveness by a factor of 50% was just over £1.5 million per annum (1981 rates). See Annex D.

The next stage in the development of collective trainers is a Brigade Tactical Trainer. This is going ahead as a result of the Battle Group Trainer success, one in Germany and the other in the United Kingdom and they incorporate the majority of the evaluation study recommendations. The major lesson to be learned is that costs of these simulators can be kept low by sensible use of computer resources and comparatively simple low cost software and yet be both acceptable to those using them and effective training devices.

INDIVIDUAL TRAINING

In the search for cost effective and efficient training it was natural for the British Army to turn to computer based instruction (CBI) as a possible training medium. A great deal has been written on the theoretical costs and savings of CBI and the criteria for applying CBI but most of this work was based on costs of contractors producing the courseware. In the United Kingdom there was initially a different philosophy for CBI development. This was to develop the lessons using instructors already employed by the military to produce the individualized training material. It was felt necessary to investigate the problems of training the instructors in this new role and assess the ease with which comparable commercial systems allowed the authors to develop their material. A pilot study was carried out during 1982 which suggested that instructors' reactions to CBI authoring were extreme — they either accepted the computer almost immediately or rejected it out of hand. The final results of the pilot study were, however, sufficiently encouraging to look for a suitable application for a full study. By coincidence the Royal Signals had embarked on an experiment at Catterick and felt that CBI could make the course more effective. It was agreed that this project should form the basis of a full research study for the whole of the British Army.

The project development was to take place in two stages. The first stage had already started and was allowed to continue. The stages were:

a. Convert the course from conventional lockstep instruction to an individualized fixed mastery variable time course (FMVT) thus students stayed in the training system until they reached the required standard at the end of each module of the course. This course was based on paper as the presentation medium.

b. If stage one was accomplished successfully convert the already individualized course to a computer based training system where this was considered to offer advantages.

Carrying out the study in the two stages allowed an evaluation to be made of the advantages, if any, of individualizing training by comparing it with the original lockstep system and then making a further comparison of computer based training against the other two systems. It was felt that this would answer the hypothesis quoted by many trainers that it was the effort concentrated into course objectives and course design and individualization of the course and not the computer which increased training efficiency. The measure of efficiency adopted was that if the training was either cheaper, faster or better it would have proved its case.

The original lock step course ran for 18 weeks and when converted to a paper based individualized course length was reduced to an average of 16.9 weeks. Since January 1984, when this validation was completed, new equipments have come into service and an increased course content was required. Between January 1984 and the present day the average training time increased to 17.5 weeks. It is estimated that the equivalent lockstep time would have been 20 weeks. A summary of the figures are in Annex E.

Comments from field supervisors showed that students who had undertaken individualized training exhibited more awareness of their environment in their field job, "FMVT students have a good theoretical knowledge of their trade and a high curiosity factor." Criticisms were "they had some difficulty in integrating into a team and lacked a sense of urgency in a live signals environment."

Conversion of the paper based modules to computer courseware started in January 1984 and a pilot run of 3 modules took place in May 1984. Internal validation of 20 students on the pilot study has shown that the time required to complete the modules increased slightly but that remediation time was reduced slightly.

Conclusions should not be drawn from such a small sample but indications are that a slight reduction in training time might result from the introduction of the computer. On balance the reduction in training time compared to the high capital and maintenance cost suggests that it would be difficult to show any savings over the paper based individualized course. A full evaluation study of the CBT course was begun in March 1985 and a report is due to be published in 1986.

PART TASK SIMULATION

The use of computer based training as a part task simulator is already showing its value. One project currently under development will train 16 operators on a system which costs less than the one high fidelity simulator originally specified. It will provide a controlled training environment and the study suggests that it will be as effective as the simulator. Another project has identified that a part task simulator costing only £5,000 would be almost as effective for training the operator controlling a weapons system as the manufacturers simulator costing £250,000.

A great deal of caution should be exercised when evaluating bids for high fidelity simulation. The lesson being learned is that in many cases the fidelity is not required and a skills analysis properly conducted can produce large cost savings by fully defining the requirement.

TRAINING IN THE FUTURE

Crystal ball gazing is a dangerous activity in an era of explosive growth in information technology and electronics but it is felt that an analysis of training needs must be made if we are going to be able to assist in the production of an effective serviceman in the future. In order to look at the training methods and media of the future it is necessary to consider how weapons systems are likely to develop. The major development which will affect our training is the increasing complexity of weapons systems and the requirement to develop the necessary skills to operate and repair them with the existing standard of recruit. Operators are having to achieve standards which do not allow for error and so commanders will demand extremely high training standards.

Training the operator is going to require more emphasis on part task simulation in the training environment and more frequent refresher training in units to maintain and confirm their skills. Evaluation of training performance will become the province of supervisors in units who already have a significant work load. One possible solution is for the operator to be able to test himself while being monitored by the weapons system computer. A built in monitoring system could assess performance and provide feedback to the operator and highlight areas of poor performance which could then be practiced. It may be possible to develop an expert system shell which is able to perform the monitoring function required.

Repair technicians are expensive to train and as equipment becomes more reliable with an increase in mean times between failures they will become less and less familiar with equipment in an operational sphere. For instance, modern communications systems equipment might only develop a particular fault every three to four years, so how can we expect our technicians to recognise them quickly when most faults will be of this type? One alternative is to provide the technician with a job aiding system based on a microprocessor which will hold the total "experience" of faults on the system. We currently envisage a system which will be used in training as an aid to the development of fault finding skills and fault

diagnosis and double as a job aiding system in the field army. A project
just starting at the School of Electronics Engineering is to investigate
the use of an expert system in electronics fault diagnosis training. The
expert system will be used to analyse the students solution to the problem,
give a probability value of it being correct and then take the student
through the optimum method of diagnosing the fault. The student will learn
by example. It is hoped that the technicians will become "experienced" in
the electronic equipment in this way.

SUMMARY

Computers used in the management of training have shown themselves to
be cost effective in the British Army but experience to date suggests that
the use of computers as a replacement for the instructor in the classroom
is in the majority of cases unlikely to improve training efficiency.
However, part task simulation, operator performance monitoring and distance
learning look likely to be cost effective and efficient and it is these
areas where computers are likely to be used in increasing numbers in both
collective and individual training.

Annex A. The Training System

Training is a continuous process which must be adaptable; it must
respond quickly and easily to the introduction of new military equipments,
operational requirements and changes in tactical thinking. The most
important aspect of any approach to training is therefore the 'closed loop'
which allows feedback from the field army to modify training. The above
model was one adopted by the British Army in the late 1960s to illustrate
the way in which maximum benefit can be achieved from training within the
resource constraints imposed on training by time and money.

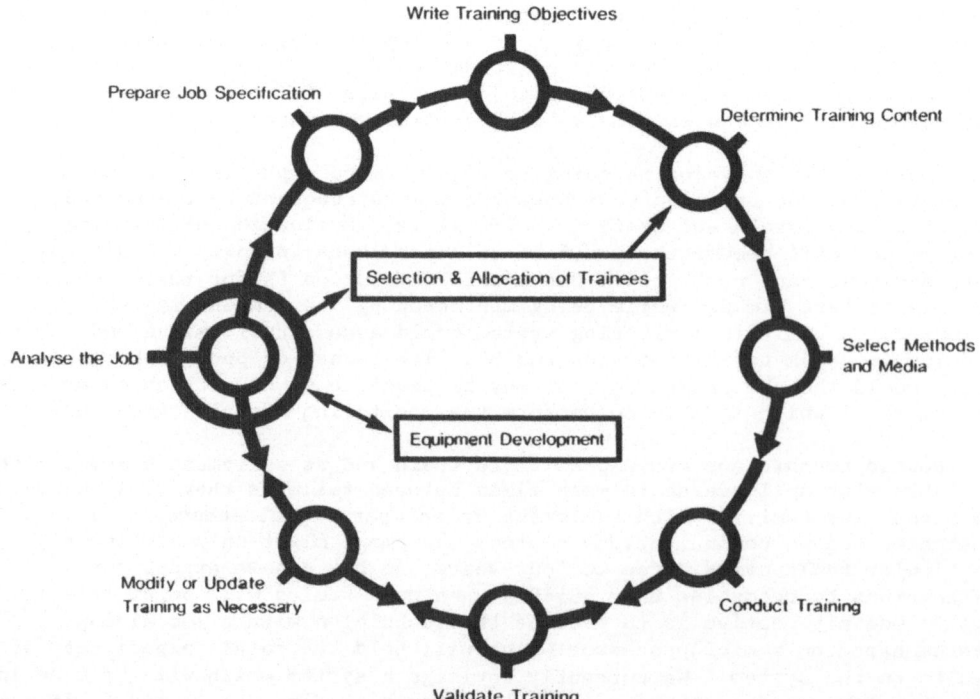

ANNEX B-1

STUDENT PROFILE

NAME	RANK	NO	UNIT	POT TRADE	COURSE
....	AT	24396551	AACOLL D COY	ET	77C

BIOGRAPHICAL INFORMATION:
DOB 24/01/61 O(M,P,E,TD+2)

SER	TEST COST	COMB SCORE	POP MEAN	POP SD	-3	-2	-1	PROFILE 0	+1	+2	+3	Z SCORE	RB
1	EPS	144	141.40	12.50	:	:	:	XXX	:	:	:	0.21	AD
2	TWP	72	61.62	10.42	:	:	:	XXXXXXXXX	:	:	:	1.00	
3	E1A	85	76.90	10.17	:	:	:	XXXXXXXX	:	:	:	0.80	
4	E2A	84	71.16	12.47	:	:	:	XXXXXXXXXX	:	:	:	1.03	
5	R1B	68	63.30	15.21	:	:	:	XXX	:	:	:	0.31	
6	E2B	81	68.62	13.26	:	:	:	XXXXXXXXX	:	:	:	0.93	
7	E3B	76	67.29	15.24	:	:	:	XXXXXX	:	:	:	0.57	
8	E1C	90	76.62	10.54	:	:	:	XXXXXXXXXXXXX	:	:	:	1.27	
9	E2C	70	61.97	17.30	:	:	:	XXXXX	:	:	:	0.46	
10	E3C	86	79.21	10.68	:	:	:	XXXXXX	:	:	:	0.64	
11	R1D	89	81.44	9.22	:	:	:	XXXXXXXX	:	:	:	0.82	
12	E2D	77	70.69	10.92	:	:	:	XXXXXXX	:	:	:	0.58	

Comment

A possible candidate to read for a CNAA degree at the Royal College of Science Shrivenham

ANNEX B-2

STUDENT PROFILE

NAME	RANK	NO	UNIT	POT TRADE	COURSE
....	AT	24396478	AACOLL C COY	ET	77C

BIOGRAPHICAL INFORMATION
DOB 24/11/60 O(MW+1) C1(+1) C(E)

SER	TEST COST	COMB SCORE	POP MEAN	POP SD	! -3 ! -3	-2 -2	-1 -1	PROFILE 0	+1	+2	+3	! !	Z SCORE	RB
1	EPS	142	141.40	12.50	! !			X				! !	0.05	
2	TES	56	49.48	10.80	!			XXXXXX				!	0.60	
3	TWP	61	61.62	10.42	!			XX				!	-0.06	
4	TEM	46	50.01	10.72	!			XXXXX				!	-0.37	
5	TED	70	64.00	10.49	!			XXXXXXX				!	0.57	
6	R1A	67	70.19	12.91	!			XXX				!	-0.25	
7	E2A	60	64.52	13.94	!			XXX				!	-0.32	
8	E1B	47	59.55	15.43	!		XXXXXXXX					!	-0.81	
9	E2B	39	63.86	14.92	!		XXXXXXXXXXXXXXXX					!	-1.67	
10	E3B	47	61.77	17.74	!		XXXXXXXXX					!	-0.83	
11	E1C	70	73.05	12.44	!			XX				!	-0.25	
12	E2C	34	59.69	16.24	!		XXXXXXXXXXXXXXX					!	-1.58	
13	E3C	75	77.56	9.85	!			XXX				!	-0.26	

Comment

Note the negative trend towards serial 9. Directed study was given at this stage and a degree of improvement in subsequent serials can be observed.

ANNEX B-3

STUDENT PROFILE

NAME	RANK	NO	UNIT	POT TRADE	COURSE
.... RA	AT	24396610	AACOLL C COY	ET VM	77C 78B2

BIOGRAPHICAL INFORMATION:
DOB 90/12/60 O(M,E) C(P,WW+1)

SER	TEST COST	COMB SCORE	POP MEAN	POP SD	-3	-2	-1	PROFILE 0	+1	+2	+3	Z SCORE	RB
1	EPS	145	141.40	12.50	!	!	!	XXXX	!	!	!	0.29	
2	TES	43	49.48	10.80	!	!	XXXXXXX	!	!	!	!	-0.60	
3	TWP	61	61.62	10.42	!	!	!	XX	!	!	!	-0.06	
4	TED	52	64.00	10.49	!	!	XXXXXXXXXXX	!	!	!	!	-1.14	
5	E1A	51	70.19	12.91	!	!	XXXXXXXXXXXXXXX	!	!	!	!	-1.49	
6	E2A	42	64.52	13.94	!	!	XXXXXXXXXXXXXXXX	!	!	!	!	-1.62	
7	E1B	34	59.55	15.43	!	!	XXXXXXXXXXXXXXXXX	!	!	!	!	-1.66	RA

Comment

The negative trend on this profile led to an early decision to reallocate (RA) from electronics (ET) to a vehicle (VM) course.

ANNEX B-4

ITEM ANALYSIS (TEST)

QUEST NO	QUEST CODE	C	MT	MQ	FV	DI	SIGNIF(5%)
1		96	67.50	79.84	62	0.61	YES
2		69	67.03	63.48	46	0.73	YES
3		57	67.02	66.84	49	0.72	YES
4		81	66.27	60.19	43	0.68	YES
5		27	56.39	52.22	45	0.90	YES
6		100	67.42	70.61	53	0.75	YES
7		66	71.14	68.41	47	0.72	YES
8		3	96.67	95.00	48	0.00	NO
9		21	65.24	67.14	51	0.74	YES
10		72	70.52	65.42	44	0.78	YES

NOTE: The Facility Values (FV) are corrected to take account of the ability of the group choosing the question whereby FV=50+(MQ-MT).

ANNEX C

SPEC EVALUATION REPORT - EXTRACT

The benefits of SPEC fall into three main categories as follows:

a. Tangible benefits whereby functions have been computerised thereby releasing staff time and effort for more important work - the specific functions are marking, test analysis and clerical tasks.

b. Facilities which directly support training in order to improve its quality i.e., training feedback and validation.

c. Observable improvements which have occurred within the period of ADP assisted quality control.

Marking and Analysis

It is estimated that SPEC is currently saving approximately 150 man days annually in distributed effort by relieving instructional staff of a significant proportion of the manual effort previously involved in testing. It is still necessary, of course, for tests other than multiple-choice to be hand marked and there is still a requirement for examiners to mark up optical cards for these tests. Nevertheless, the elimination of multiple-choice marking, and the numerical/clerical chores needed to produce merit order results list represents real savings in time. Another related benefit of SPEC in respect of the manual system has been the elimination of suprisingly frequent and substantial arithmetical errors that occurred in the adding up of student scores. This was discovered during the introduction of the system when SPEC was running in parallel with the manual system.

Clerical Aspects

The raison d'etre of SPEC is the production of the individual student profiles an the effort that would be required to produce them manually for the whole College would be in the order of 180 man days annually. This amount of time has not actually been saved because the load was too great to undertake prior to SPEC and it was only possible to produce about one sixth of the requirements. Thus the tangible saving for this item is about 30 man days. The maintenance of central test results records prior to ADP assistance involved an effort in the order of 60 man days annually. SPEC does not as yet produce consolidated results for whole courses (spread sheets) but does facilitate the operation of a master printout file which saves about half the manual clerical effort i.e. 30 man days. Further savings will be achieved as a result of the enhancement phase when the required consolidated reports will be available. Another area of savings has to do with the various review boards which meet each term to consider the academic progress of students. Prior to SPEC a clerical/typing effort of approximately 15 man days annually was required to produce consolidated lists of students together with specific scores and criteria required by the board members. This process has been greatly simplified by means of the SPEC reports and an estimated saving of about 10 man days annually has been achieved.

The total savings associated with these tangible aspects amounts to approximately one man year (about £5000) of distributed effort annually.

SPEC EVALUATION REPORT - EXTRACT

The most important consequence of this saving for the College is the release of some effort to assist with the very substantial, additional load imposed by the new TEC schemes introduced at the same time as SPEC in 1977. Thus the savings have been absorbed by TEC work.

Training Feedback and Validation

The training feedback reports provided by SPEC from time to time have highlighted specific training weaknesses. For example, the first time the system was applied to vehicle training a feedback report indicated that there was a weakness in the retention of certain aspects of carburation. Subsequent monitoring of this phase of training by equivalent tests set by E&QC revealed a positive response by the wing concerned and a correction of the weakness was observed. Similarly, in another wing, concern was expressed by supervisory staff that weaknesses were being revealed by the feedback printouts, and that they were not finding time to deal with them. As a consequence, a study was carried out of the job descriptions of the supervisors concerned in order to increase the proportion of time available for training supervision. Another interesting use of the training feedback facility of SPEC had been to survey the mathematical skills of each new intake. The printouts have been most revealing and have highlighted very significant weaknesses for both groups and individuals. For example, while topics such as Decimals and Fractions produced reasonable group scores other topics like Logarithms and Algebra produced group scores only around the chance values. These results occurred within groups of technician apprentices in which the majority had pass grades in GCE 'O' level Maths. The value of the printouts to the Mathematics Department at the College has clearly been to enable apprentices to be streamed in accordance with their individual needs.

The validation of training is essentially a long term process and it would be impossible to quantify the effect of SPEC at such an early stage. However, the function of the system is to support an internal validation loop in order to improve the efficiency of training and the requirement of SPEC is that it should promote measurements of achievement which are reliable and valid. Since the profiles are used to inform decisions taken about individual students it is particularly important that they should be soundly based. To this end the profiles are seen as the peak of a pyramid of essential prerequisites as illustrated. The base of the pyramid is represented by the valid learning objectives and a valuable feature of SPEC is that questions can be coded so that underlying objectives can be identified thus providing a check on the content validity of a given test. The next requirement is the use of test specification grids in order to prescribe both the topics and skills to be treated so as to help maintain both the validity and equivalence of tests covering a particular phase of training. The detailed test and item analysis available from SPEC enables item banking to be carried out so that tests can be assembled using questions most likely to yield reliable and valid measurements of achievement. In this way the profiles, especially as they build up, can be used with reasonable confidence for the purposes mentioned earlier.

Observable Improvements

While it would be impossible to prove conclusively the reasons for observed improvements in training it is perhaps reasonable to highlight improvements which have occurred during a period of ADP assisted quality

SPEC EVALUATION REPORT - EXTRACT

control, although not necessarily as a direct result of the SPEC system.

When the E & QC section was established in 1970 technician relegation rates were in the order of 40%. Since relegation involves repeating a whole term of the equivalent loss of productive service for the throughput of about 150 technicians per year corresponded to $(150 \times 0.4)/3 = 20$ technician/years annually. The current position is greatly improved for both Aircraft and Electronic apprentices. Current relegation rates are down to about 10% which, in comparison with the earlier figure, represents a saving of approximately 15 man years of productive service annually. This is a clear benefit because it represents a direct contribution to the skilled manpower resources available to REME. It is extremely difficult to express these savings in financial terms but the equivalent training costs would be in the order of £90K annually which is more than twice the capital cost of SPEC. To maintain these improvements would be virtually impossible without SPEC.

Another improvement has to do with the reallocation of technician apprentices to less academically demanding trades. As things stand the predictive efficiency of selection scores for various statistical reasons is only about 10% better than chance and so a considerable degree of uncertainty exists regarding the suitability of a substantial proportion of apprentices for technician training. The requirement is, therefore, that the monitoring system should be able to identify potential failures as soon as possible so that remedial action, or if necessary, reallocation can be arranged. Clearly, too much time spent on an unsuitable course represents a loss of productive service for the reallocated trade. An improvement in relation to the average term in which reallocation is carried out was achieved for both Aircraft and Electronic technicians throughout the ADP assisted period. Approximately 30 technicians are reallocated annually and currently, reallocation decisions are being taken about one term earlier than the pre-ADP period. It follows that approximately 10 man/years of productive service are being saved annually on this basis. In terms of equivalent training costs the savings would be in the order of £60K annually.

Disadvantages of SPEC

The disadvantages of SPEC within the limitations imposed by the original requirement are comparatively few. This is mainly because of the experience gained with the earlier 803 computer which enabled many pitfalls to be avoided. However, SPEC is a system which has been specifically tailored to the needs of the College and therefore there are limits to its capability. Nevertheless the adaptability of the system to other training establishments is likely to be substantial because the facilities it provides are fundamental to group training and measurement situations. The adoption of SPEC by the School of Electronic Engineering, despite its different type of organisation, illustrates the point.

Operation

As mentioned earlier the operation is more complex than originally envisaged and to some extent the complexity has been masked by the particular aptitude and enthusiasm of the present SIO 1 running the system. It is expected that the operation will be simplified by the addition of a cartridge disk during the enhancement phase.

SPEC EVALUATION REPORT - EXTRACT

Card Validation

There is still scope for improving this process since it is so vital to the whole operation. Again, the skill of the present operator tends to make the procedure seem simpler than it actually is.

Visual Display Unit

The VDU originally specified by Data General Limited in their tenderwas a Newbury Laboratories type 7005. This equipment while satisfactory in itself turned out to be incompatible with the computer and had to be modified to enable it to control the system. Despite modification there are still limitations with the 'Rub-Out' facility and the availability of lower cost print. It is understood that 20% of the purchase price in respect to Data General equipment has been withheld until these functions are provided.

Computer Dependence

The reliability and success of the SPEC system at the College has caused it to become a key part of the management/training system. If anything unforeseen happened to disable the facility, extreme inconvenience would occur to both the College and SEE. In this respect it would be useful to have a mutual back up arrangement operating a similar computer system.

ANNEX D

CALCULATION OF NET POSITIVE VALUE OF THE BGT

The Basis

The financial benefit of BGT should be measured in terms of the better value obtained from the salaries paid to officers/men during subsequent CPXs/FTXs. Using this basis, part or all of the salaries paid for the time that CPXs/FTXs took place during the twelve months after officer/soldier attendance at BGT should be reduced by the annual running cost of the BGT. The result would be the Net Positive Value of the BGT for one year.

Running Costs

The running cost of the BGT is computed by first adding the annual staff, equipment and building depreciation costs (BDC). An additional cost is the value of the contributions, normally made by officers and soldiers, to their unit, which is lost when personnel attend an exercise at BGT. This cost, known as the lost opportunity costs (LOC) should also be included in the running costs of BGT.

Assumptions

To assess the value of the benefit, some assumptions need to be made:

a. The normal productive value of an officer/soldier consists of two elements:

    (1) His individual salary.

    (2) A further element (P) which equates to the contributions the officer/soldier makes in excess of his salary.

    The second element is not quantifiable and hence, for this purpose the LOC is computed only in terms of salary.

b. It is assumed that where an officer/soldier has attended an exercise at BGT his productivity on subsequent CPX/FTX when carrying out the skills trained in and practised at BGT is increased in value by the amount of his salary.

Calculation of Net Positive Value

a. Value if improved collective training (1981 prices) is as follows:

    (1) Daily salary x (a)

    (2) Daily throughput of BGT x

    (3) Annual working days of BGT x

    (4) Length in working days of average CPX and FTX for one year where:

        -   Varies according to rank

        -   Lt Col x 1

CALCULATION OF NET POSITIVE VALUE OF THE BGT

    Maj x 2

    Capt x 3

    Sub x 6

    WO2 x 2

    SSgt x 6

    Cpl x 5

- 200

- CPX = 4 days

    FTX = 10 days

    Total = 14 days

- Total = (1) x (2) x (3) x (4) £1,740,000

b. Annual Running Cost of BGT (1981 prices) is calculated as follows:

                £

(1) Staff Lt Col x 1   85,000

    Maj x 4

    WO1 x 1

    SSgt x 1

(2) Replacement cost of equipment 8,000

(3) Vehicle cost 2,000

(4) Replacement cost of building 4,000

(5) Capitation rates for allowances

  - Personnel support costs, accommodation

  - Office support costs 25,000

(6) Lost opportunity cost 124,000

        Total 248,000

Annual Net Positive Value of BGT = A. - B.

      = £1,740,000 £248,000

      = £1,492,000

ANNEX E

STATISTICS FMVT COURSE

	SINCE 15 FEB 1982			SINCE 11 JAN 1984		
CATEGORY	OVERALL	MALES	FEMALES	OVERALL	MALES	FEMALES
NUMBER ENTERED TRAINING	630	294	336	287	163	124
NUMBER IN TRAINING	73	45	28	73	45	28
NUMBER QUALIFIED	506	217	289	202	109	93
NUMBER LOST	51	32	19	12	9	3
TRADE RE-ALLOCATION	(29)	(24)	(5)	(7)	(6)	(1)
DISCHARGE	(21)	(7)	(14)	(4)	(2)	(2)
OTHER	(1)	(1)	(0)	(1)	(1)	(0)
WASTAGE RATE	.09	.13	.06	.06	.08	.03
PASS RATE	.91	.87	.94	.94	.92	.97
COURSE TRAINING TIMES (IN WEEKS)						
AVERAGE	16.90	19.73	14.77	17.51	19.48	15.20
STANDARD DEVIATION	4.98	4.86	3.90	4.40	4.02	3.66
LONGEST TIME	35.00	35.00	26.80	27.00	27.80	26.80
SHORTEST TIME	5.60	5.60	5.60	6.40	6.40	6.80
AVERAGE NON-TRAINING TIME	1.27	1.44	1.14	2.05	2.22	1.85
	ORIGINAL COURSE 18 WEEKS			(EQUIVALENT LOCK STEP COURSE IS 20 WEEKS)		

NB: TRAINING TIMES INCLUDE 1 WEEK FOR BSS, BUT EXCLUDE NON-TRAINING TIME

TIMES FOR NON-QUALIFERS (AVERAGE IN WEEKS):

TRAINING TIMES	13.24	13.86	12.19	13.98	14.53	12.33
TRADE RE-ALLOCATION	(13.99)	(13.61)	(15.84)	(14.29)	(14.50)	(13.00)

WEAPON TRAINING AND SIMULATION

C. Saint-Raymond

Giravions Dorand Industries
Suresnes, France

General MacArthur expressed the idea that "There is no other job than ours for which the employment of ill trained personnel would lead to so important and irrevocable consequences."

This declaration is still valid today and if no one contests the necessity and importance of military training, the requirements for the latter have today become such that the training of personnel can no longer be achieved with traditional means and here again more efficient methods and modern equipment are necessary.

The problem of the Armed Forces is the following:

"To provide permanently trained personnel capable of achieving optimum effectiveness of their higher-performance weapons and ready to intervene in the shortest possible time in any theatre of operations."

To this end, while allowing for environmental, political, economical and human conditions to which we are subjected, all personnel training efforts should tend towards:

- Providing high-level instruction to allow substantial savings of munitions, operating costs (utilities, ranges, targets, travel, etc.) and wear (vehicles, engines, weapons systems, etc.)

- Shortening instruction time without affecting its level and for this purpose determining methods adapted to people of today and if possible capable of making instruction, which is necessarily repetitive and therefore likely to be boring, of an attractive nature

In the particular area of weapon instruction, simulation provides a solution particularly well suited to the problem:

- Attractive. Simulation is attractive by its nature of a "game" and its possibilities of dialoguing, evaluation and performance comparison which favours competition.

- Source of considerable saving. Simulation is such a source and constitutes a highly profitable investment when applied to weapons, since it considerably reduces the cost of "instruction munitions." For example, 48% of the French Army General Staff's training budget is presently for practice munitions.

- Efficient as an instruction means: Simulation is also efficient since it enables exercises to be repeated at little cost until the required level is obtained. And this efficiency is widely confirmed by the high level of performance achieved with real firing on firing ranges during recent operations performed by personnel trained in this manner.

Based on instruction standards determined by the Armed Forces and 30 years of experience of Giravions Dorand Industries in this area, this company has developed a range of equipment capable of providing the progressive and continuous training of personnel operating various weapon systems. This equipment covers all three conventional phases of instruction: basic, technical and tactical.

- The basic training phase corresponds to the need of familiarizing trainees with systems (fire control, command systems), the handling and operation of which require the application of strict procedures.

- The second phase is centered on the execution of firing techniques, making it possible to achieve and maintain a high level of performance evaluated by the display of effects on targets.

- The purpose of the third phase is to train technically qualified operators and teams in combat by placing them under realistic conditions of real equipment operation in the face of an equally active opponent.

According to the Giravions Dorand concept of instruction, basic training in handling and operating procedures is provided by simple low-cost interactive training-aid equipment using video techniques. This equipment constitutes the DX200 range. The first was developed for training AMX 30 B2 and AMX 10 RC tank gunners operating the COTAC automatic fire-control system. Seated in front of a video screen displaying a deliberately simplified landscape composed of synthetic images, the trainee operates a fire-control system accurately corresponding in shape and reaction to the real system.

The exercise consists of performing on targets appearing in this landscape both correctly, and as quickly as possible, the various operations of the attack sequence (acquisition, aiming, ranging, prediction, entry of corrections and firing). Each basic operation is evaluated and timed and results are clearly displayed on the screen.

Two modes of operation are possible: a manual mode, controlled by an instructor who can thus graduate instruction by calling upon programmed sequences of increasing difficulty (range, velocity and maneuvering of targets) and; an automatic mode, enabling the trainee to work alone with sequences occurring in a random manner.

The equipment is designed to allow the selection of weapon operators. In addition, the automatic execution of a commented firing sequence provides this equipment with an additional and particularly advantageous "demonstration and explanation" function.

Many versions have been derived from this basic equipment for
adaptation to other systems (fire control, aiming at air targets, operation
of radars) and more particularly for the recognition, identification and
attack of targets observed by night through a thermal-image TV camera. In
this application, the sequences produced for the trainee are no longer
synthetic images, but real images as seen by a thermal camera and recorded
and played back by a video tape recorder. A field-gun application is
presently being developed and is based on the video-disc technique.

The DX201 (COTAC fire control system simulator) ordered by the French
Army is presently in production. The DX207 (MILAN firing with the MIRA
thermal camera) has just completed trials and has been adopted by the
French Army. "Anti-aircraft" and "radar" versions have been acquired by
EUROMISSILE.

Beyond the purely military domain, this technique applicable to widely
used equipment of low operating cost can cover in particular audiovisual
and communication areas.

Technical weapon training, the second state of the Giravions Dorand
training concept, is provided by weapon simulators. Initially developed
for training in the operation of anti-tank missiles, this equipment has
since been adapted to the operation of ballistic weapons. Independent of
their application, however, these simulators share the following
characteristics:

- They are installed directly on the weapon system. They neither
  hinder nor modify the operation or use of such systems. For the
  weapon operator, they are completely "transparent."

- They are normally used in the field facing a real landscape. They
  allow simulated firings against real or synthetic targets. They
  may also be used in the classroom.

- In particular, they have the accuracy performance of the real
  weapon system, thereby eliminating from the start any possible
  source of negative-transfer training.

- Their low acquisition cost and very low operating cost enables
  them to be issued to company level, thereby ensuring continuity of
  instruction.

All these equipments have obviously evolved with time and techniques,
but are based on the same principle as follows:

By means of an optical device associated with the weapon sight, to
superimpose on the real landscape the simulated images of projectiles and
their effects. With this same optical device, to display in the absence of
real targets, synthetic targets stabilized with respect to the landscape on
which the weapon operator can train.

Initially specific to a weapon system, the weapon simulator has become
multipurpose. The simulator presently produced by Giravions Dorand
Industries provides training for several weapon systems, such as
ground-to-ground and air-to-ground anti-tank missiles, self-defense
anti-aircraft missiles and guns, short-range anti-tank weapons, etc.
Except for the optical unit adapted to the sight and computer specific to
the weapon system, all the components of these various systems are
identical (computer, image generator, TV camera and monitor, control
console), thereby minimizing investment and maintenance costs.

In addition, the search for realism has led to the use of a synthetic image technique for generating synthetic targets of changing dimensions and aspect. Their tracks or trajectories are programmable by the instructor, who can modify their characteristics at will. These targets can also be driven directly by means of a miniature control stick on the control console.

With more than 1100 equipments produced and operating in some 30 countries, the MILAN DX143 simulator has largely contributed in spreading knowledge of the Giravions Dorand concept of weapon simulation. The French Army has thus fitted its AMX 30 tanks and HOT-equipped GAZELLE helicopters with such equipment. The new multipurpose simulator has been experimented in the U.S.A. in its adaptation to the TOW and STINGER missiles and evaluated in France in its adaptation to the 20 mm anti-aircraft gun. Various installations adapted to different versions of short-range anti-aircraft weapons presently being developed have also been made.

Following technical instruction, the training of a weapon operator is not yet complete. As recently declared by a high-ranking member of the French Army General Staff, it is also necessary to make him capable of maneuvering within his unit....with the tactical intention of preparing for battle.

Combat training constitutes the third phase of instruction.

All the means used up to now for reproducing realistic conditions of combat (dummy targets and more or less complex umpiring) have never provided more than a brief representation of a real combat environment and the taking of umpire decisions has always been subjective, disputed and subject to caution.

The combat simulator today allows dual-action combat in which each participant may, with his weapons, attack an opponent having the same possibility. A "game of war" with unit against unit can be played. There are many types of combat simulators. They are all based on the use of low-power and therefore harmless laser techniques and cooperative targets carrying reflectors. The DX75 combat simulator adopted by the French Army after comparative trails, however, is fundamentally different from its competitors in its concept and operation, resulting in the high performance level for which it is known. Thus:

- As for the weapon simulator, the combat simulator is multipurpose (adaptable to any carrier) and "transparent" (in no way affecting weapon operation). Its multipurpose nature is ensured by installing the same basic components (laser transmitter, detection and reflection beacons, computer and control unit) on all carriers, the only specific component being in the form of a memory cassette plugging into the computer and containing along all information specific to the weapon system (weapon, different types of munition, corresponding ballistic tables, vulnerability area of the carrier, etc.). In addition, this cassette enables the whole of the combat sequence to be recorded for later playback and comment.

- As opposed to simulators of the same type, low-power laser transmission is not used by the DX175 for simulating the projectile trajectory, but for performing the following three functions in real time: ranging, miss distance measurement and data transmission.

- Ranging: by acquiring and locking onto a target in the manner of a radar, the laser permanently measures the range from the weapon to the target, independent of their relative motion.

- Miss distance: by comparing the position in the vertical plane through the target of the simulated projectile on its trajectory generated from firing data by the computer with that of the target given by the ranging system.

- Data transmission: from the weapon to the target in the form of encoded messages relating to the firing (time of firing, identity of the attacking unit, the munition used) and the miss distance data enabling the target to determine as a function of its own vulnerability zone the effects of the firing (destruction, attack).

The use of the laser in this form provides for the simulated attack the same degree of accuracy and range as that of the corresponding weapon.

In the case of a fire-control system with laser ranging and therefore dangerous to use for training, the ranging function is performed by the low-power laser of the simulator by means of an adaptation unit which thus renders it "transparent" for the weapon operator.

The system is completed by two peripheral elements: a multifunction umpire's gun which in particular remotely checks system operation, neutralizes or "reanimates" a vehicle and reloads a carrier with simulated ammunition and; an equipment in the form of a portable case for loading the cassette with data before an exercise and then reading and printing out on paper the results recorded during the training sequence at the end of an exercise.

The DX175 is presently in production for the French Army and the Army of a foreign country. It has been adapted to the MILAN missile and the HOT-equipped helicopter. A simplified extension of the system is being developed for training troops carrying individual weapons in precision combat against targets.

In addition, this equipment can provide the designers and experimenters of new weapons with a valuable aid, since it enables any weapon system, even if it is not yet in existence, to be simulated and experimented by merely changing a cassette.

I hope I have been able to convince you, if you were not already convinced, of the didactic and economic advantages of the simulator for weapon training. If you will allow me, however, I should like to conclude by emphasizing a few special points which I shall raise in the form of questions.

First, is the experience acquired with a simulator directly applicable to real operational conditions? This is the problem of "positive transfer."

To this question, I would answer yes without any reservations. If real firings still appear to be useful in order to "top" a period of instruction if only to overcome the apprehension of real firing, it has been demonstrated that an operator trained on a simulator only can achieve with his first firing a high level of performance (95% first-round hits after the training of MILAN and HOT anti-tank missile operators on simulators).

Second question: For weapon training, is it preferable to use classroom simulators perfectly reproducing the weapon system, its effects and the whole environment compared with lighter simulators associated with the real weapon and used in the field in a real environment?

My reply is equally clear and is based on two arguments, one economic and the other technical.

When speaking of a simulator of the first type, we are also speaking of high cost and therefore small numbers to be installed by priority in training centres. The training provided by these simulators is of a high level but once trainees have returned to their units it cannot be continued with the same means. In the case of a tank gunner, for example, he will be no longer provided with any regular training means and his performance level will quickly drop.

On the other hand, the use of a simpler and therefore less costly on-board weapon simulator issued to each unit allows, after a period of training in an instruction centre, continued training of operators at company level resulting in increased or at least maintained level of skills acquired.

My second argument is of a technical nature. For the person having to fight, it is undeniable that at the present time the best possible simulation still cannot reproduce the difficulties encountered in reality concerning detection, acquisition and attack. Only training in the field is really effective.

For these two reasons, I consider that for weapon training, and I underline the word "weapon", the on-board simulator used in the field is still the best solution.

My third question may be stated as follows: Why propose three complementary equipments for the progressive training of weapon operators when economic considerations would lead rather to the use of a single simulator capable of fulfilling all three functions?

To this I would first reply that it is not necessary to issue units with the same numbers of all three types of equipment. Thus in a company, several combat simulators may be required but a single technical simulator will suffice.

But I should like to temper my reply with the following reflection:

Although I confirm that to me it appears necessary to provide progressive instruction by means of suitable equipment, it also appears increasingly evident that with the aid of new techniques and encouraged by the dwindling of budgetary resources, the functions specific to each simulator may be partially grouped: for example, technical instruction with a combat simulator. But with this, in addition to the objection previously made concerning the number of equipments required and its economic consequences, it is necessary to check that the "all-purpose tool" effectively enables the various functions to be performed correctly and that this same tool does not become so large and sophisticated that in the end an air-conditioned building must be provided to house it.

CBT IN THE ROYAL AIR FORCE: A CASE STUDY OF TWO PART-TASK TRAINERS

M. E. Court and D. A. Sharrock

Headquarters Royal Air Force Support Command
Huntingdon, Cambs, U.K.

This paper describes two examples of computer-based training (CBT) in actual implementation in the UK Military. Although the two applications have been chosen to illustrate different approaches to the use of microcomputer based instructional delivery systems in military training, they have some features in common, in that both are used in situations where adequate "hands-on" time on the real equipment is not practical, for cost, safety or availability reasons, and both involve some form of real-time simulation. The fundamental difference between them is that the first, the Basic Radar Skills Trainer (BRST), is used as an adjunct to pre-existing larger-scale simulators, i.e., as a supplemental part-task trainer. The second, the Basic Acoustic Trainer (BAT) by contrast is the primary training device used within the course. In each case, the background to the introduction of the training device will be covered, the devices themselves described in some detail, and finally, some assessment of their effectiveness will be made.

AIR TRAFFIC CONTROLLER TRAINING AND THE BRST

The background to the introduction of the BRST was a larger-scale study of the Royal Air Force Joint Air Traffic Control Course, to investigate methods of reducing both suspension and recourse rates. The course extends over some nineteen weeks, with extensive classroom sessions being followed by practical teaching/learning and practice exercises. These latter are conducted almost exclusively on computer-based simulators, with a smaller element of live aircraft controlling. The existing simulators are based on mainframe computers, and offer a very high degree of fidelity, both physical and psychological, to the operational equipment and environment. However, these devices are highly labour-intensive, in two ways. First the instructor/student ratio is one-to-one, and second, several personnel are required to act as the 'pilots' of the simulated aircraft. These factors lead to practical problems associated with their use outside a normal working day, and hence put constraints on the amount of time which any individual student can spend on the simulator, in order to practice the skills previously taught in the classroom (and to learn those which do not lend themselves to being taught in the classroom).

In particular, in the early stages of the course, students are required to learn new procedures on the simulators without having had the opportunity to learn and practice previous, simpler, procedures to an adequate level of mastery. A detailed analysis of the overall course led to certain areas being isolated and highlighted where, sophisticated though the existing synthetic training facilities were, inadequate resources were available to meet the students' needs. These weaknesses were almost exclusively in the area of basic radar picture interpretation, and of decision-making in a relatively simple controlling situation. In addition, the existing simulators lacked many instructional features, which further reduced their suitability for extensive practice of fundamental skills and procedures. Such skills as heading appreciation, conflict prediction and avoidance, and the delaying/sequencing of aircraft prior to final approach, were identified and described in some detail. Further, by a combination of observation, analysis of training records, interviews and questionnaires, it was possible to ascribe many problems which manifested themselves in the more advanced phases of the course to a breakdown of certain of these more fundamental lower-level skills. The more advanced exercises concentrate on the integration of these and many other skills such as RT procedures, dealing with emergencies, and three-man team coordination and cooperation, into a total job performance.

The solution proposed was as follows:

- To produce a microcomputer based part-task trainer which would incorporate additional instructional support features not found on the more sophisticated trainers

- To extract from the existing simulators only those features which were required to learn the subskills covered by the proposed part-task trainer, while maintaining psychological fidelity with the subsequent training devices

- To draw up a list of criteria which any such device must satisfy. These include: low-cost, stand-alone 'turn-key' operation by student, and ease of both construction and modification of instructional material by the staff of the school

The intention was not to computerise a section of the existing course, but to provide something in addition to the facilities already available, having first ensured that adequate student time was available within the course to enable full usage of such a device to be made.

The trainer was designed around commercially available hardware, in this case a British Micro Mini 803G, with double disc drives, and a standard keyboard for courseware development. In order to make student interaction with the trainer as simple as possible, special function keys together with a numeric keypad were provided for input of commands to the trainer, and selection of menu options.

The software has all been written using in-house personnel, (the software programming flight of the training establishment concerned) and close cooperation has been maintained between the programmers, the instructors and the research workers. The device simulates the real radar and the following facilities are provided.

The radar display represents 20, 30 or 40 nautical mile radius, which are selectable during exercise preparation, and the display is updated 15 times per minute. Up to four student controllable tracks are provided, together with up to ten background tracks, which follow specific routes. The entry point of both background and controllable tracks into the display in terms of spatial positioning and entry time together with the number of each type, are selectable during exercise preparation. A small video map library is available, or alternatively the instructor can produce a map by a combination of range rings, cardinal points, a radar origin and beacons positioned at input ranges and bearings from the radar origin. Any map so produced can be added to the video-map library, and is then available for future use.

Two differences between the BRST and the main radar simulators are worthy of mention here. They concern the methods of assessing heading and relative aircraft speed, and the reason for the differences lies in the nature of displays used in each case. The existing radar simulators use actual radar displays, with long-persistence phosphor tubes, whereas the BRST uses a standard high-resolution CRT monitor. In the mainframe simulators, heading assessment of unknown aircraft is made by observation of relative directions of the current return, and the afterglow of the previous two or three returns, and relative speeds of aircraft are judged by spatial separation between these features. Since the BRST display has no afterglow, an alternative method of providing this information had to be developed. The method adopted was to provide a short 'tail' of small dots, each indicating the previous return of that aircraft's position. The direction of the tail provides the heading cue and the spacing between the dots gives relative speeds. Although only a small number of aircraft previous returns are actually displayed, in fact all previous aircraft tracks are stored, and are available for display at the end of an exercise, to provide a complete picture of all aircraft movements.

Such facilities as normal and maximum rate turns are simulated, selected by the student using special function keys, which also provide facilities such as freeze, continue and replay of an exercise. Instructional facilities offered include feedback to the student on heading errors, a replay facility, a pause facility with the option of returning to the start, or continuing with the exercise, a fast-update facility (real-time x 10), with the option of reverting to real-time, confliction detection which places a ring representing either three or five nautical miles around any controllable track, together with an audible warning (both selectable at exercise preparation) and a visual display of controlled aircraft data in the corner of the screen. The use of these facilities enables many more examples of the particular learning points of each exercise to be completed in a given time than is possible on the full-system simulators. To facilitate the production of exercises by the instructional staff, an exercise preparation program (referred to earlier) was written, enabling noncomputer trained instructors to produce and modify instructional material as early and quickly as possible. To date some twenty exercises have been produced, which are in use by students.

At present, the BRST is used in two different modes. First as a bridge between classroom instruction and the more formally assessed exercises and scenarios in the main radar simulators. In this mode students practise selected subelements of the later exercises and are encouraged to experiment with alternative solutions to the problems, while being provided with feedback from the trainer about their performance and progress. As a particular example, the use of the fast-forward facility built into the BRST enables a student to obtain rapid feedback on the accuracy of a heading or conflict prediction decision, in sharp contrast to the situation in the main simulators, where he may have to wait some five or more minutes to receive the information that his judgment was inaccurate. More effective use can now be made of the enforcedly limited time available to him on the mainframe trainers which can now be used for skill integration into complete job performance, a function for which their more complex facilities are more appropriate. The second use of the BRST is as a remedial trainer, enabling students to improve performance of selected subtasks with which they may have had difficulty during the main simulator exercises; several such remedial packages are now available, and can be used by students during free periods and in the evenings. Plans are well advanced to design pre- and post- performance tests, enabling an objective evaluation of the training effectiveness of the BRST to be accomplished. Initial indications are that since the introduction of the BRST, students are obtaining higher marks during their assessed mainframe simulator exercises, for those procedures which have had the benefit of practice on the BRST, but inadequate data is as yet available to enable a more rigorous analysis to be performed. It can at least be said with certainty that both student and instructor response to the device is totally favorable, although one must be careful not to confuse acceptability with effectiveness. Future developments of the BRST may involve its use to replace some of the existing classroom instruction by CAI, but plans for such use are at an early stage.

The second device to be described is the Basic Acoustic Trainer, used for training sonar operators in the Royal Air Force.

SONAR TRAINING AND THE BAT

The project was initiated in 1979, and essentially, it involves the development of a microcomputer based, part task device for the training of maritime reconnaissance sonar operators. Their task is to detect and classify surface and subsurface contacts. The device models the sonics processor fitted on the Nimrod MR MK2, has come to be known as the Basic Acoustic Trainer (BAT), and is currently used for the training of sonar operators in a specialist course.

Before outlining the design elements of the BAT and its effective application to present training, it is necessary to give a potted history of RAF sonar training, and to describe the operational equipment and the way in which it is used.

Air Electronics Operators (AEOps) are required to operate sonar radar and communications equipments and with the advent of the present generation of such systems, the pre-existing practice of providing a common course at basic training level, with subsequent streaming at a later stage of training, was considered financially wasteful. Therefore a policy decision was made to stream AEOps at the basic training establishment and to train a man in only those disciplines which would be required at squadron level. In this system, all students now complete a common phase which includes electronic warfare, radar and acoustics. They are then selected as sonar or radar operators and complete a detailed specialist phase.

Radar students are trained on a Radar Simulator, an expensive piece of equipment costing nearly $2 million for 6 trainers, while sonar students are trained on the BAT, which represents the sonics system, a multifunction acoustic processor. It will accept inputs from a wide range of both active and passive sonobuoys.

The complete acoustic station in the Nimrod MKII consists of 2 systems linked by a Manager or coordinator position and is operated by a team of 3 AEOps known as the 'wet team'. Each system consists of 2 CRT displays and 2 hard copy units and is capable of processing several buoys simultaneously. The operator is responsible for the control and interpretation of processed information. The interface between the operator and his equipment is the display and processor control panel which consists of a rollerball, a discrete function keyset and multifunction alphanumeric keyset.

By using this interface, the operator can request particular receiver channels and display various options, while the rollerball is used to direct the processor to various areas of VDU screen for measurement and marking functions.

Essentially the system offers 3 significant advantages over the previous equipment. First, increased processing power. Second, use of VDU's in addition to hard copy units and audio information. Third, greater freedom of analysis and more detailed analysis parameters.

While the system accepts inputs from a variety of sonobuoys, which possess their own set of processing options and display formats, it is normally the Lofar buoy which achieves the initial detection of a contact. Processed information from the buoy must be analysed by the operator.

The main function of the operator is to detect, analyze, and classify the radiated noise, called a signature, from contacts as they appear on lofargrams. A lofargram is a plot in real time of frequency against intensity of the particular sound source being monitored, and is probably best considered as an "acoustic fingerprint" of the propulsion and auxiliary system of a contact.

This description may make the task of the operator appear easy, but a number of factors complicate the analysis process, the main one being the wide variation which may occur in the "noise signature" from a given contact. These variations may be caused by the particular combination of buoy and processor options in use at the time, by alterations in target sound propagation due to oceanographic conditions, and finally changes in target sound characteristics due to range, aspect and operating mode.

With this background information available, in 1979, a number of problems remained. To put it simply:

- First, what should the student be taught?

- Second, how should he be taught?

- Third, on what should he be taught?

At this time, it was known that the student graduating from basic training required:

- First, a sound knowledge of a modern acoustic processor and of the types of processing and analysis options it offers.

- Second, to be proficient in the manipulation of the equipment.

- Finally, to possess a knowledge of targets, and their associated propulsion systems.

The operator thus needed to acquire three very basic types of skills:

- Procedural skills which involve the use of manipulative knowledge to operate the system and the completion of measurements and calculations during analysis

- Perceptual skills involving the detection of signals, the discrimination between different types of signals, and the classification of signals with respect to their origin

- Decision-making skills involving the integration and coordination of both procedural and perceptual skills for tactical planning

It was subsequently suggested that Lofargrams should be generated on a VDU and in the same format as the real equipment. This was essential as the primary display and analysis media of the real equipment were VDU's. If the same format was employed on the training equipment then basic training would transfer more easily to subsequent more advanced training. In addition, the student had to be able to interact with the system. Each student had to practice on a training device which responded to his control inputs. Mere observation of the actions of others in a prerecorded form would have been unacceptable.

The system had to work in real time. Lofargram analysis had previously been taught using static copies of lofargrams, and it was this very method that had led to the adopting of a pattern recognition strategy, rather than one of feature detection and analysis.

In order to overcome these faults a dynamic presentation was essential, and the student had to be able to observe, control and measure the development of a lofargram over time. More than one possible solution to the training problem was considered. In 1980 a Course Design Team drew up an outline specification of an acoustic trainer incorporating the above three features. It considered that some 300 hours of acoustic training was necessary and that a minimum of 100 hours should be devoted to practical training on a system simulator. Their argument for procuring such a simulator (that is a full mission simulator built by the manufacturer of the operational equipment) was based on the fact that, in the past, trained operators had had difficulty in acquiring the basic skills, as previously described, because of lack of acoustic analysis on a real time system. This training option would have cost some one and a half million pounds for the equipment alone. However it was contended that many aspects of the training could be carried out more effectively on a part task trainer rather than on a whole task simulator.

To achieve the high level of proficiency required in basic training, it was argued that students would need as much individual practice as necessary to undertake the tasks without error. Since individuals differ in the time they take to acquire a particular skill level, emphasis must be placed on the progress of the individual rather than on that of the group as a whole. This particular requirement leads to a different type of training and of trainer from that originally conceived by the Course Design Team. There was a need to acquire these basis skills, practise them in isolation, and then to integrate them. A number of training options were identified, as follows:

- To carry out basic sonar training by means of conventional classroom methods with students using copies of static lofargrams

- To purchase one or more of the real equipments and set them up in a training school

- To procure a purpose-built classroom trainer

- To purchase a minicomputer with networking facilities

- To develop a low-cost, part-task, trainer/simulator, based on a microcomputer, as a stand-alone system

The first option was ruled out on the grounds that, since acoustic processing, and therefore acoustic analysis took place over time, dynamic teaching materials rather than static were required. Option two was discounted on the grounds that the real equipment was very expensive, was not available and could not easily be used in a teaching situation even if it had been. Likewise, Option three was discounted on the grounds of both high cost and the protracted time taken by the normal procurement process. Option four was considered, but the relatively high cost, along with the need to network the system, still made this a questionable approach. The last option appeared to be the most viable and one which could be developed within existing resources.

It was proposed that for the foregoing reasons, it would be more effective to develop a microcomputer-based, part task trainer as a stand-alone system, rather than to procure a system simulator. Additionally, this approach would have a number of inherent advantages over large-scale simulators. Namely:

- Its capital cost would be very much lower.

- It would be more flexible for this stage of training in that software updates could be carried out relatively easily and quickly by in-house personnel.

- Each student could acquire the skills on an individual basis.

- Students could, if necessary, carry out remedial training on their own time.

- The part task trainer approach was adopted and the BAT will now be described.

The approach was to replace the right hand end of the system with a microcomputer, a VDU, some special purpose input/output devices and some suitable software. At the left hand end, the real world was replaced by an instructor interface, which could be as simple or as complicated as any stage of training required. It was also envisaged that in the future the instructor might be replaced, for some exercises, by a self teaching package, that is, Computer Assisted Instruction could be introduced.

The core of the BAT system is its software. There are about 10 kbytes of program, written for the sake of efficient running in 8080A assembler language and a further 10 kbytes of database. Although complicated in detail, the software has a simple overall structure which falls into 3 sections.

First, there is the interrupt routine, which has the following functions:

- It scans and buffers the key pads.

- It reads and buffers the rollerball position.

- It updates the real time clock displayed on the screen.

Second, the main program sets up and maintains the model world, and using the clocks set up by the interrupt routine, creates and outputs the display to the student. It makes frequent calls on the third section of the software, the command handler.

This builds up and validates the commands put into buffers by the interrupt routine. The completed and validated command is then used to update the model world or the display data, as appropriate. The hardware for each student station consists of a 48K microcomputer dual disk drive, printer, monitor, rollerball and special-purpose key pads, mains filter and power supply, and interfaces for the printer, key pads and rollerball.

The BAT bears a marked resemblance to the real equipment. The microcomputer is mounted in a wooden mock-up of a single Nimrod Sonics Console. While the real equipment features 2 monitors and 2 Hard Copy units, the BAT has only one high resolution monitor and one single channel hard copy unit. However, to the student, the BAT appears typical of the equipment he will later use in the air. The displays are comparable, the commands and keying sequences are identical as are the system responses. The real system interface and the BAT's interface are very similar. The rollerball works in the same way, its function is to control the various measuring devices that the operator can use which are a pair of crosswire cursors, and a set of multipoint dividers. The dividers consist of a set of short vertical lines which can be overlaid on the display and serve to measure frequency differences and harmonic relationships. The operator is not unduly aware of the one important difference. In the BAT he is dealing with a model world.

The current position is that 8 BATs are now fully operational. Priority has been given to the use of the BAT as a simulator, and use in the mode takes some 120-150 hours (that is, nearly half of the specialist phase). Nevertheless, the use of the BAT as a trainer incorporating computer assisted instruction is being progressed and will be evaluated within the next 12 months. A special purpose authoring language is being developed to allow noncomputer specialists to perform lessons on the BAT. The present training system for sonar operators would not allow a total free-flow system as output dates to the next stage of training are fixed. However, once the pattern of acoustic training was agreed, it was possible to operate a type of modified free-flow training which is a compromise between free flow and lock step.

A large library of signatures has been created and stored on floppy disk. This library has been created by the instructional staff using a simple question and answer type program.

The student starts analysing very basic lofargrams consisting of lines at various harmonic spacings; this allows the student to become familiar with the rollerball and the functions of both the alphanumeric and discrete key pads. When the student has mastered the use of the BAT interface, he progresses on to more complex signatures consisting of multiple sets of harmonically related lines and those which do not relate directly to the fundamental. Once the student has acquired all these skills, he is taught to analyze and classify contacts into categories such as:

-   Merchant ships and Warships, and to discriminate between

-   Diesel and Nuclear submarines

The BAT is an extremely flexible tool when used to teach acoustic analysis. The student is free to investigate and analyze any part of the frequency spectrum, within the confines of the processing bandwidth, rather than be limited to the size of a particular hard copy example in a library book.

Once the student has demonstrated a reasonable understanding of the principles of analysis, it is possible to expand his awareness of how the analysis task is "dove-tailed" into the crew environment. At this point several separately taught areas are integrated, the main subjects being target analysis, tactical oceanography, sonobuoys, range predictions, Doppler and fixing techniques.

A feature of the BAT in achieving flexibility with signatures is that a target (and its associated signature) can be placed within a one million square mile operating area and be programmed along a predetermined course. Other features, such as speed, signature alteration and detection range can also be programmed into an exercise, called a BATEX.

These exercises can be constructed and programmed to test, and consolidate specific objectives, and at the same time to give the student a basic understanding of the requirements of a typical maritime patrol mission.

At present, the course contains 8 BATEXs. Each one involves 2 BATs as Acoustic Stations 1 and 2 and a navigator coordinator desk. The students are mainly involved in manipulation and target data collection from the BAT and deduction of tactical information within a real time mission exercise.

A BATEX allows the student to: consolidate knowledge on oceanography, sonobuoys and range prediction, by preparing, giving and using an acoustic brief for a mission, and allows him to consolidate and integrate four separate areas: first, to manipulate equipment to obtain target data, second, to analyse, classify and deduce tactical information, third, to use Doppler techniques and other fixing methods to locate and track the target, and finally to report information concisely using correct intercom procedures.

At the same time the BATEX allows the instructor to: make an accurate assessment of a student's ability to integrate his previously acquired skills, and, to assess the student's potential ability to operate in a crew environment.

The school can thus train a student to acquire necessary academic qualifications, and a basic understanding of how to use his skills in the future working environment. That covers the use of the BAT in a simulator mode, but it is intended to use it in a different way in the CAI mode.

Here, the screen will be split in half with the top half displaying both real time and static lofargrams, while the bottom half will comprise of an information board, question board, answer board and results board. Some teaching programs have already been written and used, and more lessons are being developed (20 so far) now that the format for CAI has been agreed upon and areas for conversion have been identified.

In the CAI mode, the student will be directed to an exercise after reading a training note, and the microcomputer will assist him if he has difficulties in learning the task. The following instructional facilities will be available:

- Freeze

- Playback

- Redirection to a concept for remedial purposes

- Monitoring of the student's performance

The student will use the controls of the BAT (for example, the cursor) to identify certain aspects of a lofargram (to ensure he has learned the concept), and to make certain measurements. Multiple choice questions have been ruled out because of the facility of using the BAT's Display and Processing Panel which is much more flexible. In testing terms, students make a constructive response rather than choosing between alternatives. The computer provides the feedback to tell the student whether his answer was right or wrong.

In summary, the BAT was designed to teach the principles of acoustic analysis to AEOp students in preparation for operational service. Progress achieved so far in this project shows that it is possible to use a microcomputer as a simulator of airborne operational equipment. This provides a part-task training device which appears to be more effective and, in some cases, is much cheaper than other options. Used as a simulator, the device allows students to learn and practise a difficult procedural and analytic skill in an individualised learning context. The device is highly valued by both instructors and students. The addition of a CAI facility will, it is believed, extend the role of the BAT in terms of its flexibility although not necessarily in terms of its training effectiveness, which has already been enhanced by increased individualisation of instruction. This was achieved by the project team which not only wrote all the software but designed and built the hardware for the prototype BAT.

DEVELOPMENT OF A PROTOTYPE COMPUTER-BASED TESTING AND ASSESSMENT SYSTEM

E. J. Anastasio and R. Serotkin-Getty

Educational Testing Service
Princeton, New Jersey, U.S.A.

INTRODUCTION

   For much of the twentieth century, American education has relied heavily on large-scale, standardized ability testing; and this use of testing, as much as it can be attributed to any one set of needs, can be seen as a result of the American belief in meritocracy. Thus, testing has historically been used and supported for selection and placement decisions, assessment of school and training programs, and evaluation of educational outcomes. Within the past fifteen years, however, both testing and the testing industry have come under increasing fire. Some of this criticism, to be sure, is deserved, but much has been due to changing expectations of testing and its results as well as changing educational needs. Now, as recent developments in psychometric theory, statistics, cognitive psychology, and testing methodology converge with the availability of more sophisticated and powerful computers that are less expensive and easier to use, we are on the threshold of a technological revolution in the testing industry and can begin to meet the new expressed needs of education and training.

Recent Educational Needs and Training

   As educators struggle to meet the rising public demands for accountability and to increase the efficiency and effectiveness of instruction, they have turned more and more often to the testing industry to provide them with additional information and different types of testing. More specifically, what they have been seeking falls into several clear categories:

- More precise measurement of individual students and their achievement across all age and ability levels than conventional testing has been able to achieve.

- More detailed and diagnostic information about students, better analyses of their skills--strengths and weaknesses--and more useful reporting of that information for improved planning, policy review, decision making, and placement.

- Improved methods of handling testing information--maintaining information about students, following their progress, and utilizing that information to enhance student learning.

- A clearer link between testing and instruction and better utilization of test results for educational planning and follow-up (This is most clearly seen in the growth in popularity of criterion-referenced testing, or testing of specific instructional objectives, and mastery level testing.).

- New approaches to and more tests for licensing, certification, and job counseling and placement in the professions and trades; for personal, educational, and career assessment at all life stages; and for the improvement of educational opportunities for minorities.

Statement of Purpose

It is the purpose of this paper to outline the changes that have been occurring in the testing industry and the role in these changes played by the application of computer technology to assessment. Further, to illustrate how some of these applications are actually being used and how they might be used to enhance testing in the future, this paper also describes and reviews efforts under way at Educational Testing Service (ETS) in Princeton, New Jersey to operationalize computerized testing. And finally, a brief look into the future depicts what testing may be like in the year 2000.

THE USE OF COMPUTERS IN TESTING

Over the course of the past twenty years, the use of computers in testing has grown steadily, and the nature of that use has changed from research instrument to key component of the entire testing process--including test development, administration, analysis, and score reporting. In fact, the use of computers in testing and its expansion has closely followed the use and growth of computers themselves, each generation building on the technology of the previous one and combining previously separate capabilities (Brzezinski, 1984).

The development and availability of popular commercial microcomputers that are more powerful, more sophisticated, easier to use, and far less expensive than their predecessors, have been of particular relevance to the current use of computers in testing. Between June 1983 and June 1984, according to a recent study, the number of microcomputers being used in public schools more than doubled and as of September 1985, 92 percent of all schools owned at least one microcomputer for instructional purposes (TALMIS, 1984, 1985). Many colleges and universities have recently announced plans to acquire or to have their students purchase equipment that will result in the availability of computer resources to virtually all students at any time. With this proliferation of microcomputers in educational settings has come a virtual explosion of software and software systems for use in assessment and testing support. Systems for administration of student records and test management, item banking, and test construction--long available only to large testing organizations--are now becoming available to local institutional users. But to date, these computer applications have not directly affected students' test-taking experiences. Such changes are only now beginning as a result of other types of computer applications to testing, including actual computer test delivery.

Test Input Devices

Test input devices to replace machine-scorable answer sheets are being developed and pilot-tested. These devices, such as the ETS Keyway pad and the hand-held vocabulary tutor, enable students to enter their answers to conventional tests on small, hand-held electronic instruments that can be read by locally situated microcomputers to produce immediate score reports at test centers (Educational Testing Service, 1985; Baker, 1984).

Microcomputer Administration of Conventional (Linear) Tests

Microcomputer administration of conventional (linear) tests is becoming increasingly available. In this application microcomputers are used to present tests in a fashion that mirrors paper-and-pencil testing. Students move from one question to the next as they would in a conventional test, but use the computer to record their responses. When they have completed testing, the computer automatically scores the test--often presenting immediate on-line feedback--and, if so desired, provides various reports including score interpretation in norm-referenced or criterion-referenced frameworks. The potential benefits of such computer administration range from opportunities to individualize assessment to increases in the efficiency and economy with which information can be manipulated. Commercial test publishers have already begun to offer such software versions of popular tests (Hsu & Nitko, 1983).

Much of educational testing has traditionally been conducted using large-scale, mass production techniques that include fixed time limits and various other constraints. With this approach, an examinee's speed in completing a given test or specific types of items can seriously affect test results and the accuracy of the assessment of his or her skill levels. Computer administration, by handling testing differently, can avoid these pitfalls. For example, a computer can allow students to take tests at any time and to take as much time as they need to complete a test, while simultaneously it can keep track of the amount of time they spend on the entire test or individual components of the test. This flexibility provides additional information about examinees' skills and vastly increases understanding of their test performance. For such special subgroups as the handicapped, this ability to separately measure skill ability (power) and speed can provide test administration and test results that are more comparable to those of the majority of the population (Donlon, 1980).

In addition to eliminating timing constraints, the computer as a test administrator offers other advantages. It can provide immediate feedback to examinees--telling them their score as soon as they have completed a single question or an entire test--or it can allow them to continue answering one question until the correct answer is given (Trismen, 1981, 1982). In addition, the computer can manage the test information it gathers with greater flexibility and efficiency, producing immediate test results and tailoring reports of those results to meet a variety of needs. Finally, since computerized test administration does not rely on paper copies of tests, security of test information is increased (Ward, 1984a).

Computer Adaptive Testing

Computer adaptive testing, which retains all the advantages of computer administration, differs from conventional testing in that different examinees receive different test questions, chosen by the computer to tailor the difficulty of the test to the skill of each examinee. There are various ways in which this is done, but generally the following procedure is followed: one or more questions from the pool of those available is selected for each examinee, and when this item has been answered, the computer makes an estimate of the examinee's ability. Based on this estimate, the computer selects the next question that is most appropriate--more difficult if the question was answered correctly, easier if it was not. When this second question is administered, ability is re-estimated and the entire procedure is repeated until the desired number of questions has been given (fixed length tests) or ability has been measured to within a desired range of accuracy (variable length tests). Adaptive testing can thus be seen as measuring ability by a converging procedure where the change in question difficulty from step to step becomes smaller and smaller until the actual level of ability is pinpointed (Wainer, 1983; Weiss & Kingsbury, 1984).

Item Response Theory (IRT), now feasible for use with microcomputers, is the relatively recent advance in psychometric theory that provides the mathematical framework that is used to select the most appropriate questions to be given at each point and to produce scores that are comparable for all examinees. Further, it serves as the basis for identifying atypical responses caused by guessing or carelessness, both of which might produce misleading assessment in conventional tests (Lord, 1980; Wainer, 1983; and Weiss, 1983).

The primary benefit of adaptive testing is its ability to provide more efficient measurement over a broader range of ability. Traditional norm-referenced testing is composed principally of moderately difficult questions designed to provide accurate measurement for the majority of subject populations. Out of a concern for testing efficiency and test length, relatively few difficult questions, which can identify individuals whose ability level is extremely high, or easy ones, which identify those with minimal skills, are generally included. Computer adaptive testing, on the other hand, makes it possible to provide a pool of questions that can include enough easy and difficult questions for good discrimination across the entire range of abilities for which the test is intended. At the same time, since each individual receives only the questions that are likely to provide substantial information at his or her level of ability, the test can be significantly shorter than comparable conventional tests--between 50 to 80 percent--and still provide the accuracy of the best of those tests (Urry, 1977).

Because of their individualized or "tailored" nature, adaptive tests present a number of additional advantages over paper-and-pencil and linear computer delivery of conventional tests:

- Because of time saved through shortening the tests, new sections to assess a broader range of abilities can be introduced.

- The same "branching" strategies that direct students to appropriate questions can be used to route them to appropriate tests and around inappropriate ones.

- Since each student receives an individualized selection of test items, test security is enhanced and the tests can be used repeatedly to measure student progress without duplicating themselves.

Despite its potential benefits, adaptive testing does present some problems. It may require more powerful microcomputers than those found in many educational settings. In addition, it is easier to use with assessment of broad aspects of developed abilities, such as reading comprehension and mathematics, than it is with achievement testing in specialized content areas. Further, it requires a larger pool of test questions and more extensive data on those questions than conventional tests (Green et al., 1984). Finally, although it is very useful in testing examinees with a wide range of ability levels, it does not offer a substantial advantage over conventional tests in assessments of candidates

with a narrow range of ability. Thus, its most promising applications lie
in professionally developed, large-scale standardized testing, such as
aptitude batteries for selection and placement and professional licensing
and certification examinations (Ward, 1984a).

Diagnostic Testing

Diagnostic testing, in contrast to adaptive testing, seeks to break
down broad ability areas and identify in detail the specific components of
an individual's strengths and weaknesses in those areas. The major goal of
diagnostic testing is to provide information about what skills a student
needs to learn or develop further and about those skills he or she has
which can be used to develop additional learning and remediation. Ideally,
such tests should incorporate theories of knowledge and instruction, based
on which testing can then provide teachers with suggestions for
instructional approaches that are likely to prove effective with each
student. In diagnostic testing, adaptive techniques are used not to
measure skills in which students are competent or in which they are totally
lacking, but to quickly hone in on and identify a student's strengths and
weaknesses, information not normally provided by conventional testing or
adaptive testing.

Computer delivery of diagnostic tests makes it possible to develop
profiles of student skills, and to keep track of student outcomes. It also
makes possible a faster determination of skill areas that need to be
explored and makes available a wider range of assessment techniques than a
counselor using a series of conventional tests could provide. Further,
diagnostic testing that utilizes the interactive capabilities of a computer
makes it feasible to assess student techniques and approaches to problem
solving. And by leading students through complex operations, it can
pinpoint the specific sources of errors or weaknesses in these skills
(McArthur & Choppin, 1984; Bejar, 1984).

As the testing application most recently affected by computers,
diagnostic assessment is currently the focus of a great deal of research
and development effort. More experience with the computer's ability to
analyze, classify, and determine relationships and networks of errors, will
enable instructors to extract an increasing amount of useful information
not only about actual student errors but about their reasoning processes as
well. Thus, combined with the growing body of knowledge gained from
research on artificial intelligence and cognitive development, computer
adaptive diagnostic testing has the potential to vastly change
education--enabling teachers and trainers to tighten the connection between
assessment and instruction and to determine, plan, and utilize the
instructional strategies that are best suited to each individual student
(Ward, 1984a; Bejar, 1984).

IMPLEMENTATION OF A COMPUTERIZED ADAPTIVE TESTING SYSTEM: THE ETS/COLLEGE
BOARD COMPUTERIZED ADAPTIVE TESTING PROGRAM

In order to facilitate the timely and accurate collection of
information about students, Educational Testing Service (ETS) and the
College Board have been collaborating on the development of a
microprocessor-based system to administer and score both conventional and
adaptive tests. The first application of this system to practical
measurement situations has been the development of a computerized adaptive
test of skills in college reading, English, and mathematics. The test,
which has been undergoing field trials for about a year, was designed to
enable post-secondary institutions to determine whether students have the
requisite skills for college-level work or would need remedial studies to
develop those skills.

What It Is

The ETS/College Board Computerized Adaptive Placement Test consists of four independent modules--Reading Comprehension, Sentence Skills, Arithmetic, and Elementary Algebra. Consistent with current emphasis on English and mathematics instruction, its contents were designed to emphasize question types that require reasoning and problem solving. (Sample questions are reproduced in Appendix A). The test is of the fixed-length variety noted earlier. In each test module, all students are required to answer the same number and categories of questions, but since this is an adaptive system, the difficulty of the questions or items administered to each student varies according to that student's ability level. Despite this difference in individual questions answered, however, the distribution of questions according to their type, their content, and the kind of cognitive processing they require is strictly controlled so that all students are tested in an equivalent manner. In the Arithmetic and Elementary Algebra modules this distribution system has been modified somewhat for further adaptation to student skills. In the Arithmetic module, for example, although all students receive questions drawn from all of the categories utilized, the number of questions from each varies systematically with the level of skill of the examinees. Thus, students with minimal arithmetic skills are given more of the basic operational questions and fewer of the more difficult applications and problem-solving items. This proportion of questions shifts progressively as the level of skills increases, thereby allowing students to be examined more precisely at the more appropriate levels. The Elementary Algebra Module is similarly constructed, and one of the system's possible formats allows for this module to be completely bypassed by students for whom it is inappropriate.

ETS/College Board experience in developing and administering the New Jersey College Basic Skills Placement Test and the extensive data on placement practices collected by the New Jersey Basic Skills Council provided the basis for determining what levels of skills should be included. The test is intended to yield accurate measurement from the lowest to the highest level of skills that any of the colleges in the New Jersey program now use for setting cut scores in basic skills placement decisions.

In addition to the actual test modules, the system includes an introductory sequence that incorporates complete instructions, a sign-on procedure, background questions, and familiarization screens. Thus, because the system is self-explanatory, no verbal orientation of students is necessary prior to testing. Further, the system was designed to be easy to use and does not require prior experience with computers. In fact, once the student has keyed in personal identification information, only two keys are used to respond to the entire program. The background questions included in the introductory sequence serve several purposes; as currently designed they provide students with practice in answering questions on the computer as well as basic information for research on the test. However, the information supplied can be used to supplement student reports, and the user institution can designate its own set of questions to be given in addition to, or in place of, those that the system routinely includes.

Hardware and Software Considerations

The system supports fully intermixed text and graphics, including figures, mathematical symbols, italics, and special symbols. Responses can be multiple-choice or free-response, using a variety of response protocols. As noted, both linear (conventional) and adaptive item selection and scoring are supported. Virtually any kind of testing can be handled, simply by specifying the appropriate item selection, scoring, and reporting rules, and then "scripting" the flow from one test to the text. Thus, in the Computerized Adaptive Placement Test, the system can easily be adapted to present any combination or order of the test modules that a school desires.

To achieve this flexibility without incurring the overhead of major software revisions each time a new test is used with the system, the item selection, scoring, and reporting functions are isolated from the main test administration portion of the software. The needed modules are then pieced together under a central test administration driven, which handles display functions, response recording, and overall flow.

Further, the software was designed to be portable so that it can be operated on a variety of microprocessors. Portability was achieved by using an operating system (P-system) which is available for several hardware systems, and is likely to be available for new systems as they are developed. Easy portability was also achieved by isolating all the hardware-dependent software (such as the graphics module), so that it can be replaced easily without affecting the main portion of the test administration system. Currently, the system is designed to run on IBM personal computers located at training/testing sites and can be used in a variety of testing programs.

System Design

All of the essential components of a computerized, adaptive-testing system have been developed and integrated into the ETS/College Board program. These consist of an item banker, item calibrator, test authoring system, test pre-evaluator, test administration system, and test interpretation generator.

The Item Banker   The item banker allows the test developer to enter, store, and edit both item text and statistics in a way that makes rapid retrieval and display possible.

The Item Calibrator   The item calibrator calculates conventional item statistics and estimates item response theory parameters so that only the best and most appropriate items will be selected for each student.

The Test Authoring System   The test authoring system permits the test developer to specify any conventional or adaptive testing strategy that is desired. In adaptive testing this means determining the strategies that the system will use to select items for each student (including branching) and the scoring procedures that will be used to yield the most information.

The Test Pre-Evaluator   The test pre-evaluator evaluates the properties of tests before they are administered. This is done through simulations that estimate the performance of adaptive tests, based on data obtained from conventional test items.

The Test Administration System   The test administration system administers the tests and records the data. It is this part of the total system that controls the selection of items presented to students and the branching design that is followed.

A Test Interpretation Generator   A test interpretation generator converts the test scores to the scale used in reporting and produces a narrative text interpretation of the individual's scores. For the ETS/College Board project, three aspects of the examinee's performance are reported for each test module: the estimated number right true score ("Total Right Score"), which indicates how many questions the examinee would be expected to answer correctly if it were feasible to administer the entire pool of questions to that person; the confidence interval ("Range"), which estimates the precision with with the examinee's ability has been assessed; and the percentile rank, which compares the examinee's ability with that of a reference population. Currently, the test interpretation system provides for generation of reports in three ways (see sample reports in Appendix B):

- An abbreviated report of the individual's scores can be represented on the computer screen at the completion of the test (B-1).

- A full individual report, which includes the three types of information described above as well as a narrative interpretation of the meaning of these scores, can be displayed or printed as soon as the test is completed (B-2).

- Results for all students tested can be collected and printed in rosters (B-3), or summary statistics for the group can be reported (B-4).

How the ETS/College Board Test Works

One of the hallmarks of the ETS/College Board adaptive test is its speed and ease-of-use for students. Its flexibility and automatic individualization for students are helpful to test coordinators and supervisors. A scenario of the test's use may be helpful in conceptualizing these benefits:

- A student arranges to take the test by signing up in advance or simply walks in and takes the test if a computer is available.

- Since no verbal orientation is necessary, the student can immediately sit down and begin the test program at a supervisor-prepared terminal. (This is a simple process--the supervisor can prepare 10 computers within 10 minutes.)

- After the student reviews the test familiarization and introductory sign-on sequence and answers the optional set of background questions, the tests are presented by the computer.

- Each test begins with a random choice made by the test administration system among four or five "starter" questions, which are of middle difficulty level relative to the range of difficulty covered by the test.

- If the examinee answers the first question correctly, the next question will again be chosen randomly, this time from among several of the most difficult questions available. If the examinee instead gives a wrong answer, the question will be chosen from among the easiest available. Since this "jumping" from middle difficulty to either very easy or very difficult questions makes it likely that a student will quickly give at least one correct and one incorrect answer, the system begins early in the test to converge on the appropriate level of difficulty.

- As the test proceeds, a continuing re-estimation of the examinee's skills is made after each question, based on all the information available to that point. The estimate is used to look up, in a table prepared in advance, what next question will provide the most information: that question is then administered, and the

computer repeats the procedure until the desired number of
questions have been answered. Since these estimates are performed
while examinees are reading and responding to a question (only
about 4 seconds are required for the necessary calculations), no
noticeable delay occurs between the presentation of successive items

- Since each item is chosen based on a student's response to a
  previous question, all questions must be answered and none may be
  omitted. Further, although examinees can change an answer when
  responding to an item, they are not permitted to backtrack to
  change a response to a previous item. (In an adaptive test, it is
  not sensible to permit backtracking, since at a later time the
  estimate of an examinee's ability may be different, and thus the
  best question to administer next would also be different.)

- Upon completion of all four tests, the computer displays the
  on-screen report of the examinee's percentile ranks. At this
  time, the individual student report can also be printed, and a
  counselor or test supervisor can discuss the results with the
  student.

- At the conclusion of a testing day, supervisors can have rosters
  and summary reports printed.

Pilot Testing and Student Reactions

Field-testing was begun at three colleges during the spring of 1984 and
has been expanded to other campuses throughout the past year. Most
students, including those who reported no previous experience with
computers, have been able to use the system successfully, and their
reactions have been very positive. They particularly like the absence of
time limits on the test and not having to grid ovals on answer sheets.
Further, examinees find the test more "interesting," less intimidating, and
more appropriately challenging (neither too difficult nor too easy) than
conventional tests. In fact, almost 75 percent of all students surveyed
preferred the computer-administered test to a paper one, while only 10
percent preferred a paper test (Ward, 1984b).

Faculty and staff at pilot sites have also had favorable reactions to
the system, citing its individualization and immediacy of feedback; its
simplicity and ease of use; and the fact that students are not overwhelmed
by questions beyond their reach.

Advantages of the ETS/College Board Test System and Computer Adaptive
Testing

The adaptive capability of the ETS/College Board system has a number of
pronounced advantages over both conventional linear testing and
paper and-pencil test delivery. Most notably, these advantages include the
following:

The Adaptive Test Yields Measurement as Accurate as that Provided by
Conventional Tests Requiring more than Twice as many Questions. Since
students are given only those questions most appropriate to determining
their ability, the tests do not need to include as many items, and testing
time is consequently shorter. Although estimates have ranged as high as an
80 percent reduction in the number of items required to obtain
reliabilities comparable to those of conventional test scores, this figure
may be somewhat high. The length of the ETS/College Board test--chosen for
enhanced reliability rather than maximum time-savings--represents an
approximately 55 percent reduction in test length.

<u>Students' Ability can be Measured More Precisely with Adaptive Testing, Especially for an Examinee of Lower or Higher Ability than Average, even when Conventional Tests are Derived from the Same Pool of Items.</u> Again, this is because the computer adaptive testing system can select those questions that are most closely matched to a student's actual ability level and that will yield the most information about that student (Stocking, 1984). Further, data gathered in pilot tests of the ETS/College Board system indicate that the adaptive testing process and its computer delivery do not alter the nature of the skills that determine test performance or the level of skills an individual is estimated to possess (Ward, 1984b).

<u>Computer Adaptive Testing Allows Greater Flexibility in Evaluation.</u> With the ETS/College Board Adaptive Testing Program for College Placement this flexibility is apparent in four general areas:

- Testing can be done in groups, by student appointment, or on a "walk-in" basis, anytime during operating hours of the testing facility, subject only to computer availability. Thus, students can be tested as needed and do not have to wait for periodic group administration of tests.

- Tests included in the system and actually administered to students can be varied by the user institution and presented in any order. The system permits branching between as well as within test modules, with a student's performance on one test determining whether or not that student will be given a second test (e.g., skipping the algebra test with lower ability students).

- Besides being able to administer both conventional and adaptive tests, the system can handle a variety of item types, including free-response and multiple-choice items. As computer technology and research evolve, additional item types are being developed and will also become available to the system.

- Many adaptations and enhancements to the system can readily be made to fit user needs. For example, it would be relatively easy to add an on-screen time clock, incorporate feedback on incorrect items, and revise the general data handling capabilities to accept additional information, do specialized summaries, reports, etc.

<u>The Scoring and Reporting Capabilities of the Computer Adaptive Test Make it Convenient for Staff to Administer.</u> The provision of immediate score reporting in the ETS/College Board system also permits counselors to advise and place students as soon as they have completed testing.

<u>Students are Less Threatened and Less Bored, and Many Report Feeling More Motivated and Challenged by the Testing Process.</u> Students participating in the ETS/College Board field studies who were aware of the adaptive nature of the test even reported a sense of competing against the computer, especially when they felt they could judge whether they had answered correctly or incorrectly.

<u>Test Security is Enhanced and not Compromised by Repeated or Staggered Administration.</u> Because students receive individualized sequences of test questions, even two examinees with nearly identical skills receive different versions of the test. Further, since there are multiple questions that are similar in their measurement characteristics and these are randomly selected, the tests can be given repeatedly to measure student progress without individual items becoming known and familiar.

Current Availability and Applications of the ETS/College Board Computer-Adaptive Testing System and Placement Test

Many enhancements of the ETS/College Board Testing System are possible and would require not more than a few hours or days to effect. Examples of these modifications include recombinations of the four test modules, branching around tests, replacement of standard background questions with others desired by an institution, and the addition of a specialized text to the individual reports printed for students. Other types of "tailoring" of the system would involve more substantial effort but are also possible, including but not limited to: micro-to-mainframe communications, different types of reports, placement recommendations, and delivery through microcomputer networks and multi-use systems such as VAX. In short, because of its flexible design and portability as well as its history of success in the field, the ETS/College Board system is currently available and adaptable to a wide variety of applications. Although the current placement test was developed primarily as a basis for determining the time students begin their college careers, what level of course work is appropriate for them, there are also additional ways in which it can serve the evaluation needs of students and institutions.

Applications of the ETS/College Board Computer-Adaptive Test Include the Following:

- Admissions Testing and Applicant Screening. The adaptive placement test is ideally suited to open-admission institutions such as community colleges which may wish to ensure that students have certain minimum level basic skills and will be able to participate in even the lowest level remedial programs at the school. In addition, the test could provide an "early warning" to identify students who are likely to encounter difficulties in their college work, creating the possibility of timely intervention by counselors or instructors as well as special follow-up attention for such "at risk" students.

- Placement of Students in Appropriate Classes. The placement of students in appropriate classes for regular college level work or for some level of developmental or remedial studies is the original planned application of the test.

- Monitoring of Student Progress within a Developmental Course. If a course is intended to teach the basic skills that the test measures, the student's acquisition of those skills should be reflected in changes in his or her scores. This monitoring could serve several functions. It could be an option made available for the student's benefit in determining how well he or she is doing--scores might be made available only to the student in this case, or it could serve the instructor--indicating how well an individual or a group of students is progressing. The computer-adaptive test is especially well-suited for this purpose because a student taking the test for a second time will not receive exactly the same set of questions; therefore practice effects will be less important than they are in conventional testing.

- Measuring End-of-Course Mastery. The test could be used to determine whether students completing a developmental course have mastered the skills the class was intended to teach and are ready to go on to higher level work.

- Monitoring Class/Curriculum Success. The ETS/College Board test can also be used as a way to establish standards across a diverse set of full- and part-time faculty teaching the same courses. It can be used to determine whether students are actually being exposed to similar content and similarly benefitting, as well as whether the courses offered are actually effective in developing the required skills for advanced learning.

- Provision of Better Counseling. Because of the computer's ability to supply immediate test results, students are able to benefit from more timely and informed counseling. Further, when test scores can be transmitted directly from the testing center to a registration office, students will not experience delays in scheduling appropriate classes. One possible modification of the ETS/College Board test might be to combine the adaptive testing with the computer's capacity to present counseling information, course-related information, and advisement information in letter form.

- Off-Site Access. The ability to deliver off-campus placement testing by computer (either via stand-alone micros or via links to a central system on the main campus) gives potential students easier access to the college registration and placement process and reduces the cost of administration.

- Improved Articulation Between High Schools and Colleges. Where a test such as the ETS/College Board placement test is used at the secondary school level to diagnose the college readiness skills of college-bound students, academic deficiencies can be identified and remediation in the areas of skill and knowledge required for college study can be prescribed. Further, the test could be used to indicate areas in which improvement is needed before college entrance exams are taken and to counsel students about college entrance.

Applications of the ETS/College Board Computer-Adaptive Testing System Itself Include the Following:

- Adaptation to Other Widely Used Tests. Currently, ETS is exploring the possibility of using the computer-adaptive testing system for several of its other major test programs. The system, however, is flexible enough to be useful for any test directed at examinees with a broad range of abilities.

- Use for Local Criterion-Referenced Testing and State Assessments. Because of the growing interest in the integration of testing and instruction, educators are demanding customized tests tied to their own instructional objectives and are interested in item banking. The computer-adaptive testing system could be used to support the development and administration of these localized tests. The system level subject area and skill and content area, from which the customized collections may be drawn to produce local criterion-referenced tests. The adaptive-testing technology would be used to adapt the mix of items administered to individual students. In addition, these items could be combined with questions to test achievement of state-mandated minimum competencies and thus be used to evaluate student progress and course and unit mastery while simultaneously meeting state assessment requirements. Further, test results could be used by teachers to plan instruction, and by counselors and teachers for placement and grouping of students. Such integration of testing would improve testing efficiency and reduce duplication of effort. Such tests could cover objectives in the basic skill areas (reading, mathematics, and learning skills) as well as common core subjects such as history, biology, algebra, and foreign languages.

- Diagnostic Adaptive Testing. In another project jointly sponsored by ETS and the College Board, a diagnostic testing system has been developed to complement the computerized adaptive test for assessment and placement. The diagnostic tests provide information to students and teachers that can serve as the basis for planning instruction, including: strengths, weaknesses, and patterns of error; specific instruction required to master needed skills; and suggestions of appropriate instructional materials for use in developmental work. In short, where adaptive testing for assessment of ability and achievement provides scores that can be used to assign students to classes or determine whether they are prepared for further study, adaptive diagnostic testing identifies specific problem areas and provides prescriptions for meeting each student's needs (Forehand et. al., 1982; Educational Testing Service, 1985).

The first prototype of the ETS/College Board diagnostic testing system, now being field-tested, concentrates on students in remedial programs at the college freshman level. It is intended to serve institutions that admit students with a wide and largely unknown range of readiness for college level instruction. The exercises it contains may be used while students are in remedial education programs, or before they enter an instructional program in an effort to improve their preparation. It will diagnose student weaknesses in the traditional basic skills--English (including written communication), reading, and mathematics--as well as more general learning skills, such as listening, note-taking, vocabulary development, memorizing, and using reference sources. In all, there will be 25 tests. (For a complete list, please see Appendix C.)

A flexible length test, the ETS/College Board diagnostic test builds on the technology and patterns of the previously described placement test. At the beginning of most of the test modules, a student is presented with one or more "challenge" items of a mid-difficulty level. These challenge questions combine skills in realistically complex ways. Students who do not perform well on challenges are then routed to "probes," questions which assess constituent skills and determine why an error has been made; students who do well skip the probes and may be presented with challenges of increased difficulty or moved on to other test modules. Using the challenge/probe format, the system can provide students with corrective feedback--explaining why selected answers were incorrect--and provide them with a strategy for selecting the correct answer. The system can also diagnose their specific problems and, through branching, provide additional practice in a particular area as well as avoid boring more advanced students by routing them around unnecessary testing areas.

No attempt was made to impose uniformity across the diagnostic testing tasks. Rather, the item types, assessment techniques, and branching strategies that seemed to be most effective for each task were employed. Thus student response modes range from multiple-choice to student-constructed responses, rearrangement of complex materials, essay writing (essays are printed out for instructor review), and interactive sequences. Some test modules are timed and some are not. Some provide students with second chances to answer items and give explanations of correct choices; and some utilize common misconceptions for incorrect answers in order to diagnose patterns of error. (Samples of the variety of exercises used are contained in Appendix D.)

Similarly, reporting systems are tailored to each module to provide appropriate feedback in terms of success, specific misconceptions, and basic misunderstandings. The reports give encouragement wherever possible and offer suggestions for instructions. (Samples of the types of reports produced for students are contained in Appendix E, and those for instructors are in Appendix F.)

Although the ETS/College Board prototype of computerized diagnostic testing was designed for use with college freshmen in remedial or developmental programs, the system can be utilized in a number of different areas. It could be used in the freshman or sophomore year of high school to diagnose and prescribe remediation in skills and knowledge required for college--focusing on those tested in college entrance exams--so that an accompanying program of study could be implemented before graduation. In addition, the system can be adapted to diagnose skills at higher levels of ability, for example, identifying engineering students' skills in calculus. Other applications of the system might include use with English as a Second Language (ESL) programs, diagnosis and remediation for graduate level admissions testing, and combined training and assessment systems. In short, computer-adaptive diagnostic testing can be used wherever accurate, individualized information is needed for instructional follow-up.

- Military Applications. Both adaptive testing and computerized diagnostic testing are particularly well-suited to military training needs and the determination of an examinee's abilities to benefit from training and to succeed on the job. Adaptive testing would provide assessment of skills in less time and with fewer items, immediate scoring, improved test security, and a simplified system of replacing items. Diagnostic testing would pinpoint weak areas and suggest strategies for improving so that training would be more successful. Further, the ETS/College Board system with its inherent flexibility and ability to accept new tests and operate on commercially available hardware would be especially useful in this area.

<u>Issues in Adaptive Testing Still to be Resolved.</u> Although ETS has succeeded in developing a system for effectively presenting adaptive and diagnostic testing on popular commercially available microcomputers, several issues remain to be resolved through further field tests and research and development. These include the following:

- Methods of incorporating additional feedback and instructional information.

- Improved branching techniques, especially for branching based on types of errors in diagnostic testing.

- Improved computer assessment of student-constructed responses, including computer assessment of student essays (Ward, 1984a).

- Improved methods of assessing and producing the large numbers of high quality items needed for adaptive testing, including the ability to calibrate such items by computer rather than by large-scale administration to student populations (Wright & Bell, 1984).

- Development of more complex psychometric models to support diagnostic instruments and provide their framework.

- Better integration of assessment results and instructional programs.

- Methods of isolating and eliminating questions that are not effective for selected groups of students, such as non-native speakers of English, minorities, etc.

- Methods of automating test construction.

- Improved methods of incorporating the graphics required for some items into the system.

- Methods of presenting complex item types that involve extensive text materials, such as long reading passages.

- Balancing the advantages of adaptive testing against the cost of its initial implementation.

- Risks associated with hardware and software malfunctions.

- Procedures to guarantee the accessibility of the computer and software only to authorized individuals.

TESTING IN THE YEAR 2000

As the rate of change in computer technology and psychometric and cognitive theory continues to accelerate, the world of testing is also bound to be affected--technical advances in videodisc applications, improved computer graphics, voice input and output capabilities, and computer networks have already begun new avenues for improved testing, and they will continue to do so in the future (Baker, 1984). As the costs of more powerful, easy-to-use microcomputers continue to fall, making them available to a wider audience, the demand for computer applications to education, training, and assessment for more levels and purposes will increase (Brzezinski, 1984). Thus it becomes possible to envision a world where the following situations may be commonplace:

- Elementary and secondary school students follow continually updated individualized educational plans based on adaptive testing that is incorporated in their computerized learning programs. Results of testing and student progress are automatically monitored on state and local levels by various computer networks.

- Students working alone and with counselors focus their career interests and learn about various job opportunities through adaptive career guidance products. Using computers, they can test their levels of interest and ability against those of successful people involved in their chosen careers, and through videodisc presentations, can observe people at work in those careers.

- Students can file initial applications and take corporate and industry placement and certification tests on local microcomputers. These might include simulated video exercises, with which potential employers could measure an applicant's responses and reactions to actual on-the-job situations and his or her potential for success and retention in training programs.

- Job training programs will be computer-driven multimedia packages, and their pace will be adapted to individual student progress based on unobtrusive continual diagnostic assessment incorporated in the programs.

- Students interested in higher education will learn about schools and programs of interest through computer programs and will automatically receive information from the desired institutions by having their names added to computerized search service data bases. They will register and study for college entrance exams using microcomputers that will also help them diagnose and remedy deficient skills and estimate their performance on the tests. When they are ready to take the examinations themselves, they will do so on computers and receive their scores immediately. Simultaneously, the scores will be transmitted to the desired institutions, and admission decisions could be given within a short time and transmitted to the student via computer.

- When students have completed required education and training programs, they will take professional and occupational certification, licensing, and recertification examinations on computers and then keep their skills honed and up-to-date through computer-delivered, adaptive continuing education programs.

REFERENCES

Baker, F.B. (1984). Technology and testing: State of the art and trends for the future. "Journal of Educational Measurement," "21(4)," 399-406.

Bejar, I.I. (1984). Educational diagnostic assessment. "Journal of Educational Measurement," "21(2)," 175-189.

Brzezinski, E.J. (1984). Microcomputers and testing: Where are we and how did we get there? "Educational Measurement: Issues and Practice," "3(2)," 7-10.

Donlon, T.F. (1980). "An exploratory study of the implications of test speededness" (GRE-76-9P). Princeton, NJ: Educational Testing Service.

"Educational Measurement: Issues and Practice" (1984). "3(2)."

Educational Testing Service (1985). "ETS Developments," "30(4)."

Forehand, G.A., Rice, M.W., & Wilder, G.Z. (1982, November). "Development of diagnostic testing procedures for skills of written communication." Unpublished proposal, research in progress. Princeton, NJ: Educational Testing Service.

Hsu, T., & Nitko, A.J. (1983). Microcomputer testing software teachers can use. "Educational Measurement: Issues and Practice," "2(4)," 15-30.

Lord, F.M. (1980). "Applications of Item Response Theory to practical testing problems." Hillsdale, NJ: Erlbaum.

McArthur, D.L., & Choppin, B.H. (1984). Computerized diagnostic testing. "Journal of Educational Measurement," "21(4)," 391-397.

Stocking, M. L. (1984). "Two simulated feasibility studies in Computerized Adaptive Testing (CAT)." Paper presented at the annual meeting of the American Educational Research Association, New Orleans, LA.

"TALMIS Report: The K-12 Market for Microcomputers and Software" (1984). Chicago, IL: TALMIS, Inc.

"TALMIS Industry Update" (1985, September). New York, NY: TALMIS, Inc.

Trismen, D. (1981). "The development and administration of a set of mathematics items with hints." (ETS Research Report 81-5). Princeton, NJ: Educational Testing Service.

Urry, V.W. (1977). Tailored testing: A successful application of Latent Trait Theory. "Journal of Educational Measurement," "14," 181-196.

Wainer, H. (1983). On Item Response Theory and computerized adaptive tests. "The Journal of College Admissions," "28(4)," 9-16.

Ward, W.C. (1984a). Using microcomputers to administer tests. "Educational Measurement: Issues and Practices," "3(2)," 16-20.

Ward, W.C. (1984b). Computerized adaptive testing program for college placement, preliminary report: Spring 1984 pilot testing. Unpublished paper describing pilot test results of the ETS/College Board Computerized Adaptive Testing Project. Princeton, NJ: Educational Testing Service.

Weiss, D.J. (1983). New horizons in testing: Latent Trait Theory and computerized adaptive testing. New York: Academic Press.

Weiss, D.J., & Kingsbury, G.G. (1984). Application of computerized adaptive testing to educational problems. "Journal of Educational Measurement," "21(4)," 361-375.

Wright, B.D., & Bell, S.R. (1984). Item banks: What, why, how. "Journal of Educational Measurement," "21(4)," 331-345.

APPENDIX A

COMPUTERIZED ADAPTIVE TESTING PROGRAM FOR COLLEGE PLACEMENT

EXAMPLES OF TEST QUESTIONS

Reading Comprehension

This test measures your ability to understand what you read.

Read the statement or passage and then choose the best answer to the question. Answer the question on the basis of what is stated or implied in the statement or passage.

Myths are stories, the products of fertile imagination, sometimes simple, often containing profound truths. They are not meant to be taken too literally. Details may sometimes appear childish, but most myths express a culture's most serious beliefs about human beings, eternity, and God.

The main idea of this passage is that myths

   are created primarily to entertain young children
   are purposely written for the reader who lacks imagination
   provides the reader with a means of escape from reality
   illustrate the values that are considered important to a society

Two underlined sentences are followed by a question or statement about them. Read each pair of sentences and then choose the best answer to the question or the best completion of the statement.

EXAMPLES OF TEST QUESTIONS

<u>The Midwest is experiencing its worst drought in fifteen years.
Corn and soybean are expected to be very high this year.</u>

What does the second sentence do?

    It restates the idea found in the first.
* It states an effect.
    It gives an example.
    It analyzes the statement made in the first.

Sentence Skills

This test measures your understanding of sentence structure—of how sentences are put together and what makes a sentence complete and clear.

Select the best version of the underlined part of the sentence. The first choice is the same as the original sentence. If you think the original sentence is best, choose the first answer.

Ms. Rose <u>planning</u> to teach a course in biology next summer.

    planning
    are planning
    with a plan
* plans

Rewrite the sentence in your head, following the directions given below. Keep in mind that your new sentence should be well written and should have essentially the same meaning as the sentence given you.

Being a female jockey, she was often interviewed.

Rewrite, beginning with

<u>She was often interviewed</u>. . .

The next words will be

    on account of she was
    by her being
* because she was
    being as she was

Arithmetic

This test measures your ability to perform basic arithmetic operations and to solve problems that involve fundamental arithmetic concepts.

Solve the following problems and choose your answer from the alternatives given. You may use the paper you have been given for scratchwork.

EXAMPLES OF TEST QUESTIONS

All of the following are ways to write 20 percent of N EXCEPT

    0.20N

    $\frac{20}{100}$ N

    $\frac{1}{5}$ N

* 20 N

Which of the following is closest to $\sqrt{10.5}$?

* 3
  4
  5
  8

Three people who work full time are to work together on a project, but their total time on the project is to be equivalent to that of only one person working full time. If one of the people is budgeted for 1/2 of his time to the project and a second person for 1/3 of her time, what part of the third worker's time should be budgeted to this project?

  $\frac{1}{3}$ * $\frac{1}{6}$

  $\frac{1}{4}$ $\frac{1}{8}$

<u>Elementary Algebra</u>

    This test measures your ability to perform basic algebraic operations and to solve problems that involve elementary algebraic concepts.

    Solve the following problems and choose your answer from the alternatives given. You may use the paper you have been given for scratchwork.

If a number is divided by 4 and then 3 is subtracted, the result is 0. What is the number?

* 12
  4
  3
  2

16x − 8 =

    8x
    8(2x − x)
* 8(2x − 1)
    8(2x − 8)

If $x^2 - x - 6 = 0$, then x is ▶

    * −2 or 3
      −1 or 6
      1 or −6
      2 or −3

APPENDIX B-1

COMPUTERIZED ADAPTIVE TESTING PROGRAM FOR COLLEGE PLACEMENT

ON-LINE REPORT OF INDIVIDUAL STUDENT'S PERCENTILE RANKS
(As Presented on Computer Screen at End of Testing Session)

This completes the testing. Your scores are as follows:

TEST	PERCENTILE RANK
READING COMPREHENSIVE	60
SENTENCE SKILLS	53
ARITHMETIC	72
ELEMENTARY ALGEBRA	41

A percentile rank of 60 on a test means that your score is higher than those of 60% of a statewide sample of students who completed the test. You will receive a printed report explaining your results more fully.

Please press RETURN to clear the screen.

APPENDIX B-2

COMPUTERIZED ADAPTIVE TESTING PROGRAM FOR COLLEGE PLACEMENT

PRINTED INDIVIDUAL STUDENT REPORT

REPORT FOR: Warton, Ralph W.

ID: 333-22-1111   BIRTHDATE: Nov. 21, 1964

TEST RESULTS	TOTAL RIGHT SCORE	RANGE	PERCENTILE RANK	TEST DATE
READING COMPREHENSION	32	25-38	6	07/24/84
SENTENCE SKILLS	29	25-33	<1	07/24/84
ARITHMETIC	36	29-43	11	07/24/84
ELEMENTARY ALGEBRA	40	32-48	26	07/24/84

   Each test you completed was chosen from a group of 120 questions. The TOTAL RIGHT SCORE shows how many of these you could expect to answer correctly if you took a test made up of all 120 questions.

   Any test score is an estimate, not an exact measure of your skills. The RANGE tells you how accurate your score is. If you took a test a second time, you could expect your new score to fall somewhere within the RANGE that is shown.

   The PERCENTILE RANK compares your score with the scores of entering college students who completed a test of basic skills in a statewide assessment program. A PERCENTILE RANK of 6, for example, means that your score is higher than those of 6 percent of the students who completed the test.

<u>Answers to Background Questions:</u>

Years studied English in high school:	3
Years studied mathematics in high school:	3
Studied algebra in high school:	Yes
Sex:	Male
Self description:	Omit
English first language:	Yes
Disabling condition:	Deafness or other hearing impairment
Father's education:	High school diploma or equivalent
Mother's education:	High school diploma or equivalent

APPENDIX B-3

COMPUTERIZED ADAPTIVE TESTING PROGRAM FOR COLLEGE PLACEMENT

ROSTER OF TOTAL RIGHT SCORES FOR A GROUP OF STUDENTS

ROSTER FOR: Alamont Community College

ROSTER OF: Total Right Scores

FOR: All Students Tested 07/24/84 through 07/25/84

ORGANIZED BY: Student Name

NUMBER OF STUDENTS: 8

NAME	ID	READING COMPREHENSION	SENTENCE SKILLS	ARITHMETIC	ELEMENTARY ALGEBRA
ANDERSON, EDGAR W.	989-89-8989	14	60	40	35
BOWERS, JANET C.	099-89-0909	112	108	66	64
EVANS, THOMAS J.	555-66-9999	68	80	37	24
GRAGE, JULIA	777-66-7777	120	120	92	80
HARRAT, SUSAN T.	767-67-6767	62	82	104	118
RATTNERY, HANSON V.	241-35-6778	30	32	40	32
WARTON, RALPH W.	333-22-1111	32	29	36	40
WINFIELD, WILBUR C.	333-44-5555	114	118	116	120

APPENDIX B-4

COMPUTERIZED ADAPTIVE TESTING PROGRAM FOR COLLEGE PLACEMENT

SUMMARY STATISTICS REPORT

SUMMARY REPORT FOR: Alamont Community College

REPORT OF: Total Right Scores

FOR: All Students Tested 07/24/84 through 07/25/84

	READING COMPREHENSION	SENTENCE SKILLS	ARITHMETIC	ELEMENTARY ALGEBRA
115-120	1	2	1	2
110-114	2	0	0	0
105-109	0	1	0	0
100-104	0	0	1	0
95 - 99	0	0	0	0
90 - 94	0	0	1	0
85 - 89	0	0	0	0
80 - 84	0	2	0	0
75 - 79	0	0	0	0
70 - 74	0	0	0	0
65 - 69	1	0	1	0
60 - 64	1	1	0	1
55 - 59	0	0	0	0
50 - 54	0	0	0	0
45 - 49	0	0	0	0
40 - 44	1	0	2	1
35 - 39	0	0	2	1
30 - 34	2	1	0	1
25 - 29	0	1	0	0
20 - 24	0	0	0	1
15 - 19	0	0	0	0
10 - 14	0	0	0	0
5 - 9	0	0	0	0
0 - 4	0	0	0	0
NUMBER OF STUDENTS	8	8	8	8
MEAN SCORE	72.5	78.6	66.4	64.1
STANDARD DEVIATION	37.9	36.1	33.2	38.5

APPENDIX C

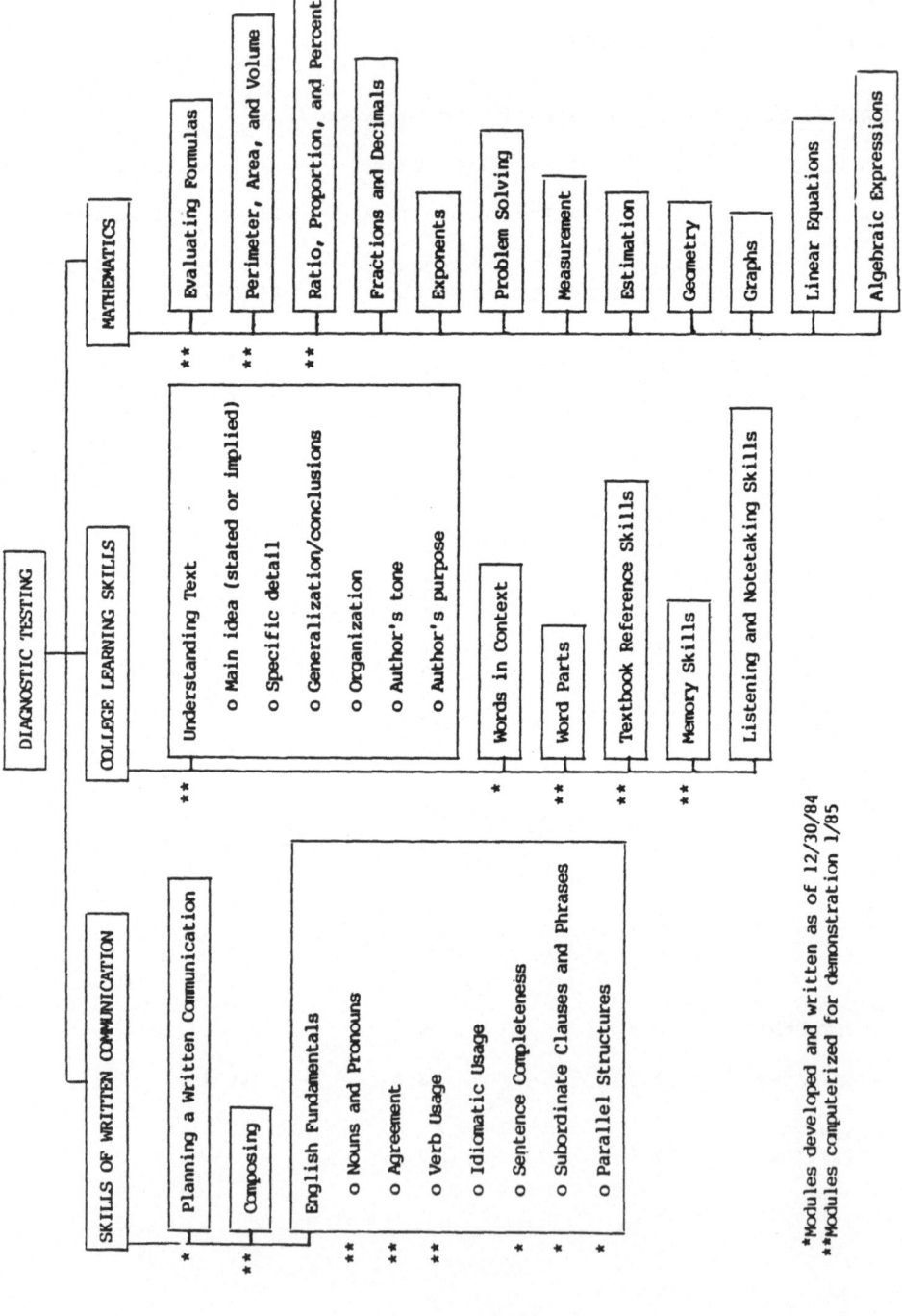

APPENDIX D-1

STUDENT WRITING

Choice

Your assignment now is to develop a two-paragraph essay.

The essay has been started as follows:

When I was a kid I had a cousin who drove his father's car, in a back lot and an alley, however. His name was Claude, and at that time he was twelve like me. He seemed to know what was going on. I thought he was sophisticated.

Below are four ways of rewriting the beginning of the essay. Choose the way of rewriting it that presents the ideas most clearly and directly.

(A) I once had a cousin who drove his father's car. That showed me he was sophisticated.

(B) Being twelve at the time about which I am speaking, my cousin Claude already drove his father's car. He only drove it in the back yard and an alley, however, impressing me by this that he was sophisticated and really knew what was going on.

(C) When my cousin Claude and I were twelve, he drove his father's car. He only drove in a back lot and an alley, but that convinced me he was sophisticated.

(D) My cousin Claude drove his father's car, which brings up the idea that he was sophisticated. He always knew what was going on, and drove it (I mean his father's car) in a back lot and an alley, even though he was only twelve. I was also twelve at the time.

APPENDIX D-1

STUDENT WRITING

<u>Feedback</u>

(A)...

    This is not a good choice because it leaves out important information (such as Claude's age and where Claude drove the car). Make a different choice.

(B)...

    This choice is wordy. It is not stated as directly and clearly as it should be. Make a different choice.

(C)...

    A good choice.

(D)...

    This is not a good choice. It rambles from point to point. The information about Claude and the writer should be organized more clearly and directly. Make a different choice.

APPENDIX D-2

STUDENT WRITING

Choice

When my cousin Claude and I were twelve, he drove his father's car. He only drove in a back lot and an alley, but that convinced me he was sophisticated.

* * * * * * * * * * * * * *

The essay now begins with the two sentences above. Which of the following questions should the writer answer in developing the next few sentences of the essay? Choose (A), (B), (C), or (D).

(A) What were some of the things the writer liked to do when the writer was twelve years old?

(B) How, in his driving and other ways, did Claude seem sophisticated?

(C) How long had the writer known Claude and what earlier experiences had the two of them shared?

(D) Who among the friends of the writer seemed more sophisticated than Claude?

APPENDIX D-2

STUDENT WRITING

Feedback

(A)...

    Starting off in this direction, the writer would probably stray too far away from the topic that has been started. Make a different choice.

(B)...

    A good choice. This is the question your reader will want answered.

(C)...

    This information, while it might be interesting, is not related directly enough to the topic that has been started. Make a different choice.

(D)...

    This choice would start a new and unrelated topic. Make a different choice.

APPENDIX D-3

NOUN AND PRONOUN USAGE

Challenge 1 (Nouns)

1. The twelve ___(1)___ in the English department agreed on standards for grading all of their ___(2)___ ___(3)___.

(1)	(2)	(3)
instructor [b]	Students [e]	essay [b]
instructors	Student's [f]	essays
instructors' [g]	Students'	essays' [g]

2. Five more ___(1)___ ___(2)___ were signed this morning.

(1)	(2)
players [e]	contract [a]
player's [f]	contracts
players'	contract's [c]

3. This ___(1)___ founders were willing to face challenges and take ___(2)___.

(1)	(2)
nation [d]	risk [a]
nations [e]	risks
nation's	risk's [c]

4. ___(1)___ paper has an article about the four ___(2)___ escape from prison.

(1)	(2)
Today [d]	inmate [d]
Todays [e]	inmate's [f]
Today's	inmates'

5. Three ___(1)___ and a proofreader are working on the ___(2)___ annual report.

(1)	(2)
typist [a]	treasurer [d]
typists	treasurers [e]
typist's [c]	treasurer's

6. In the ___(1)___ opinion, the four best ___(2)___ in the class are Mark, Alicia, Wanda, and Julio.

(1)	(2)
coach [d]	athlete [b]
coaches [e]	athletes
coach's	athlete's [c]

APPENDIX D-4

PLURALS (WITH SINGULAR POSSESSIVES FOR CONTRAST)

Probe 1A (Plurals)

1. Behind the garage they discovered a nest of _____.

    wasp   [a]
    wasps
    wasp's   [c]

2. He has been building that sailboat for at least four _____.

    year   [b]
    years
    year's   [c]

3. Earl found his jacket in _____ car, where he had left it.

    Marian   [d]
    Marians   [e]
    Marian's

4. She found seven more _____ when she examined the computer printout.

    error   [b]
    errors
    error's [c]

5. All the board _____ agreed with the proposal.

    member   [b]
    members
    member's [c]

6. Perhaps we will learn more about the accident on _____ news.

    tonight   [d]
    tonights   [e]
    tonight's

7. Several _____ were made by the study committee.

    suggestion   [b]
    suggestions
    suggestion's [c]

APPENDIX D-5

SINGULAR AND PLURAL POSSESSIVES

Probe 1B (Possessives)

1. My oldest _____ temper is very short.

                brother   [d]
                brothers [e]
                brother's
                brothers' [g]

2. The five _____ decisions were reported in considerable detail.

                judge   [d]
                judges   [e]
                judge's [f]
                judges'

3. The ball popped out of the left _____ glove.

                fielder   [d]
                fielders [e]
                fielder's
                fielders' [g]

4. This _____ opinion of the new album is entirely different from mine.

                reviewer   [d]
                reviewers [e]
                reviewer's
                reviewers' [g]

5. The Mexican and Canadian _____ schedules have been arranged.

                ambassador   [d]
                ambassadors [e]
                ambassador's [f]
                ambassadors'

6. All of those duties should not be one _____ responsibility.

                person   [d]
                persons [e]
                person's
                persons' [g]

7. The two rescue _____ heroic efforts were praised by the fire chief.

                worker   [d]
                workers [e]
                worker's [f]
                workers'

APPENDIX E-1

DIAGNOSTIC TEST OF TEXTBOOK REFERENCE SKILLS

SAMPLE SUMMARY REPORT FOR (Student Name)

You had no problems with the following areas:

    author identification
    copyright data
    using the table of contents
    using the glossary

You made at least one error in the following areas:

    using the subject index
    using the name index

When you were asked to skim the text to find particular information you got the right answer for five our of the seven problems. You took an average of three minutes to find the correct answer on the five items you got right. You should work on using chapter headings to find answers more quickly.

* * * * * * * * * * * * * *

(Example or optional information entered by local institution.)

You may want to improve your textbook reference skills by looking at the following books in The Learning Resource Center (LRC) _____, _____, _____. The LRC also offers a "Computerized Learning Skills Development Package" that might be helpful for you.

The Learning Resource Center is located at 115 Greene Hall and is open from 9:00 a.m. to 9:00 p.m. Monday – Friday.

APPENDIX E-2

DIAGNOSTIC TESTS IN MATHEMATICS

RATIO, PROPORTION AND PERCENT

SAMPLE STUDENT REPORT

NAME: Henry Jones

You did well in the following areas:

Meaning of ratio

Sample problem: ■ ■ ☐ ☐ ☐

In the figure above, what is the ratio of the number of shaded boxes to the number of boxes?

Writing ratios in fraction form

Sample problem: Express a ratio of 7 to 4 in fraction form.

Equivalence of ratios

Sample problem: The ratio of 1 to 12 is equivalent to the ratio of 2 to?

You need to review the following areas:

Solving ratios and proportions

Sample problem: If $\frac{1}{50} = \frac{x}{100}$, then x =

Meaning of percent

Sample problem: $\frac{3}{10}$ of a number is what percent of that number?

APPENDIX E-3

DIAGNOSTIC TESTS IN MATHEMATICS

RATIO, PROPORTION, AND PERCENT

SAMPLE STUDENT PROBLEM ANALYSIS SUMMARY

NAME: Henry Jones

Following are the numbers of the questions you answered incorrectly. Please refer to your Problem Analysis Workbook for the solutions: 3, 11, 12, 19

<u>Note to Reader:</u> The Problem Analysis Workbook will have material like the following illustrative item:

If $\frac{150}{100} = \frac{6}{y}$, what is the value of y?

Solution: $\frac{150}{100} = \frac{6}{y}$

$150y = 6(100)$
$150y = 600$
$y = \frac{600}{150} = 4$

APPENDIX F-1

SAMPLE TEACHER REPORT: COMPOSING

TEACHER REPORT FOR PAULA PLANT

(At challenge level, student passed only skills A, B, & C; at probe level, student passed part 3 of E but failed D, F, and parts 1 and 2 of E)

Overall performance in the context of creating and revising paragraphs shows basic knowledge of the following skills:

    Developing an idea
    Organizing information
    Structuring paragraphs

Needs to develop the following skills:

    Transitions and connections
    Sentence coherence and variety
    Word choice

<u>Transitions and connections</u> Was unable to make logical and effective transitions and connections among related ideas. Needs to learn how to use transitional and connective elements correctly.

<u>Sentence coherence and variety</u> Was unable to place modifiers correctly. Was unable to restructure sentences to achieve variety. Demonstrated ability to eliminate short, choppy sentences through sentence combining in isolated items. Was not successful on similar items in a composing context.

<u>Word choice</u> Was unsuccessful at choosing "the right word" for precision, effect, and/or tone.

APPENDIX F-2

SAMPLE TEACHER REPORT: ENGLISH FUNDAMENTALS

TEACHER REPORT FOR PAULA PLANT

Nouns and Pronouns

    Formed plurals correctly.
    Needs to learn how to form the plural possessive.

    *   *   *   *   *   *   *   *   *   *   *   *   *   *

    Correctly used nominative, objective, reflexive, and possessive pronouns. Correctly used who and whom.

Agreement

    Understands basic rules for subject-verb agreement but needs to learn rules that apply to special cases, such as indefinite pronouns as subjects, compound subjects joined by or, and infinitive phrases as subjects.

    *   *   *   *   *   *   *   *   *   *   *   *   *   *

    Understands and can apply the principles of pronoun-antecedent agreement.

Verb Usage

    Was unsuccessful in some aspects of verb usage. Particular skills needing attention are described below:

    Use of ed Understands use of ed to indicate past tense but made some errors in the use of ed when asked to produce (rather than select) the correct form.

    Use of ing Used ing incorrectly in items dealing with this skill alone; made some ing errors in terms involving several skills.

    Use of do Needs to learn how to use the form of do and how to form verb phrases with do as the helping verb.

    Use of be Knows how to use the forms of be correctly but does not always apply this knowledge in combination with other skills.

    Use of appropriate tense Needs to learn the formation and use of the tenses.

Sentence Completeness

    Identified and corrected most sentence fragments presented one at a time. Missed fragments consisting of subordinate clauses standing alone.

    *   *   *   *   *   *   *   *   *   *   *   *   *   *

APPENDIX F-2

SAMPLE TEACHER REPORT: ENGLISH FUNDAMENTALS

Was able to join sentences correctly without creating run-ons but was not able to mark off complete sentences in an unpunctuated paragraph.

<u>Subordinate Clauses and Phrases</u>

Successfully created correct sentences containing subordinate elements, using a sentence combining technique.

<u>Parallel Structures</u>

Needs to learn how to create parallel structures within sentences.

APPENDIX F-3

DIAGNOSTIC TESTS IN MATHEMATICS

RATIO, PROPORTION, AND PERCENT

SAMPLE INSTRUCTOR REPORT

Instructor Report: Group Strengths and Weaknesses

Group Identification: Mathematics 001, Section A

Number of Students in Group: 26

Subject Area	Number of Students		
	Need Review	Satisfactory	Not Assessed
Meaning of ratio	18	8	0
Writing ratios in fraction form	15	11	0
Equivalence of ratios	16	10	0
Solving ratios and proportions	19	7	0
Application of ratio and proportion	13	11	2
Meaning of percent	17	9	0
Fraction/percent equivalence	20	3	3

APPENDIX F-4

DIAGNOSTIC TESTS IN MATHEMATICS

RATIO, PROPORTION, AND PERCENT

SAMPLE INSTRUCTOR REPORT

Instructor Report: Listing of Students Needing Review, By Area

Group Identification: Mathematics 001, Section A

Number of Students in Group: 26

Students Needing Review	Area(s)
Jones, Henry	Solving ratios and proportions Meaning of percent
Smith, Karen	Meaning of ratio Writing ratios in fraction form
Truscott, William	Equivalence of ratios
West, Philip	Application of ratio and proportion Fraction/percent equivalence

Etc.

APPENDIX F-5

DIAGNOSTIC TESTS IN MATHEMATICS

RATIO, PROPORTION AND PERCENT

SAMPLE INSTRUCTOR REPORT

Instructor Report: Group Misconceptions

Group Identification: Mathematics 001, Section A

Number of Students in Group: 26

Misconception	Number of Students Showing the Misconception at Least Once
Reversal of numerator and denominator	21
If $a/b=c/d$, then $d=b-a$	19
If $a/b=c/d$, then $d=a/c$	22
If $a/b=c/d$, then $b=c/d$	16
If $a/b=c/d$, then $ac=bd$	23
If $a/b=c/d$, then $a+c=b+d$	9
If $a/b=c/d$, then $a+c=b+c$	12
If $a/b=c/d$, then $a+d=b+c$	13
If $a/b=c/d$, then $a+c=b+d$	18

IMPLEMENTATION OF COMPUTER BASED TRAINING: A SYSTEM EVALUATION AND LESSONS LEARNED

J. Y. Yasutake

Air Force Human Resources Laboratory
Lowry Air Force Base, Colorado, U.S.A.

INTRODUCTION

Following a series of preliminary studies in the early 1970s, the United States Air Force embarked on a major research and development effort to design, demonstrate, and evaluate a computer-based instructional system at a major technical training center. The system called the Advanced Instructional System (AIS) was developed to demonstrate the feasibility of managing and administering individualized instruction for up to 2,000 students daily in four technical training courses. A major state-of-the-art advancement was an integrated computer-based support capability which provided a full range of Computer-Based Instruction (CBI) functions including course development and presentation, resource allocation and scheduling, and individual student management. A unique feature was the Adaptive Model, which produced student prescriptions based on trade-offs between learning requirements, student characteristics and resource availability. To support the integrated CBI system, a higher-order language called CAMIL (Computer-Assisted/Managed Instructional Language) was developed. Hardware support was provided by a CYBER 73-16 with 10 management terminals and 50 interactive terminals. The purpose of this paper is to describe the background of the AIS, summarize the evaluation data, and discuss current efforts underway as a result of lessons learned from the AIS demonstration program.

BACKGROUND

Descriptions of the genesis of the AIS and of the total concept are available elsewhere (Nunns, 1982; Rockway & Yasutake, 1974). Below is a brief description of the program.

Four courses were chosen to demonstrate the AIS capabilities. These were the Inventory Management (IM), Material Facilities (MF), Precision Measuring Equipment (PME), and Weapons Mechanic (WM) courses. They represented approximately 1,500 hours of instruction and were selected because of the differences in course lengths, training content, technical complexity, student aptitude requirements, and the fact that they were relatively high-flow courses. During the demonstration period the four courses had a student flow of approximately 7,000 per year.

Prior to the AIS program these courses were taught in a conventional group-paced classroom environment. As the AIS segments were implemented, the classrooms were converted to learning centers with a variety of self-paced instructional materials. The role of the training cadre was changed from that of platform instructors to learning center managers and training facilitators.

Self-paced instructional materials were developed to replace conventional classroom instruction. For approximately 25% of the course content, optional tracks were developed. Some options used different presentation modes (e.g., printed texts and audio-visual presentation) while others differed in the strategy of presentation (e.g., the amount of redundancy). It was the availability of these options that allowed a test of the effectiveness of the Adaptive Model.

Computer support was provided by a Control Data Corporation (CDC) Cyber 73-16 with 10 management terminals (each consisting of a document reader, printer, and minicomputer) and 50 interactive terminals (plasma display and keyboard). A primary component of the software was CAMIL (Computer-Assisted/Managed Instructional Language), a higher-level language specifically designed to facilitate both CMI (Computer-Managed Instruction) and CAI (Computer-Assisted Instruction) using a common integrated data base.

The configuration of the AIS at the time of system evaluation was essentially that of a large-scale, self-paced CMI (SP/CMI) system. The CMI capabilities included the standard features such as test scoring and analysis, student rosters, student progress records and various course evaluation reports. In addition, two major unique features were designed and evaluated as to their effectiveness to enhance training. The first was the Individualized Instructional Assignment (IIA) capability and the second, the Student Progress Management (SPM) system. In brief, the Individualized Instructional Assignment (IIA) provided each student with a specific prescription for the next sequence of instruction. The prescription was driven by a heuristically based Adaptive Model. A simplified diagram of the primary components of the model is provided in Figure 1. IIA selected an instructional sequence (from available alternatives) which was predicted to maximize student performance. Input data included past performance, student characteristics, and resource and lesson availability.

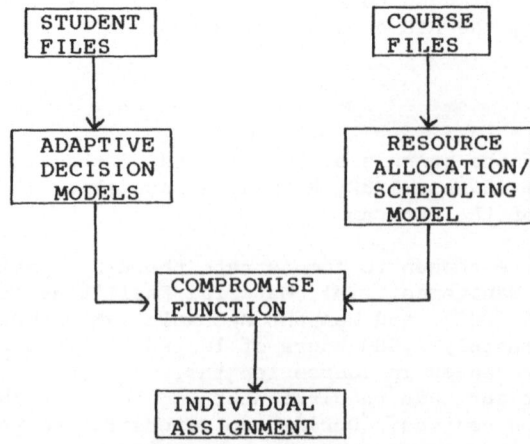

Figure 1. Adaptive Model

The Student Progress Management (SPM) capability maintained records of the rate of student progress and produced predicted completion times for segments of training as well as the entire course. Each student was able to track his/her own progress and establish individual goals to meet the predicted completion time. Predictions were based on student aptitude, past performance, and historical data on past students with similar profiles. Where necessary because of extraneous circumstances (e.g., illness), instructors were able to revise the computer-generated predictions.

EVALUATION OF AIS

Issues in Evaluations of Large-Scale Systems

A well-controlled evaluation of a large-scale system represents a particularly difficult task because of real-world constraints. Initially, consideration was given to freezing the content of the four courses during the AIS demonstration and test phase and to have a parallel control group (conventional classroom) and an experimental group (self-paced, CMI) within each course. In this manner, it would have been possible to introduce various conditions in the experimental group and compare outcomes with the control group. However, real-world limitation (e.g., facilities and equipment) precluded such an approach. Rather, a decision was made to use a "pre" and "post" paradigm. Thus, for each course "pre" data were collected on course length, attrition rates, test scores and field supervisor ratings for a 1-year period to AIS implementation. These data served as a baseline for comparisons with data gathered after AIS segments were implemented. Although this approach was followed to the extent possible, changes in field requirements during the course of the demonstration dictated changes to training content. Thus, an issue of comparability of the pre- and post-course versions needed to be resolved. This issue was handled by carefully analyzing course content of the two versions (i.e., conventional and AIS) and making comparisons only with subsets of the courses which were common to both.

Evaluation Approach and Results

From the beginning of operations to the completion of the formal system evaluation, well over 20,000 students were graduated from the self-paced CMI courses. Two major categories of evaluation data were collected during this time. In the first category were the recurring and periodic assessments of training effectiveness as measured by student time savings, achievement, student and instructor attitudes, and field supervisor ratings. These data were gathered systematically over a 3-year period to determine the extent to which instruction was functioning to meet stated training goals. The second major category of evaluation was the Integrated Systems Test (IST). Of particular interest during this test was the effectiveness of the Individualized Instructional Assignment (IIA) and student progress management (SPM) capabilities. Extensive data were also gathered regarding the reliability of computer hardware and software. The intent was to ensure that the contractual specification under which the AIS was developed had been met.

    <u>Training Effectiveness Evaluation</u> Four separate indices were used to assess the effectiveness of training: (1) Student training time savings; (2) achievement on paper and pencil tests; (3) student attrition rates; and (4) field supervisor rating of the adequacy of training to meet job requirements. These data were collected at various times during the 4-years that the AIS demonstration was in effect.

(1) Student Time Savings: Calculations of savings in student time were made based on the extent to which students met criterion under self-paced CMI versus conventional instruction. Calculations were made only on segments of the course which were common to both. Table 1 shows the time savings for each of the four courses. As can be seen, time savings ranged from 24% to 35%.

(2) Paper-and-Pencil Test Scores: Within-course achievement was measured by comparing test scores for instructional content common to both pre- and post-AIS implementation. Because of the difficulties in determining test item commonality, data were compared only for the Inventory Management course. Results shown in Table 2 indicate that test achievement under the pre- and post conditions were quite similar.

(3) Student and Instructor Attitudes: Upon completion of the course, each student completed a 40-item attitude questionnaire. The questionnaire was designed to assess attitudes toward various aspects of the self-paced CMI-supported instruction. On two occasions, instructor attitudes were also measured. In general, 80-90% of the students reacted favorably to their experiences. In contrast, instructors were generally negative. An interesting comparison between instructor and student attitudes toward similar items is depicted in Table 3. These findings are in general agreement with those of other studies (Carson et al., 1975; Seidel, Rosenblatt, Wagner, Schulz, & Hunter, 1978).

(4) Academic Attrition: Although data on attrition were collected, it was recognized that they were not necessarily indicative of instructional quality. Various factors such as field demands and changes in student quality influence attrition. Nevertheless, the data were collected to determine whether any unexplained fluctuations occurred after AIS implementation. Table 4, adapted from the Orlansky and String report (1981), shows that after an initial decrease, there was a trend toward increased attrition.

It is interesting to note, however, that during the same time period, attrition rose in all courses being taught at the training base.

(5) Field Supervisor Ratings: Approximately 6 months after students completed training, follow-up questionnaires were sent out to the field to obtain supervisor opinions of the performance of graduates. Table 5 shows the results. The data indicated that supervisor ratings were favorable regarding the performance of the graduates of the self-paced CMI courses.

Table 1. Student Time Savings
SP/CMI

Course	% Savings
IM	35
MF	24
WM	31
PME	31

Table 2. Conventional vs SP/CMI Test Scores

	Conventional %	SP/CMI %
Block 1	82	89
Block 2	83	83
Block 3	84	87
Block 4	80	84
Block 5	83	87

Table 3. Student (S)/Instructor (I) Attitudes

COURSES	PRE SP/CMI	SP/CMI YEAR 1	SP/CMI YEAR 2	SP/CMI YEAR 3
IM	1.2	.7	1.4	3.0
MF	3.7	1.8	3.2	2.7
WM	1.6	1.6	3.9	4.5
PME	16.5	10.8	6.4	15.3
All Other Courses	4.0	2.8	3.0	4.5

Table 4. Academic Attrition (%)

Student Question		S (N=363)	I (N=46)	Instructor Question
				COMPARED TO CONVENTIONAL INSTRUCTION.
COMPARED TO LECTURE, SELF-PACED COURSE IS BETTER WAY TO LEARN.	D N A	15% 28% 56%	57% 22% 22%	STUDENTS LEARN AS WELL UNDER SELF-PACING.
THE INSTRUCTOR WAS AVAILABLE WHENEVER I NEEDED HIM.	D N A	6% 9% 85%	30% 30% 39%	UNDER SELF-PACING, I HAVE LESS TIME TO SPEND WITH STUDENTS.
PREFER FUTURE AF COURSES TO BE OF THIS TYPE.	D N A	14% 26% 60%	59% 26% 15%	STUDENTS SEEM TO LIKE SELF-PACING.
THE PROGRAMMED INSTRUCTION WAS BORING.	D N A	56% 31% 13%	13% 28% 59%	SELF-PACED MATERIALS ARE BORING.

D = Disagree
N = Neutral
A = Agree

Table 5. Field Supervisor Rating of Performance

	IM (N=310) %		MF (N=235) %		PME (N=78) %		WM (N=147) %	
E	29	(27)	25	(21)	45	(13)	18	(15)
VS	38	–	39	(48)	26	(31)	31	(35)
S	28	(72)	33	(28)	19	(52)	47	(50)
M	4	–	2	–	9	(2)	5	–
U	1	(1)	1	(3)	1	(2)	0	(1)

E = Excellent
VS = Very Satisfactory
S = Satisfactory
M = Marginal
U = Unsatisfactory

( ) = PRE SP/CMI GRAD EVAL

Integrated Systems Test (IST)

As may be recognized, the training time savings discussed above could in large part be attributed to the instructional design process in self-pacing the four courses. A major goal of the Advanced Instructional System demonstration was to determine whether individualized instruction (i.e., prescribing instruction based on individual difference measures) could enhance training. Thus, the IST was designed to determine the extent to which using the Adaptive Model for Individualized Instructional Assignments (IIA), and setting individual goals by use of the Student Progress Management (SPM) capability, could contribute to time savings above and beyond those attributable to self-paced/CMI.

A more detailed account of the IST may be found in a report by Lintz, Pennell, and Yasutake (1979). The discussion here is focused on the two major experimental issues; namely, the effectiveness of the IIA and the SPM. The IM course served as the main vehicle for investigation of the IIA. Data on SPM were collected for all four courses.

The evaluation design to study the effects of the IIA and SPM is depicted in Table 6.

Condition A – self-paced CMI version of the course with a predetermined sequence of instruction.

Condition B – assigned modules which were "best" for that student based on personal characteristics and past achievements. "Best" was defined as the module that could be passed successfully in the shortest time.

Condition C – the same as A, except that students were given target completion times and a chart to track their daily progress toward that target.

Condition D – the same as B with SPM added.

Table 6

Condition	Phase I (12 Weeks) SP/CMI	Phase II (12-17 Weeks) CMI & CPM
Single-Track	A	C
IIA	B	D

Table 7. Time Savings

CONDITION	COURSE	PHASE I SP/CMI % Savings	PHASE II SP/CMI+SPM % Savings
Single-Track	IM	Baseline Data	10%
	MF		6%
	WM		13%
	PME		5%
IIA	IM	3%	13%

Table 7 shows the results. The data indicated that approximately 3% above and beyond the savings due to SP/CMI could be attributed to Individualized Instructional Assignments (IIA) where students were given alternate, instructional segments as a function of their individual characteristics. An additional 7% to 10% savings were attributable to the Student Progress Management (SPM) system, which established differential course completion targets for individual students as a function of their background and aptitude. Although both of these figures are statistically significant, whether they are practically significant may be questionable (i.e., is it operationally effective to add individualized assignments and student progress management to a self-paced course?).

It was disappointing that the magnitude of the IIA evaluation findings was not greater, although these results might have been expected due to the nature of the experimental conditions. At any rate, the research community still has much to learn about the transition of research findings regarding individual differences from carefully controlled small-scale experiments to large scale dynamic "real-world" environments.

LESSONS LEARNED

As a result of the experiences from the development, demonstration, and evaluation of the AIS, several observations can be identified as "lessons learned." Some are reaffirmations of findings from other similar experiences.

Instructional Aspects

Well designed self-paced materials can provide training equivalent to that of conventional classroom instruction, in less time. Self-paced materials provide variety in instructional presentation techniques (e.g., use of multimedia) and have a mixture of learning activities to sustain interest.

The state of knowledge regarding individual differences is still not advanced enough to have practical, significant impact on design of instruction. The computer software necessary to execute a sophisticated model of adaptive instruction carries a considerable cost in terms of system complexity. Further research is essential to make individualized instruction more cost effective.

Instructional goal setting lies a very powerful motivational mechanism and can impact learning progress considerably.

The cost of self-paced instruction lies more in the instructional design and revision process than in instructional delivery. More efficient authoring capabilities and instructional development procedures are needed.

Organizational Aspects

The transition of a nonconventional instructional system into an operational environment is a very complex process. Many factors including management and instructor commitment, and administrative and logistics support mechanisms, are critical to sustain a new system. The developing agency needs to serve as a transition agent considerably beyond the system development phase. Further study investigating the factors required to enhance transition of new systems into existing environments is required (McCombs, Back, & West, 1984).

Instructor roles are changed dramatically under self-pacing. The selection and training of instructors and redefinitions of instructor roles in self-paced instructional environments require further study.

CURRENT RESEARCH AND DEVELOPMENT EFFORTS

During the 4-year demonstration period, well over 20,000 students were graduated from the four AIS courses, with training time savings representing more than 1,500 man-years. In terms of cost-avoidance, the training time savings helped to amortize the cost of system development. Although the training effectiveness data were largely favorable, questions regarding the costs associated with a large mainframe approach led to a decision not to implement AIS as an operational system, but to explore more cost-effective alternatives for future use. There was wide recognition of the powerful CBI capabilities existing in the AIS software and the fact that this capability should be captured using a more modularized and transportable approach. The more recent advances in computer hardware/software technology and particularly the emergence of mini-micro computers have made such an approach technically feasible. These advances, together with many of the lessons learned from past efforts, have guided the direction of much of our more recent and current efforts in CBI research and development.

Instructional Support Software (ISS)

The development of the ISS was initiated in 1982. The functional requirements for ISS were established as a result of a review of the basic AIS capabilities and a survey of DOD agencies to identify any additional capabilities which were viewed as being desirable. The approach was to make ISS modular and transportable to a wide range of mini-/micro-computer configurations using a standard DOD language called Ada. The intent in modularizing the functional capabilities was to allow specific subsets (e.g., CAI, CMI Graphics, resource allocation and course authoring) to be executed separately or together as a totally integrated system. The basic ISS is now completed and running on a Vax 11/780. Demonstration of the capability of specific subsets of the ISS to execute on a micro-computer has also been completed. Both capabilities are now under operational test. Once the ISS is stable, it is anticipated that it will be a part of a standard DOD CBI capability. A further description of the ISS may be found in a paper by Marshall (1983).

CAI Handbook

Often, training managers are faced with the issue of whether CAI is appropriate for their particular training situation. To assist them in making informed decisions, a CAI handbook was recently completed (Richardson, Lamos, & West, in press). This handbook provides an introduction to the concept of CAI, describes various factors to be considered, and provides decision aids to assist users in systematically analyzing their requirements.

Personnel Roles in Nonconventional Instruction

Past experiences clearly indicate the need to redefine the role of the instructional cadre in nonconventional instructional (NCI) environments. A study analyzed such requirements and developed recommendations for an instructor training curriculum (McCombs & Lockhart, 1984). In brief the ideal role for an NCI instructor was determined to be that of a counselor, modeler, evaluator, diagnostician, remediator, implementor, and planner.

Automated Task Analysis Authoring Aid (ATA3)

Task analysis as the front end of the Instructional Systems Development process is a necessary, yet often tedious, requirement. Several efforts have been accomplished to provide analysts with various aids to assist in their job. The ATA3 is an initial attempt based on procedures developed by DeVries, Eschenbrenner, and Ruck (1980), to provide an interactive, menu-driven system for conducting task analysis on-line. The intent is to facilitate timely task analysis by using computer support. Preliminary indications are that with continued improvements, the aid will be very useful.

Intelligent Computer-Assisted Instruction (ICAI)

Recently AFHRL has initiated a systematic long-range research and development thrust to investigate the potential of artificial intelligence to job aiding and training. Current efforts are involved in preliminary investigations of expert systems and the establishment of an ICAI test-bed. It is anticipated that these efforts will eventually lead to the development of a portable ICAI system.

CONCLUSIONS

Computer-based instruction in military applications has been demonstrated to be a viable and effective alternative and supplement to more traditional means of training. The early promise of its potential is reaching fruition. Yet, there are still many issues to be resolved and new applications to be explored before its capabilities are fully exploited. A great challenge still remains for the research community in this area.

REFERENCES

Carson, S. Graham, L. Harding, L. Johnson, K. Mayo, G. & Salop, P. (1975). "An evaluation of computer-managed instruction in Navy technical training" (NPRCD-TR-75-38). San Diego, CA: Navy Personnel Research and Development Center.

DeVries, P. Jr., Eschenbrenner, A. Jr., & Ruck, H. (1980). "Task analysis handbook" (AFHRL-TR-79-45(II), AD-A087 711). Brooks AFB, TX: Air Force Human Resources Laboratory, Manpower and Personnel Division.

Lintz, L. Pennell, R. & Yasutake, J. (1979). "Integrated system test of the Advanced Instructional System (AIS)" (AFHRL-TR-79-40, AD-A081 854). Lowry AFB, CO: Air Force Human Resources Laboratory, Technical Training Division.

Marshall, A. (1983). Development of a transportable CBI system. "Journal of Computer-Based Instruction," "10(3&4)", 66-69.

McCombs, B., Lockhart, K. (1984,). "Personnel roles and requirements for nonconventional instruction in Air Force technical training" (AFHRL-TP-84-40). Lowry AFB, CO: Air Force Human Resources Laboratory, Training Systems Division.

McCombs, B. Back, S. & West, A. (1984, August). "Self-paced instruction: Factors critical to implementation in Air Force technical training - A preliminary inquiry" (AFHRL-TP-84-23). Lowry AFB, CO: Air Force Human Resources Laboratory, Training Systems Division.

Nunns, W. (1982). "Advanced Instructional System: Applications for the future" (AFHRL-TP-81-45, AD-A117 144). Lowry AFB, CO: Air Force Human Resources Laboratory, Logistics and Technical Training Division.

Orlansky, J., & String, J. (1981). Computer based instruction for military training. "Defense Management Journal," 46-54.

Richardson, S. Lamos, J. & West, A. (in press). "CAI decision handbook" (AFHRL-TP-84-46). Lowry AFB, CO: Air Force Human Resources Laboratory, Training Systems Division.

Rockway, M. & Yasutake, J. (1974). The evolution of the Air Force Advanced Instructional System. "Journal of Educational Technology System," "2(3)," 217-239.

Seidel, R.J., Rosenblatt, R., Wagner, H., Schulz, R., & Hunter, B. (1978). "Evaluation of a prototype Computerized Training System (CTS) in support of self-pacing and management of instruction" (HUMRRO FR-ED-78-10). Alexandria, VA: Human Resources Research Organization.

EVALUATING NEW TECHNOLOGY: FORMATIVE EVALUATION OF INTELLIGENT COMPUTER ASSISTED INSTRUCTION

E. L. Baker

University of California, Los Angeles
Los Angeles, California, U.S.A.

Evaluation processes are touted to be productive mechanisms for the improvement of educational systems and products. And there is hard evidence of the utility of evaluation in actually improving technology based products and efforts in instructional development. Evaluation is known as well as to contain a strong negative potential. Evaluation can identify weaknesses in such a way as to inhibit exploratory behavior and risk taking on the part of researchers and developers. Playing it safe may be seen to be the winning strategy. Evidence of evaluation utilization studies suggests that when the focus of the evaluation is classification or accountability (good vs. bad; useful vs. wasteful), the openness of R & D project personnel to evaluation processes is inhibited. Formative evaluation, on the other hand, is evaluation whose specific function is to identify strengths and weaknesses for the purpose of improving the product or system under development (Baker, 1974; Baker and Alkin, 1973; Markle, 1967; Baker and Soloutos, 1974). The trick, of course, is in determining what should be studied, in what context the evaluation should take place, when evaluation processes are most useful, and in skilled hypothesis generation about what improvement options logically and feasibly may be implemented. In addition, the identification of weaknesses (no matter how benign the intentions of the evaluation may be) creates a documentary trail that might be misused by project managers or funding agency monitors.

These issues take on special dimensions when the evaluation addresses the effectiveness of new technology. All technology development of necessity focuses on the initial problem of system operation: Can the envisioned delivery system work at all, as opposed to the refinement of what the system's merits may be or what effects might be planned or imagined. The boundaries between technology development and science become especially blurred. The creation of technology may be a pleasant side-effect for the creator, whose perception of his/her main task may be knowledge production. Intellectual exploration is a premium for new technology development, and evaluation processes can be seen to inhibit or be irrelevant to invention.

Recent writing in the field of evaluation planning has emphasized a stakeholder perspective in evaluation implementation. Simply put, this means that interested parties must have an opportunity to understand and to shape the nature of the evaluation questions and methods so that they will be more invested in the process and more apt to use any results generated (Byrk, 1983).

With this discussion as context, a preliminary model of evaluation was designed to be adapted especially to the problem of new technologies. This paper will detail the features of this model and illustrate their use in the problem of evaluating intelligent computer assisted instruction, a particularly difficult area characterized by weak boundary conditions. From this illustration, specific recommendations with regard to design of ICAI systems will also be made.

FEATURES OF A MODEL FOR THE FORMATIVE EVALUATION OF NEW TECHNOLOGIES

The Information Must Provide an Enhanced Documentary Base for the Processes of New Technology Development

A characteristic of new technology is lack of documentation describing the process leading to the development of the systems or product. The purpose of a strong documentary base is to provide the trace of developmental processes so that the field can improve overall. Aggregating across a series of case histories of projects can allow the inference about productive strategies to be made. In addition, a good documentary base can inform about dead-ends in substance as well as in developmental processes. Since most R & D reporting is based upon positive findings, it is difficult to avoid useless, but unreported paths.

This lack of documentation exists for a variety of reasons. First, the process of early design of technology is complex, iterative, and non-linear. All of us are familiar with documents of development which retrospectively rationalize and make "neat" processes that are chaotic, or at best, hard to track. Furthermore, the metacognitive awareness required of designers to document their own processes while at the same time working on problems of interest present an almost insurmountable attention burden, even if there were predisposition on the part of the research and development personnel to do so. Solving the problems at hand appears to be more important. Contributing to an abstraction such as "R & D processes" attracts less compelling energy, despite the intellectual apprehension that the field overall can be improved by a "lessons learned" perspective. Another inhibition is the precedence of proprietary knowledge, well known in the private sector, but of potentially increasing import in a public R & D environment characterized by competitive procurement policies.

In an attempt to meet this overall goal in instructional technology, some "case histories" were prepared 20 years ago (see D. G. Markle, 1967) and an historian was even on the payroll of another large R & D facility. But these persons can be pestering and diverting as media reporters, trying to get the idea of what's going on without true understanding of the processes involved. In new technology development, the problem is obviously exacerbated.

Fully participating formative evaluators provide another model, however, if they are linked early on in the development process and if the R & D management and staff understand the intent is to assist as well as to document process. How this can operate will be detailed in a later section of this paper.

The Information Must Use State-of-the-Art Evaluation Methodology, i.e., Both Quantitative and Qualitative Approaches

One of the reasons evaluation processes have been received with healthy skepticism is that they appear to be so content-free, on the one hand, and methodology-driven, on the other. The history of evaluation, as in any new mode of inquiry, is replete with "new" models that propound a particular

methodological view of the world. A good deal of the discredit done to
evaluation has occurred with the support and consent of its most famous
practitioners, who advocated one or another highly quantitative design and
analysis method as the preferred mode for solving all evaluation problems
(see Baker, 1983 for a list).

Obviously, analytical approach and evaluation design should be driven
by what information is required by whom by when, by the credibility needed
by the information analysts to do their job, and most importantly by the
nature of the project or activity under review (Cronbach, 1980). Such
precepts would suggest an eclectic approach, mixing journalistic,
documentary and effectiveness information as appropriate.

The Information Must Provide Policy Feedback to the Supporting Agencies

This feature assumes that the funding source is the contracting agency[1]
and that the formative evaluation is not a totally in-house activity. What
kinds of policy feedback are appropriate? That depends in part on the
nature of the formative evaluation team selected. Clearly, issues of
project management might be a necessary concern. However, it is more
likely that the substance to which the technology is directed, i.e.,
instruction, is a more useful area for feedback. At minimum, the formative
evaluators should attend to the fidelity of the process by the project to
the project's stated goals and procedures and to the kinds of contractual,
monitoring, and other oversight arrangements that might be useful in the
future. Furthermore, the evaluation report can consider specifically the
features or tasks that might be included in the specification of future
activities of the sort evaluated.

The tension of providing such information in a way that does not undo
either the project activities under study or the receptivity of future
projects to evaluation cannot be ignored. A fine line needs to be walked,
keeping track of both the professional ethics applicable to contracting
agency relationships (telling the truth) and to maintaining positive
connections to the target R & D communities.

The Information Must Provide Timely and Useful Alternatives for the Formative Evaluation of the Project(s) Under Study

This platitude takes serious effort to implement. It depends in no
small measure on being informed accurately and intimately with the state of
development of the project; and in the evaluation staff's sensitivity to
the form as well as the substance of findings that might be useful to the
project staff. This requirement also depends strongly on the level or
stage of development of the technology activity. Early on, certain
suggestions can be made and have potentially large effects. However, early
on, the evidentiary base of such recommendations is likely to be weak.
Later on, good evidence of project benefits and weaknesses can be more
fully drawn; however, modification of the technology may be considerably
less likely, may cost more, and so on.

The Information Must Provide Generalizations that can be Tested in the Design of Other Similar Technology-Based Efforts

Findings and recommendations must be cast in a way to make sense to the
project staff, with sensitivity to the needs, experience, and feasibility of
recommendations. But to be useful, particularly in the science policy
arena, these recommendations must address concerns of larger audiences:
other funders, other project designers, and the R & D community at large.
This means that recommendations must range across technical, management,

---

[1]see Figure 1, page 161

and effectiveness dimensions, and very well may break set with some of the project personnel's own point of view regarding technology policy.[2] Again, a tension between meeting the precept and maintaining friends in the community is obvious.

THE FORMATIVE EVALUATION OF ICAI

Background

The formative evaluation of ICAI projects was initiated with the intent to build instructional psychology into the design of ICAI efforts. This decision was apparently based upon the notion that ICAI had developed sufficient strength of underlying technology, tools and science so that attention could be turned to improving the effectiveness of the project(s) with research-based principles drawn from instruction. This approach was in no way intended to distract project staff from their various preoccupations with cognitive science, but rather to broaden, where appropriate, their knowledge and attention to instruction and performance assessment approaches. For instance, would the general fixation on guided discovery and student initiated instructional demands be explored? If so, what trade-offs in efficiency and effectiveness with exploratory behavior might result?

A first task, then was to decide on an overall evaluation plan. We decided that we wanted to look at multiple efforts. However, to avoid the specter of an implicit comparison (which project was best or worst?), we intended to select projects at different stages of development. We wanted a project that was just starting out, a project that was well under development, and a project that was in some state of maturity.

Project Selection

The process of project selection itself deserves a paper but briefly the criteria intended and the criteria enacted differed dramatically. Like the location in real estate, cooperation was the overriding standard for selection. We also were interested in a distribution of content for ICAI, different target student groups, and to some extent different ideology or approach. In the process of exploring projects for participation, we were: 1) asked why should any one agree to such an evaluation? 2) told that ICAI, although the announced target of the particular project, was not at all of interest, it was merely a mechanism to secure funding; and 3) that evaluating a project might be a good marketing device, thus participation was solicited (and rejected.) The actual sites for ICAI efforts chosen for evaluation in this project include:

1. A project at a profit-making firm

2. A project at a university

3. One of the "tried and true" ICAI efforts: WEST

Project One has a target population of maintenance technicians and is designed to assist in learning maintenance on complex xerographic equipment. Project Two has a target student group of freshman liberal arts students learning introductory PASCAL programming skills. Project Three is designed for upper elementary students and is intended to teach numerical concepts and some strategic level learning.

---

[2]see Figure 2, page 161

Project One

   The ICAI maintenance task was at an incipient stage during the start of the evaluation project. Project staff met both with R & D personnel and with those who, at another site, will be responsible for integrating ICAI in ongoing training environments. The incipience of the project was somewhat protracted. At best, it appeared possible to solicit information via structured interview, to track documentation, and to observe, from a relative distance, the ICAI design process. An essential goal of the design team was science. The training staff had shorter-term concern and were interested in the potential for the formative evaluation to create evaluation designs and criterion measures that would assist them in the evaluation of the training in this ICAI implementation and, by extension, to future support of other ICAI projects.

   One difficulty in meeting this goal was the approach to development employed, a common enough one, rapid prototyping. In the words of one expert, that ". . . is formative evaluation at its best: make, try it out, and fit it." On the other hand, how one knows the "it" works, other than "runs" is problematic. A bottom up process may foster the acceptance of whatever effects occur, rather than encouraging the design and revision of the ICAI to meet explicit performance specifications. Performance specifications here means those outcomes, learning, and proficiencies demonstrated by target students rather than the system.

   The decision on this project interacted with the fixed time limit for the evaluation (planned for one year.) Artful scheduling permitted a brief extension at no cost, but we do not anticipate having a ICAI implementation to test, make suggestions about, or even applaud before the end of the contract. Documentation and interviews were the fall-back strategy.

Project Two

   Our hopes for Project Two were high. The ICAI researcher met and conversed openly about the potential for the evaluation to assist in his goals for the project. We agreed on a design that would permit: 1) the specifications of dependent measures; 2) a test of the generalizability of the ICAI; 3) a set of replications, one in the university environment in which it was developed and another at UCLA, to test the exportability of the system.

   This project proceeded in amiable good cheer. But problems existed as well. First, the ICAI part of the project, a tutor, was still on the drawing board, although the researcher was open to consider how such a tutor might best be built. Nonetheless, what was available for evaluation was the analyzer of the PASCAL program rather than the tutor. That limitation may change in sufficient time for the evaluation team to make an assessment of the tutor function. Second, the set of specifications for criterion tasks stimulated a revision of the performance measure (on student programming ability) by the researchers, rather than the wholesale adoption of our recommendations. Nonetheless, progress is possible here too. Last, the off-site replication was replete with the inevitable surprise. UCLA UNIX environment and time-sharing procedures created system transfer problems. Thus, the 150 student subject pool shrank to less than 10% of that number because of loading times that ran from one half hour to three hours at peak use. (Students were not particularly interested in doing their homework at 3 a.m. at the computing facility.) However, comparative cross-site data will be generated, and recommendations for strengthened criterion measures and tutor characteristics will be made. As a side effect, a proposal for the design, analysis, and interpretation for instructional improvement of a relational database on student performance data, protocols, and individual difference measures was developed and is presently under review.

Project Three

We turned to WEST because at one level it is a known commodity. We developed criterion measures assessing both content (math) and strategic (game playing skills). We believed WEST permitted us to "play" at alternative instructional strategies and have planned variations where children will be experimentally divided into groups where they will engage with WEST under various experimental variations. Disabling the tutor is one focus: What does the AI add? Alternatives such as a job performance aid to model the information provided in the "coach" will be tested. We have also developed dependent measures that assess math performance in a broad way, and will also look at how well or what pieces of strategic thinking WEST produces. It is also our intent to look at individual difference predictors of outcome performance. This project was not without its problems as well. The WEST software was developed over time, patched and not well documented. Good assistance has been secured from the software developers to assist our staff's interest in modification to introduce experimental variations. But minor annoyances persist. Delivery dates for hardware were not met; the schedules for running 75 children as subjects, fixed during the start of the school year, needed constant modification, due to hardware delays. Thus, findings from this work are not available.

However, in WEST we have an opportunity to explore the instructional power of our ideas against a set of clear external performance criteria. We have as well the mixed blessing that WEST belongs to everyone, so that the threat of psychic investment is not a problem. Last, since no agency is looking at WEST as an instantiation of its own research policy, agency interest is less high, but still of sufficient level to make our efforts useful.

Other Tasks

One goal of the evaluation project was to use our findings from empirical work and documentation to permit the design of specifications for an AI instructional editor. This work is now less based on the linear flow of information from our project than the overall integration of ICAI experience from technical experts and the knowledge the evaluation team has about instruction and measurement options.

Recommendations

Our recommendations are of necessity highly tentative. It does appear that a focus on good dependent measurement is an area of real weakness in ICAI activity. We recommend that future activity be required to use measures that have content and psychometric validity.

In the instructional realm, it is clear that AI types may need to choose or at least agree to a more direct instructional approach for some of the goals of ICAI systems. The trade-off between developing the earth shattering perfect student model(s) vs. focusing the system on producing (not just tracking) learning must be directly considered.

In reviewing funding agency roles, three recommendations are imperative. First, the formative evaluation period for contracts must be undertaken with the knowledge that everything will take more time than it should, and that evaluation can not be done effectively when the "its" to be built reside in the heads of R & D personnel.

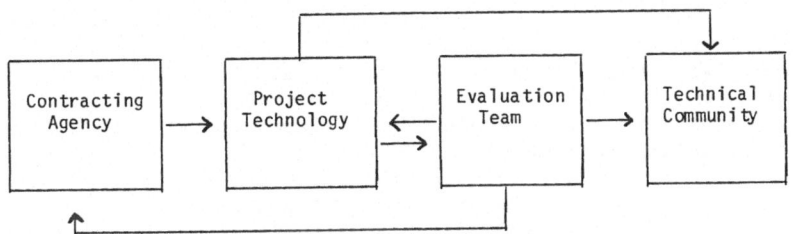

Figure 1. Model of Relationships for the Formative
Evaluation of New Technology

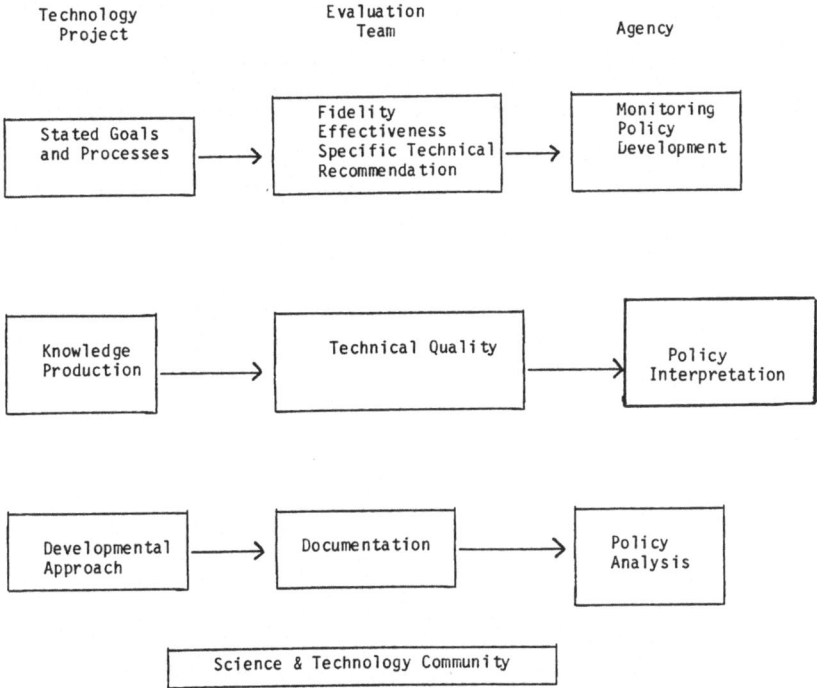

Figure 2. Evaluation Model Information Flow

Second, since cooperation and credibility turn out to be so important, agencies must be much more aggressive in insuring understanding and linkage between research project and evaluation personnel. Good will between groups is simply not sufficient to sustain the effort.

Third, agencies, must design their procurements such that they meet the intent of researchers (to expand science) and to provide support for attending to the effectiveness and efficiency of the ICAI project.

REFERENCES

Baker, E.L. & Alkin, M.C. (1973). Formative evaluation in instructional development. "AV Communication Review," "21(4)".

Baker, E.L. (1974). Formative evaluation of instruction. In J. Popham (Ed.), "Evaluation in education," McCutchan.

Baker, E.L. & Soloutos, W.A. (1974). "Formative evaluation of instruction." Los Angeles: UCLA Center for the Study of Evaluation.

Baker, E.L. (1983). "Evaluating educational quality: A rational design." Invited paper, Educational Policy and Management, University of Oregon.

Byrk, A. (Ed.) (1983). Stakeholder-based evaluation. "New Directions for Program Evaluation." Vol. 17. San Francisco: Jossey Bass.

Cronbach, L.S., et. al. (1980). "Toward reform of program evaluation." San Francisco: Jossey Base.

Markle, D.G. (1967). "An exercise in the application of empirical methods to instructional systems design." (Final report: The development of the Bell system first aid and personal safety course, American Institutes for Research, Palo Alto, CA.) New York: American Telephone and Telegraph Company.

Markle, S.M. (1967). Empirical testing of programs. In P.C. Lange (Ed.), "Programmed instruction." The Sixty-sixth Yearbook of the National Society for the Study of Education, Part II. Chicago: NSSE.

ONLINE HELP: DESIGN ISSUES FOR AUTHORING SYSTEMS[1]

T. M. Duffy and M. D. Langston

Carnegie-Mellon University
Pittsburgh, Pennsylvania, U.S.A.

INTRODUCTION

   Computer-based instruction (CBI) has been heralded as an educational panacea since the early applications of the 1950s. Many believed that computers would see widespread instructional use, presenting high quality educational materials with pacing and feedback geared to the individual student. In fact, CBI has not been so widely used. At first it seemed that the high cost of computer systems prevented users from investing in CBI. In recent years, however, hardware costs have dropped dramatically and microcomputers have invaded homes, schools, and businesses. Users are exploiting computer resources for database management, accounting, and word processing. But they are still not using the computer as an educational tool, except perhaps for general "computer literacy" instruction. In a recent survey of Texas Instruments and IBM microcomputer users, for example, not one person indicated that he or she used educational software (Duffy & Kelly, 1985). Publishers still consider educational software to be a high risk investment. Even in the American military, where much of the basic research on CBI has been conducted, computers seldom see active duty in the classroom.

   A major reason for CBI's limited success is that producing high quality materials is difficult and expensive. Developing dynamic, highly interactive instruction requires considerable programming skills as well as substantial instructional planning. The designer must understand not only instructional principles, but also the strengths and weaknesses of computerized delivery. He or she must integrate research on everything from screen displays to interface design in order to produce successful CBI. The combined programming and design effort adds significantly to production costs. Producing just one hour of high quality CBI demands 200 to 400 hours for TICCIT, 77 to 714 hours on PLATO, and 475 hours for the IBM 1500 Instructional System (Fletcher, 1984; Orlansky & String, 1979).

---

[1]Portions of this chapter were presented at the NATO Symposium on Computer-based Instruction in Military Environments, Brussels, Belgium, April, 1985.

Cost is only one problem for CBI development, however. Another is the need for many kinds of expertise in the design process. We have only recently begun to train enough instructional designers and to develop strategies for a coordinated team approach involving both the designer and the subject matter expert. Now, with CBI, still another kind of expertise is necessary: computer programming. Too often, in fact, programming takes the spotlight in CBI development and overshadows concern for the quality of instruction, including effective sequencing and presentation strategies (Merrill, 1983; Reigeluth & Stein, 1983). Typical CBI is an unimaginative collection of drill-and-practice exercises, often preceded by on-screen "pages" of textual instruction. While the programs presented in other chapters of this volume are innovative and exciting, they are certainly the exceptions, not the rule.

In the last few years, several authoring tools have appeared in an attempt to reduce production costs and return the focus of development to instructional design. A sampling of such tools is described in a recent issue of the Journal of Computer-based Instruction (1984, #3). These tools are generally high-level authoring languages which include special commands relevant to instructional programming--commands, for example, to create branches or check answers. Their main purpose is to facilitate the coding process; insofar as they are successful, they reduce the emphasis on programming and leave more time for attention to instructional principles.

However, simple aids to coding cannot, in themselves, promote more effective instructional design. To achieve that goal, an authoring system should be devised which aids the entire instructional design process as well as coding. The United States Department of Defense is engaged in developing such a system, one which would not only simplify the production process but also encourage the principled design of instruction.

The success of an authoring system--or any computer system, for that matter--depends largely upon two things: the system's capacities or power and the user's ability to exploit those capacities. Computer systems are becoming more powerful as a natural consequence of technological improvements. Users, however, are not faring so well. Fischer, Lemke, and Schwab (1985) report that according to their data, users only take advantage of about 40% of a complex system's capabilities. Users are often unable or unwilling to explore the full powers of a system because they cannot find the information that would enable them to do so, either in the printed documentation or as part of an online help system. Indeed, the inadequacies of computer documentation and its often adverse effects on system use are legendary.

Developers of authoring aids are beginning to recognize that making their tools easier to use is an important goal. Fairweather and O'Neal (1984) describe recent authoring tools and systems as not only very powerful but also ". . . menu driven, highly prompted, and completely helped," suggesting the new emphasis on usability. However, the help in these authoring tools is usually restricted, consisting of a page or so of help information on each command describing its format and function. In other words, it is typical of the help provided by most computer systems, perhaps best exemplified by the UNIX help facility (Norman, 1981).

In the remainder of this chapter, we review the research and present the issues involved in designing effective online help systems. Of necessity, the review and much of the discussion focus on broad considerations for help systems, issues that are relevant to any application software. At various points, however, we look specifically at what the research implies for authoring languages or systems.

Defining the Audience

The general goal of a help system, regardless of application, should be to provide the typical user with all the information he or she needs to efficiently operate the system. Furthermore, help should be available without disturbing or limiting the user's activities. The goal cited by Fenchel and Estrin (1982) seems especially appropriate: the optimal help system will allow any application with which the user interacts to describe itself.

Historically, the design of help systems has focused more on avoiding disruption than on providing complete information, mainly because until recently most users were highly trained computer specialists. Such users required only minimal help since they had broad experience and were surrounded by other highly trained users. If the help information was incomprehensible, a user could simply ask a colleague. Under these conditions, even the most inadequate help system is tolerable as long as it is unobtrusive. Draper (1984) found, for example, that the UNIX "man" and "key" system is easy to use for those with considerable UNIX experience.

However, thanks to the increased availability and affordability of computers, a growing number of users are just learning about computer systems. The problems of these "naive" or "novice" users have led to a more widespread interest in the role and the design of help systems. One response to the naive user group has been the development of online introductory tutorials such as Apple's "Apple Introduces Apple." Most such tutorials cover initial user activities. While they provide users with some hands-on experience, they seldom aid with anything beyond the basics. Therefore, they are not likely to assist users in exploring the system's full capabilities.

Today, most developers of help systems have the naive user in mind during the design process. However, another equally important and rapidly-growing user group has appeared: the computer sophisticated user who is naive only to the particular application program or the subject matter for which the software was designed (accounting in the case of spread sheets, for example). Whereas the novice user arose out of the general proliferation of computers, the "experienced novice" is a product of the proliferation of application software. An experienced novice is familiar with computers and with some software, and so has little need for the basic introductory tutorials. However, he or she needs more than the rudimentary command-level descriptions that might suffice for computer programmers. The experienced novice is not a programmer; he or she is interested in using computer resources to solve a particular problem in a discipline other than computer science. For example, the user of authoring software might be either a subject matter expert or an instructional designer who wishes to use the computer as a tool to produce educational materials.

The user of widely-varying application programs, whether a novice or an experienced novice, must have two kinds of information at hand. First, he or she must learn the specific functions and command structure of each piece of software. Second, as application programs become more sophisticated and offer more support for complex problem-solving in specialized areas, the user will have to understand the major strategies of problem representation and problem solving within each domain.

An adequate help system for a sophisticated application program must provide assistance with both kinds of information. For an authoring system, such help would include not only command level explanations, but guidance with strategies for more macro design tasks (designing the assessment, for instance, or linking presentation and practice) and help in understanding the instructional model underlying the system. That is, if the software is a tool to aid authoring, then the help must extend beyond the command level to authoring tasks and the instructional design model. The subject matter, not just the program itself, must become a factor in creating the help.

The changes in the user population and the software market raise new issues for the design of online help systems. After a brief survey of experimental help systems, we will examine several of these issues in the remainder of this chapter and conclude by presenting recent research findings which suggest that the design of the information contained in the help system is a critical concern.

Prototype Help Systems

While designers and computer companies are recognizing the importance of helping the user, and virtually every commercial program has some sort of help system, there is a paucity of research on the design of help systems. A number of individual researchers have done general surveys of the field (Houghton, 1984; Relles & Price, 1981; Relles, Sondheimer, & Ingargiola, 1981; Sondheimer & Relles, 1982) or have worked on relatively isolated aspects of help systems (Carroll & Kay, 1985; Fenchel & Estrin, 1982; Pollack, 1985; Rich, 1982; Shrager & Finin, 1982; Temin, 1982). Several sustained research efforts into basic human factors issues relevant to online help have come from Don Norman and the User Centered System Design Group at the University of California (Norman & Draper (Eds.), in press); Ben Shneiderman and his colleagues at the University of Maryland (Shneiderman, 1980, 1984); and Phil Hayes and the COUSIN interface group at Carnegie-Mellon University (Ball & Hayes, 1980; Glasner & Hayes, 1981; Hayes, 1982).

Much of the research to date has been concerned with the development of experimental prototypes. Specifically, many of the development efforts have been channelled into the following nine prototype help systems:

1. A Help System for the SIGMA Message System. Designed by Rothenberg (1975, 1979) at USC, this is perhaps the most complete and most sophisticated help system proposal, providing dynamic access to the help data base, help based on a user profile and linked to the command line interpreter, both interactive and textual tutorials, and integrated on and offline help.

2. Thumb. Thumb is a system for locating materials within texts such as online manuals. Developed by Price (1982), Thumb creates a "passage tree" or functional outline of an online document, allowing the user to locate and retrieve only those passages relevant to his or her needs. Thumb aids the user by providing extensive cross-referencing and access tools. Prototypes implemented at NASA and BNR.

3. A Help System for SARA. This system is a software engineering tool. Developed by Fenchel and Estrin (1982), the system provides pointers to the help database according to command line input, responds to syntactic errors, provides further detail on request, and simplifies the entry of help information by the programmer of a new application.

4. A Help System for Consul. Consul is an experimental message system. Developed by Mark (1982) at USC, this system is model-driven, responding to help requests by consulting online

models of user behavior and system capacity, and mapping between the models. It accepts natural language input and responds with assistance to any system command that cannot be executed. It provides a system acquisition aid to assist programmers in providing help information on each new application.

5. A Help System for the COUSIN Interface. Developed by Hayes (1982) at Carnegie-Mellon University, this system is based on the ZOG menu system, providing static and dynamic help generated from online descriptions of each tool documented, which are provided by the tool designers.

6. DOCUMENT. DOCUMENT is an online documentation system to support the full spectrum of programs available through the National Magnetic Fusion Energy Computer Center. Developed by Girill and Luk (1983), this system is noted for the sophisticated methods of accessing the help data base. The DOCUMENT system allows full integration of on and offline materials, contains an acquisition aid for documenters to insure consistency across help texts, responds to omitted parts of a command line with appropriate options, and varies the level of presentation according to user profile information.

7. An Experimental Help System for UNIX Print Commands. This system was developed by the UCSD group at the University of California (Smolensky, Monty, & Conway, 1984). They have examined the use of a quick-reference facility based on a task-oriented documentation format with this system.

8. The Document Examiner. The Document Examiner is an online reference manual. Developed by Walker (1985), the Document Examiner includes dynamic cross referencing, a system of "bookmarks" to help users return easily to previously-examined sections of the document, an advanced screen display strategy using three windows, and complete integration of online and offline documentation.

9. An Experimental Help System for UNIX Directory and File Commands. This system was developed by Borenstein (1985) at Carnegie-Mellon University. Borenstein's three-window display includes a separate help menu window that is constantly updated in response to the user's activities and a text window which allows the user to view the help information without sacrificing his or her current context (an incomplete command line, for example).

Unfortunately, few of these prototypes or their design features have been formally evaluated. Therefore, while the developers' conceptions of effective help have been embodied, we have little evidence of how effective or valid the underlying concepts are. The primary focus has been building the prototypes based on a best guess about proper responses to the major issues. These issues or factors are:

1. The degree to which the help is dynamic or based on an analysis of the context

2. The mechanism for accessing help

3. The structure of the database

4. The amount and kind of information presented to the user

Before considering these factors, we note that despite the general lack of empirical evaluation, the prototypes reflect an encouraging consensus about the minimal components of an optimal help system. Designers seem to agree that every help system should contain features reflecting five basic capabilities:

1. Static Help. This is the basic query-driven help. The user requests help via a command or menu and receives the appropriate textual information.

2. Dynamic Help. This is context-sensitive help. The user encounters a problem or is uncertain how to complete an activity, and receives information based on the current state of his or her interaction with the system.

3. Tutorials. Tutorials are for new users of an application. Many current online tutorials are simply textual explanations of the facilities, though there is a growing interest in interactive tutorials.

4. Error Handling: Error handling is automatic calls to the help system on the presence of an error condition or the detection of inefficient user operations, such as using several commands where one would suffice.

5. Integration of Online and Offline Documentation. This is the ability to use the help files to produce the offline manual, enabling the writer to update both at once.

FACTORS IN THE DESIGN OF HELP

Dynamism

The "dynamism" of a help system is the degree to which it can assess and respond to the user's needs of the moment. Dynamism, sometimes referred to as "context-sensitivity," is a continuum along which help systems can range. At the simplest level is the traditional, static help system in which the user must fully specify the help topic through a query or menu selection. At the other end of the continuum is an intelligent system which possesses both a model of the user and an expert model, and can fully diagnose the user's problem. Between these extremes are systems in which help is presented to the user based on the system's analysis of various features: the current command line, the prior command sequence, or a profile of the user's prior experience (see Rothenberg, 1979 and Mark, 1982).

The kind of online assistance most widely available is the lower end of the continuum or static help, which in its most primitive form is simply an online manual accessible by keywords or menus. Static help is particularly useful for users who want to expand their knowledge of the system or are looking for information on a specific command, and is generally considered the minimum for an online help system. Its major weakness is its inability to offer assistance directly related to the present state of the user's activity. The user must already know what help he or she needs or engage in a trial-and-error process to find out.

A second weakness is that the system cannot select in advance the category of help information needed--examples, say, or command syntax--or offer alternative strategies. The system does not "know" what the user is doing and hence will usually provide an information dump on one command along with pointers to the most closely related commands. These two weaknesses are, of course, the classic problems with the UNIX help system.

Reliance on static help alone will be inadequate for an authoring system to be used by both subject matter experts and instructional technologists. We cannot assume that either group will be familiar with the particular instructional model and strategies for design that the system embodies, so the static help should be augmented by some form of dynamic help. Dynamic help occurs when at least some portion of the current context is used to guide the help response. It attempts to provide the information most likely to aid the user at the moment, together with pointers to further information. Dynamic help can be provided from the same database as the static help. However, the ideal system will reconfigure the presentation of help information, particularly the help categories and the degree of explanation, according to its analysis of the user's needs.

As we move along the continuum toward more dynamic help, we engage in a tradeoff between the inferencing supplied by the user and that supplied by the help system. Dynamic help at any level is based on some amount of inferencing about what the user wants to do and because of that will be subject to errors of inference. Help based on a mistaken inference can be as bad as no help at all. The user must spend valuable time trying to escape from unwanted or inappropriate help before he or she can locate the needed help. The likelihood of inferential errors increases as we attempt to make the system more intelligent.

Many designers agree that the minimal amount of dynamic help would allow the user to engage the help system at any point in the interactive dialogue and receive a brief explanation of his or her options at that point (Relles & Price, 1981; Relles et al., 1981; Wasserman, 1981). At least this kind of dynamic help should be available for an authoring aid. Such a capacity requires that the help system be supplied with system state information and some record of a user's command history.

While assistance with the user's next possible commands seems a feasible level of help for an authoring system, moving any further toward the AI end of the continuum seems unwarranted except for experimental purposes. We do not know enough about the instructional design process to provide the system with an adequate basis for effective inferencing. The development of an intelligent system would require both an expert model and a model of the user. The system must be able not only to detect errors or suboptimal strategies (that is, deviations from the expert model), but also to infer the faulty reasoning that led to the error by consulting a user model in order to supply the appropriate help.

At the present time, we simply do not have a user model, or even data which could be used to generate one. We could not locate any data on what we consider to be two critical, minimal components of a user model: 1) assessing and contrasting the goals and strategies of the two primary user groups (subject matter experts and instructional technologists) and 2) evaluating expert and novice behavior in each group.

<u>Access</u>

Current help systems use three basic mechanisms for accessing help information. First, the help options may always be visible on the screen. For static help this would be a menu based system best characterized by ZOG and COUSIN (see Hayes, 1982). For dynamic help systems, the help would also be in a menu display but available in a separate window and constantly updated in response to the user's choice of commands. The WordStar help menu is perhaps the best available example of this dynamic, visible help (<u>WordStar Reference Manual,</u> 1983). In general, designers assume that this visible presentation of help options is best for novice users. When a novice is first using WordStar, for example, he or she can always have available the list of next possible commands. Then, as expertise develops, he or she can hide the help selections and make more of the workspace available for composing.

The second means of accessing help is through a query system. In this case, help options are not presented on the screen; rather, the user must request help explicitly. For static help systems, the user must request information on a specific command as in the UNIX "key" and "man" systems. For dynamic help, the user simply requests that the help options be presented. The same information constantly available in the "visible" help system is available only on request. Such a "hidden" menu system is exemplified by the TOPS-20 system used at CMU (Bond, Hayes, Janik, & Swaney (Eds.), 1982).

Finally, the system may present help when it infers that the user needs assistance, usually by recognizing that a system error has occurred. Error handling by online help systems requires, at a minimum, that a trigger to the help system be attached to the machine state or the command interpreter, so that the presence of an error condition or a command which cannot be executed generates a call to the help system. Both Rothenberg's (1975) Tutor and Fenchel's help system for SARA (Fenchel and Estrin, 1982) propose such a mechanism. Ideally, the system would also contain a history of the user's activities so that it can determine how much help the user probably needs. Rothenberg's system also contains such a user profile.

The availability of powerful multi-window computing environments with varying access devices (icons, mice, etc.) makes the issue of user access mechanisms much more complex than a simple three-alternative, keyword-menu-automatic choice. To our knowledge, no research has been done exploring the implications of these new technologies for user access. Indeed, only Rothenberg (1979), Borenstein (1985) and Walker (1985) have employed advanced displays and windows, but none reports any testing of alternative access or display strategies based on the technology.

INFORMATION REQUIREMENTS

Level of Explanation

Most help systems, regardless of design, only provide help with individual commands, usually in the form of an online reference manual. While this may be adequate for operating systems, where the application goals vary widely, it appears completely inadequate for targeted application programs. Authoring languages, for example, are meant to aid users in creating dynamic and highly interactive instruction. Yet typical help systems would not provide assistance in integrating a series of commands to accomplish that goal. The help is on individual commands, not on strategies for using the commands in a larger context. As we mentioned earlier, even if an authoring language advertises the availability of menu-driven help systems, the commands on the menus tend to be at the micro editing level and the author is left to his or her own devices to determine strategies for moving through these commands.

We have argued that the help system must provide at least three "levels of explanation" in an authoring system or other sophisticated application program. The lowest level is help with individual commands, which is almost always organized by the command structure, including the format and options. O'Malley et al. (1983) have proposed that even at the command level, the help information might be made more responsive to the user's needs by organizing it around tasks the user performs (his or her goals) rather than the command set.

In fact, the UCSC group (Smolensky, Monty & Conway, 1984) has embodied a task-oriented approach in a command level help system for the UNIX print commands (printing tasks). Their "task attributes" include such categories as printing method, formatting, and portion of files printed. They recommend the development of an "attribute encyclopedia", which brings together under task-oriented headings all the information relevant to one aspect of a task (formatting, for example). Their task-oriented help is based largely on reorganizing and reformatting the command descriptions. For example, rather than listing the options for a command alphabetically, the task-oriented information lists the options by their functions. To our knowledge, the UCSD group has not tested this task-oriented format against a command-oriented format.

At the next level, the help must set the command into the context of the application's larger framework. In the case of an authoring system, the user is employing the individual command as part of the larger goal of creating a component of instruction. The help should relate the command to the design of the component. Such help might include, for example, strategies or examples of how to create different assessments, practice presentations, feedback, or animated segments (assuming, as seems reasonable, that completing each of these tasks will require a lengthy command sequence).

The third level of help information would assist the user in the instructional design process. Any system that aids instructional design will embody some model of the instructional design process and "good" instructional techniques. In an authoring language or system, the model will be reflected in the macro commands available (and not available), the ease of linking components of instruction (for instance, presentation, practice, and assessment), and the contingencies between the components and the overall instruction (that is, front end analysis, objectives, delivery, and assessment). The help system would simply make the model explicit, providing "system overview information" and instruction design advice. The model would show the relationships between the user's current task domain and other tasks or data bases in the authoring system. In a dynamic state, this overview information would also provide the author with a summary and an evaluation (relative to the model) of the instruction developed to that point.

Extensive evidence in the cognitive science and problem solving literature suggests that an individual's strategies for using a system are guided by an internalized model of that system. His or her effectiveness in problem solving will be largely dependent on how accurately that "mental" model corresponds to the actual workings of the system. Rumelhart and Norman (1981) have demonstrated the importance of such a functional model in the use of the UNIX screen editor. In one condition, they provided subjects with the reference information on the editor commands and examples of the application. Subjects in a second condition received the same information along with a description of how the text editor worked--that is, a model of the system. Subjects in the latter condition were significantly more successful in carrying out editing tasks.

Amount of Information Presented

One of the worst problems for users of static help systems is the deluge of information they often receive when they ask for help. The system usually provides a large text containing much information that is irrelevant to the user's current needs. The user must scan through the text to find the target information, often a lengthy and frustrating process. Two solutions have been proposed to this problem: controlling the level of detail presented and controlling the kind or category of information presented.

Level of Detail

When the user wants only to check the syntax or options for a command, presenting an abbreviated form of the help information seems appropriate. O'Malley et. al. (1983) at UCSD suggest that for these situations, two kinds of static help be available:

1. Full explanation, which for any entry contains all the information presently available in the online manual

2. Quick reference, which contains in each entry the correct syntax for the command, the options which may be supplied with it, and a brief explanation of its use

The quick reference facility would also contain pointers to the full entries on relevant topics. Bannon and O'Malley (1984) evaluated a quick reference facility on the UNIX system in their University of California research lab, finding that users liked it and made fewer calls to "man" for full explanations after the quick reference facility was implemented.

Categories of Information

An alternative strategy is to present only a particular kind of information on a command or task. That is, a help entry might contain many categories of information (command format, option definition, applications, cross references, examples, bugs, and others). Rather than providing a condensed version of all this information, we could allow the user to select the categories he or she needs, or have the system infer the appropriate categories. If the user only needs to understand the command format, for example, he or she could receive only that information.

One way to implement the control of information categories is to organize the help data base on a "hypertext" model (Nelson, 1974). Hypertext-oriented data bases consist of small, richly-interconnected pieces of information which can be accessed and combined in a variety of ways. The pieces of a help text (syntax summary, options, examples, others) can be stored as separate data base items and accessed either individually or by a routine that formats them into a reference manual entry. The COUSIN help system (Hayes, 1982) uses such an organization, as does the prototype system developed by Borenstein (1985). Such a data base facilitates cross-referencing while improving the likelihood that a particular help request will yield only the information required.

Tutorials

While help systems present many different categories of help information to a user, few systems provide what might be considered a critical help -- tutorials. Tutorials differ from other help categories because they involve interaction with the user. The user actually works through a problem or example using the computer. The ideal tutorial system would in fact allow the subject to use a real-world problem as the basis for the tutorial. Alternatively, the user could complete the tutorial in one window while he or she works on ongoing activities in another window.

Tutorials seldom appear in help systems, most likely because the best tutorials require interactive programs. A few interactive tutorials are available which introduce particular systems or software, such as "Apple Introduces Apple" and the Lotus 1-2-3 tutorials (Posner, Hill, Miller, Gottheil, & Davis, 1983). While these products, as well as the tutorials found in most hard copy documentations, make clear the importance of tutorials, we have been able to identify only one experimental help system that included interactive tutorial assistance, the proposed Tutor module for the SIGMA message system (Rothenberg, 1975; 1979). We present a brief summary of its proposed features to suggest the directions that future development in interactive tutorials might take.

In Rothenberg's Tutor module, the online tutorials would perform three functions: 1) introducing new users to the operation of the system; 2) allowing users to expand their knowledge of system capabilities; and 3) intervening with assistance when the user seems to be attempting something he or she does not yet know how to do. The module was designed to combine textual with interactive tutorials. The user would read about the system briefly and do exercises with it, able to "try" certain procedures within a special protected environment which prevents the sending of practice messages and the alteration of data. Commands issued within the protected environment would be executed as far as possible without damage to data or the system state; the consequences of the commands beyond that point would be simulated. The Tutor module would also provide an authoring language for creating interactive lessons.

AN EVALUATION OF A HELP SYSTEM

Most of the work in designing help systems has focused on the issues of dynamism and access, while few have attended to the quality of the information presented. Providing increasingly dynamic help is a movement toward an intelligent system and many system designers, especially programmers, are interested in that goal. The access issue is nicely circumscribed and therefore readily amenable to human factors analysis. The quality of the information, by contrast, is difficult to assess and is not explicitly a computing variable, which may account for the sparse attention paid to it. However, a dissertation recently completed by Nathaniel Borenstein at Carnegie-Mellon University provides data suggesting that the quality of the information may be the critical variable in the design of a help system.

Borenstein (1985) designed a prototype help system called ACRONYM for the UNIX operating system. We will not consider the details of the data base structure and access mechanisms here, but will focus on the human-computer interface which was a primary concern of Borenstein's evaluation. For the prototype system the screen was divided into three parts. The command line window was in the bottom portion of the screen; a menu of help options appeared in the middle of the screen; and a brief help text could be presented in the top part of the screen. Of the different experimental conditions described below, only ACRONYM contained the multi-window display.

Two help access conditions appeared in the evaluation. In the first, a context-sensitive condition, the command line was parsed and the menu and text displays were modified to reflect the options available to the user at a given point in the command sequence. For example, if the user typed "rm", the options and arguments for "rm" would be displayed in the top part of the screen and a menu of further information would appear in the middle portion, including "examples," "options," "delete a directory, rmdir," and "what is a file." In this condition, the user could also request help for a particular command by using "man" or "key" in the bottom command line. The second help condition was the traditional UNIX static help system. That is, the user could only receive help by requesting it via "man" or "key".

A second variable was the help text presented to the user. In one condition the text was the standard UNIX "man" text in which commands are described in terms of the name, format, description, cross references, bugs, and relevant system files. The function, options, and any examples of the command are all presented in the description section. The alternative text condition was basically the UNIX help information presented in Sobell's (1984) A Practical Guide to the UNIX System. The alternative help text, then, was not idealized nor was it customized for this particular study. However, it was in general more clearly written than the "man" text and was divided into more even and more functional chunks of information. For example, the command summary, options and examples each appeared in a separate section. In contrast to the standard UNIX manual entries, there was always an example. Information beyond the basic description was presented in a separate "additional notes" category.

Borenstein combined these two variables to create three experimental conditions: standard UNIX (static help and UNIX documentation); simplified text (static help and the Sobell text); and ACRONYM (both static and dynamic help, the Sobell test, and the three-window display). A fourth condition was meant to set the standard for the maximally effective help: a human tutor condition in which subjects could ask the tutor any question, but the tutor could not use prior knowledge of the tasks to respond.

All of the subjects were experienced computer users; however, one group was experienced with UNIX while the other was not. The subjects were given 12 tasks to complete using the standard UNIX help system and 12 tasks to complete using one of the three experimental help systems. Experienced and inexperienced users received different tasks reflecting their different levels of expertise.

The average time per task for experts and for novices is presented in Table 1. When entered into a regression analysis to remove task and subject variability, the data for experts and novices supports essentially the same conclusions. The simplified text made up about half the difference between the standard UNIX help and a human tutor. The provision of dynamic help, with its menus and command summaries, did not seem to aid performance over and above the simplified text. There was no performance difference between the simplified text and the ACRONYM conditions for either the experts or novices, though subjects did show an affective preference for the ACRONYM condition, perhaps because the display allowed them to continue working while help information appeared in a separate window.

Table 1. Mean Normalized Time (Sec.) to Complete a Task
(from Borenstein, 1985)
(The experts and novices received different tasks.)

	EXPERT	NOVICE
STANDARD UNIX	168	167
SIMPLIFIED TEXT	116	115
ACRONYM	139	103
HUMAN TUTOR	103	60

Borenstein's results indicate that the quality of the help text is far more important than the mechanism by which the help text is accessed, and this conclusion holds for both experts and novices. The data do not indicate the nature of the "quality" variable that led to the significant effects. However, the effects apparently are not due to simple readability. Borenstein found the readability of both Sobell (1984) and "man" texts to be at approximately the 10th grade level according to several standard readability formulas. More likely "quality" variables are the action-oriented style of writing; the use of meaningful headings and the more even chunking of information; and the more performance-oriented contents of the information presented.

SUMMARY

Throughout this chapter we have emphasized the importance of a multi-level help system that goes beyond simple command descriptions to include assistance with goals and strategies within the application domain--in this case, automated authoring. The help system should be dynamic in at least some degree, basing its presentation of help options on the user's current activity. We would also suggest that an adequate help system would include a mechanism for controlling the amount of information presented on a help request and an interactive facility to allow users to try out different features in a procedural fashion. Finally, the textual information contained in the help data base must be carefully designed and structured to make the necessary assistance both accessible and understandable for maximum user efficiency.

REFERENCES

Ball, E. & Hayes, P. (1980). Representation of task-specific knowledge in a gracefully interacting user interface. "Proceedings of the First Annual National Conference on Artificial Intelligence" (pp. 116-120). Palo Alto, CA: Stanford University.

Bannon, L.J., & O'Malley, C. (1984, March). Problems in evaluation of human-computer interfaces: A case study. "User centered system design: Part II, collected papers from the UCSD HMI project" (LaJolla, CA) (ICS Report No. 8402, pp. 67-73). San Diego: University of California, Institute for Human Information Processing.

Bond, S.J., Hayes, J.R., Janik, C.J., & Swaney, J.H. (Eds) (1982, August). "Introduction to CMU TOPS-20." Pittsburgh, PA: Carnegie-Mellon University, Communications Design Center.

Borenstein, N.S. (1985). "The design and evaluation of online help systems." Ph.D. thesis, Carnegie-Mellon University, Pittsburgh.

Carroll, J.M., & Kay, D.S. (1985, April). Prompting, feedback and error correction in the design of a scenario machine. "Proceedings of the Computer-Human Interaction 1985 Conference on Human Factors in Computing Systems" (San Francisco) (pp. 149-153). New York: The Association on Computing Machinery.

Draper, S. (1984, March). The nature of expertise in UNIX. "User centered system design: Part II, collected papers from the UCSD HMI Project" (La Jolla, CA) (ICS Report No. 8402, pp. 19-27). San Diego: University of California, Institute for Human Information Processing.

Duffy, T.M., & Kelly, P. (1985, June). "An analysis of the use of the Texas Instruments, Inc. professional microcomputer." Pittsburgh, PA: Carnegie-Mellon University, Communications Design Center.

Fairweather, P.G., & O'Neal, A.F. (1984). The impact of advanced authoring systems on CAI productivity. "Journal of Computer-based Instruction," "11," 90-94.

Fenchel, R.S., & Estrin, G. (1982, March/April). Self-describing systems using integral help. "Institute of Electrical and Electronic Engineers Transactions on Systems, Man and Cybernetics," "smc-12(2)," 162-167.

Fischer, G., Lemke, A., & Schwab, T. (1985, April). Knowledge based help systems. "Proceedings of the Computer-Human Interaction 1985 Conference on Human Factors in Computing Systems" (San Francisco) (pp. 161-167). New York: The Association on Computing Machinery.

Fletcher, J.D. (1984). Intelligent instructional systems in training. In S.A. Andriole (Ed.), "Applications in artificial intelligence." Princeton, N.J.: Petrocelli Books, Inc.

Girill, T.R., & Luk, C.H. (1983, May). Document: An interactive, online solution to four documentation problems. "Communications of the ACM," "26(5)," 328-227.

Glasner, I.D., & Hayes, P.J. (1981, November). "Automatic construction of explanation networks for a cooperative user interface" (Technical Report CMU-CS-81-146). Pittsburgh, PA: Carnegie-Mellon University, Department of Computer Science.

Hayes, P.J. (1982). Uniform help facilities for a cooperative user interface. "American Federation of Information Processing Society Proceedings of the National Computer Conference" (pp. 469-474). Montvale, NJ: AFIPS Press.

Houghton, R.C. (1984, February). Online help systems: A conspectus. "Communications of the ACM," "37(2)," 126-133.

Mark, W. (1982). Natural-language help in the consul system. In "American Federation of Information Processing Society Proceedings of the National Computer Conference" (pp. 475-479). Montvale, NJ: AFIPS Press.

Merrill, D. (1983). Component display theory. In C. Reigeluth (Ed.), "Instructional design theories and models: An overview of their current status." Hillsdale, NJ: Lawrence Erlbaum and Associates.

Nelson, T.H. (1974). "Dream machines." South Bend, IN: The Distributor.

Norman, D.A. (1981, November). The Trouble with UNIX. "Datamation," "27(12)," 139-150.

Norman, D.A., & Draper, S.W. (Eds.). (in press). "User-centered system design: New perspectives in human-machine interaction." Hillsdale, NJ: Lawrence Erlbaum and Associates.

O'Malley, C., Smolensky, P., Bannon, L., Conway, E., Graham, J., Sokolov, J., & Monty, M.L. (1983, December). A proposal for user centered system documentation. "Proceedings of the Computer-Human Interaction 1983 Conference on Human Factors in Computing Systems" (Boston) (pp. 5-8). New York: The Association on Computing Machinery.

Orlansky, J., & String, J. (1979). "Cost effectiveness of computer-based instruction in military training" (IDA paper P-1375). Arlington, VA: Institute for Defense Analysis.

Pollack, M.E. (1985, April). Information sought and information provided: An empirical study of user/expert dialogues. In "Proceedings of the Computer-Human Interaction 1985 Conference on Human Factors in Computing Systems" (San Francisco) (pp. 155-159). New York: The Association on Computing Machinery.

Posner, J., Hill, J., Miller, S.E., Gottheil. E., & Davis, M.L. (1983). "Lotus 1-2-3 user's manual" (Computer program manual). Cambridge, MA: Lotus Development Corporation.

Price, L.A. (1982, March/April). Thumb: An interactive tool for accessing and maintaining text. "Institute of Electrical and Electronic Engineers Transactions on Systems, Man and Cybernetics," "smc-12(2)," 155-161.

Reigeluth, C., & Stein, F. (1983). The elaboration theory of instruction. In C. Reigeluth (Ed.), "Instructional design theories and models: An overview of their current status" (pp. 335-379). Hillsdale, NJ: Lawrence Erlbaum and Associates.

Relles, N., & Price, L. (1981, March). A user interface for online assistance. "Proceedings of the Fifth International Conference on Software Engineering" (pp. 400-408). New York: Institute of Electrical and Electronic Engineers.

Relles, N., Sondheimer, N.K., & Ingargiola, G. (1981). A unified approach to online assistance. "American Federation of Information Processing Society Proceedings of the National Computer Conference" (pp. 383-387). Montvale, NJ: AFIPS Press.

Rich, E. (1982). Programs as data for their help systems. "AFIPS Proceedings of the National Computer Conference" (pp. 481-485). Montvale, NJ: AFIPS Press.

Rothenberg, J. (1975, May). "An intelligent tutor: online documentation and help for a military message service" (Technical Report ISI/RR-74-26). USC-Information Sciences Institute.

Rothenberg, J. (1979). Online tutorials and documentation for the SIGMA Message Service. "American Federation of Information Processing Society Proceedings of the National Computer Conference" (pp. 863-867). Montvale, NJ: AFIPS Press.

Rumelhart, D.E., & Norman, D. (1981). Analogical processes in learning. In J. Anderson (Ed.), "Cognitive skills." Hillsdale, NJ: Lawrence Erlbaum Associations.

Shneiderman, B. (1980). "Software psychology: Human factors in computer and information systems." Cambridge, MA: Winthrop Publishers.

Shneiderman, B. (1984, September). "Human factors issues of manuals, online help, and tutorials" (Technical Report CS-TR-1446). College Park: University of Maryland, Department of Computer Science.

Shrager, J. & Finin, T. (1982). "An expert system that volunteers advice" (American Association for Artificial Intelligence-82, pp. 339-340).

Smolensky, P., Monty, M.L., & Conway, E. (1984, March). Formalizing task descriptions for command specification and documentation. "User centered system design: Part II, collected papers from the CSD HMI project" (La Jolla, CA) (ICS Report No. 8402, pp. 51-63). San Diego: University of California, Institute for Human Information Processing.

Sobell, M. (1984). "A practical guide to the UNIX system." Menlo Park, CA: The Benjamin/Cummings Publishing Company.

Sondheimer, N., & Relles, N. (1982, March/April). Human Factors and user assistance in interactive computing systems: An introduction. "Institute of Electrical and Electronic Engineers Transactions on Systems, Man and Cybernetics," "smc-12(2)," 102-107.

Temin, A.L. (1982). "The question-answering module in an automated natural language help system for the text-formatter scribe." Thesis proposal, University of Texas at Austin.

Walker, J. (1985, April). Implementing documentation and help online. (Tutorial conducted at the Conference on Human Factors in Computing Systems). San Francisco, CA.

Wasserman, A. (1981). User software engineering and the design of interactive systems. "American Federation of Information Processing Society Proceedings of the National Computer Conference" (pp. 387-393). Montvale, NJ: AFIPS Press.

"WordStar reference manual" (Computer program manual) (1983). San Rafael, CA: MicroPro International Corporation (Release 3.3).

A USER-MAINTAINED DATABASE FOR TRAINERS IN MILITARY ENVIRONMENTS

A. Meyers

University of Alberta
Edmonton, Alberta, Canada

TRAINERS DATABASE PROJECT

The increasing rapidity with which our technology is changing is putting pressure on trainers to develop programs to provide the personnel who will handle this technology. Instructional materials rapidly become obsolete as changing technologies demand new software.

To keep pace with these changes an inexpensive, comprehensive, database is needed to provide up-to-the-minute information on training information, materials, and personnel. Such information is especially useful where a training course is to be set up on short notice and where technical experts, rather than trainers, are to teach the course.

In October, 1982 an article was published in the Training and Development Journal describing a project underway at the Department of Industrial and Vocational Education of the University of Alberta in Canada to develop a computer-based data collection system for trainers in business, industry, and government, and inviting interested organization to participate in its development and testing.

Over 80 organizations in North America responded to the invitation including a number of military organizations in Canada and the United States. Additional inquiries were received from Europe, Asia, and Africa.

The project involves creating a database of databases about training to which data can be added, removed, updated, and searched by users who know almost nothing about computers. Further, the data can be transmitted to the database over the telephone via DATAPAC/TELENET/TYMNET networks from a terminal or microcomputer located in the user's own home anywhere in North America (or the world, where other networks can be accessed). To avoid chaos, any user may add data or search the database, but modification of the contents is restricted to the person who entered them.

TELIDON Capability

The feasibility of storing and retrieving Teletex data (e.g., TELIDON graphics) is assumed since they are transmitted as ASCII characters acceptable to the database. Investigation of this capability will be undertaken when funds become available.

Project Status

The present status of the project is that the database works well and needs mostly to be filled with information to be fully operational.

PURPOSES OF THE DATABASE

The purposes of the databases are:

- To serve as a clearinghouse for information on training trainers

- To make more effective use of training funds by incorporating user experiences in judging the appropriateness of personnel, materials, meetings, and courses for an organization's needs

- To serve as a means for users to confer individually or in conference as a special interest group

- To provide immediate access to safety procedures during actual emergency situations

DESCRIPTION OF THE DATABASE

The Trainers Database consists of series of databases housed in a host computer (an Amdahl 5860 operating under the Michigan Terminal System [MTS]) located at the University of Alberta. The Database Management System (DBMS) is SPIRES, developed at Stanford University to handle very large databases and originally designed to maintain their library collection (over 5,000,000 volumes).

The databases that make up the Trainers Database include:

- ARTICLES Database - a description of articles on training put out by in-house organs that due to their limited audience are not usually contained in standard indexes to periodical literature.

- BOOKS Database - a list of books useful to trainers. To avoid a redundant list of thousands of items, large collections of materials, such as the catalog of the National Information Center for Educational Media (NICEM), would be listed here rather than having its contents listed in the MATERIALS Database. User-evaluations of the catalog's contents, however, would be entered in the EVALUATION Database.

- CHEMICALS Database - a description of emergency procedures to be used in the event of chemical spills.

- COURSES Database - a description of training courses offered by business, industry, and government.

- DIRECTORY Database - a list of names, addresses, and fields of interest of training personnel and organizations.

- EVALUATION Database - user-supplied evaluations of the courses, materials, meetings, etc., described in the Trainers Database.

- MATERIALS Database - description and availability of training materials.

- MEETINGS Database - a global list of upcoming meetings of interest to trainers.

- USERS Database - a directory of the IDs of users of the Trainers Database listed by their fields of interest (to provide anonymity).

    Anonymity of Users - anonymity was implemented at user's request for two reasons:

    (1) To prevent the names of the users being placed on mailing lists without their permission.

    (2) To encourage the free exchange of ideas during database conferences of special interest groups. It was felt that unclear ideas (useful in brainstorming sessions) are less likely to be expressed when one's superior might be a participant and aware of the source.

    Although the user is free to identify oneself, the practice has prevailed of not doing so. The database is a means of conducting business and users have found that anonymity tends to keep conversations business-like.

In addition to the databases above, search access (only) is available to the ERIC Databases issued by the United States Department of Education: Current Index to Journals in Education (CIJE) and Resources in Education (RIE).

APPLICABILITY OF THE DATABASE FOR MILITARY USE

This Symposium notes that "In a future military environment of (1) fewer persons to select from, (2) potentially lower entry skills, and (3) a sophisticated weapons environment," Computer-Based Instruction (CBI) offers the promise of "a cost-effective way of individualizing instruction."

Accepting that "although military hardware is reducing in cost, courseware costs are assumed to be increasing," Instructional Resource Sharing has been suggested as an approach to reducing courseware costs.

The Trainers Database shows promise as a cost-effective means of sharing resources. User-friendly software, for example, permits clerical personnel rather than more expensive computer-support personnel to perform data entry operations.

Additional cost savings through improved productivity are possible for developers and users of training materials in that the database:

- Enables developers to communicate with each other enhancing cross fertilization of ideas for materials

- Makes more effective use of training funds by incorporating user experiences in judging the appropriateness of personnel, materials, meetings, and courses for an organization's needs

- Enables small businesses to compete in the training material by eliminating the need for costly advertising to reach the trainers market

- Serves as an incentive to organizations to produce quality instructional material for in-house use since there is a possibility of recouping their development costs by selling the material to outside organizations

Identifies organizations with similar interests, encouraging collaborative projects

DESIGN CONSIDERATIONS

Historically, end user contact with data in databases has largely been accomplished through intermediaries and usually limited to retrieval. Efforts have been going on over a number of years, however, to achieve closer contact between end users and their data. The result has been an increase in the number of end users who want to know how to search databases for themselves, an increase in the number of programs designed to help them learn, and an increase in efforts to design retrieval programs that will require little knowledge about computers on the part of the end user.

Summit (1967), described Lockheed's early efforts "to allow a user who is neither knowledgeable about not interested in computers to obtain useful results from a large file of document descriptions (citations) in a rapid, convenient, and effective manner." (p. 51)

Faibisoff (1981, p. 347) wrote that "as the price of computer terminals becomes more affordable...we may expect the end user to use the terminal to access all types of information," while Meadow (1979, p. 52) anticipated Faibisoff's statement, noting, in addition, that the end user will "actively and knowledgeably participate in the process...Getting the job done right will come to dominate getting it done economically."

Bellardo (1981), wrote on the idea of dispensing with intermediaries noting that "the heyday of the intermediary may be over soon. Enhancements which will make on-line systems much easier to use, and which will allow multifile and even multisystem use with a single command language will encourage direct access by end users. Intermediaries will be needed only for the difficult searches. Even difficult searches will be easier in many cases, with new free test and controlled vocabulary aids, database selection guides, etc. Still needed, however, is further research in effective training and education by both humans and computers, and more study of the effectiveness of the computer functioning as an intermediary compared to human intermediaries." (p. 210)

Haines (1982) describing an experiment to determine the need for developing an end-user search capability among researchers at Eastman Kodak, showed that "end-user searching is feasible and valuable for end-users with sufficient interest and a need to consult the literature frequently." (p. 18)

Swanson (1982, p. 38) noted that "the demand for instruction in the use of on-line databases is expected to increase...as end users start doing searches for themselves."

Codd (1982), noting the increasing demands being placed on programmers to design new programs, and seeking a means of reducing the need for such programs suggested that one "put end users into direct touch with the information stored in computers." (p. 109)

Radhakrishnan, et. al. (1982) described the design of "an interactive data retrieval system which is used for the study of commodity market data" (p. 23). Designed for "casual" users, it makes use of queries as the main form of interrogating the database with menus as backup aids. System-acceptable keywords are required as input.

Efforts toward improving contact between user and data can follow two routes: user-designed databases and user-maintained databases.

In the former, persons familiar with database management systems (DBMS) can design their own databases. However, Blair (1982), writing on the topic of creating one's own database on a microcomputer suggested a very cautious appraisal of that approach, balancing throughout the article the two realities that while excellent DBMS applications packages exist, and that "a relative newcomer to microcomputers could, with concentrated effort, design a usable file structure...just one deviation from instructors can be calamitous" (p. 11).

In the latter, persons completely unfamiliar with computers can access data by following instructions that are user-friendly. It is this method that has been employed in the database described in this paper.

While the database described in this paper offers a number of advantages, it has one major drawback: The main premise in constructing this database was that it would be maintained by a naive user, roughly defined as a person who knows nothing, and who cares to know nothing, about computers. To develop competence in such a user, the number of options had to be reduced to a few basic operations. The tradeoff is that while the user learns quickly to perform the limited range of operations, the user is denied access to the more sophisticated capabilities of the system.

Accepting that reservation, however, the database presents some interesting features:

Generation/Maintenance by a Naive User

Following Nickerson's statement (1969, p. 514) that "the need of the future is not so much for computer-oriented people as for people-oriented computers," the user is often required to do little more than enter a number from 1 through 10 from a menu. Prevention, detection, and remedy of errors are provided for by automatic procedures built in at appropriate points.

Database Control

To avoid chaos, access to the database for purposes of entering or searching for data is available to all users, while access to manipulate data is limited to the user who entered the data. The contents of the entire database are accessible to the Database Coordinator who can be reached by users via a message through the computer.

Convenience of User

Writing on man-computer interaction, Nickerson (1969, p. 505) noted that "all users tend to be impatient with redundancies in the language and with noninformative computer-to-user messages." Blair (1982), writing on man-microcomputer interaction stated "humans tend to get bored with repetition." (p. 83)

To overcome these problems of user impatience, a choice of two speeds of operation is offered: abbreviated instructions or full instructions.

A second procedure to reduce impatience is a choice of two speeds of searching: direct insertion of search terms known to be system-acceptable, or browsing a directory to find system-acceptable search terms. The faster method is presented first.

As a further convenience, the option to explain procedures or operations is a menu item, rather than a query, thus making it available for the newcomer yet avoidable by the experienced user.

User Access

Using a telephone interface the database can be immediately accessed from a terminal anywhere in North America via the DATAPAC, TELENET or TYMNET networks. Microcomputers with an RS-232 interface should have no problem accessing these networks.

For the user with no computing hardware, low cost, lightweight, portable units consisting of a telephone interface and a keyboard are commercially available. Using the home telephone and the television set as the respective input/output devices, the database can be easily accessed from the user's own living room. The results can be either viewed and printed out immediately (where a hard copy terminal is used) or viewed immediately and the hard copy mailed (where a video screen is used).

Timely Data and Immediate Dissemination

Newly entered data are retrievable the next day. Once the data are available, they are available to all users virtually simultaneously.

Access to Other Databases

Other databases can be accessed through this database provided the contents are input in a system-acceptable format. Arrangements can be made via message to the Database Coordinator (a menu choice).

Consolidation of Effort

The same procedures are used for each database. Thus, all the databases can be accessed at one sitting by selecting each desired database from the menu one at a time and implementing an operation (add/remove/search/update).

Low Cost of Operation

Reduced cost to the user of the database is a major consideration (though lowest in our priorities) in designing the database so that users with limited budgets can have access to it.

DESIGN AND OPERATION OF THE DATABASE

The general design of the database is an inverted tree with branches narrowing choices until the requested answer is found. A loop facility enables the user to return to the beginning of any branch or to the beginning of the tree itself. A simplified flowchart (Appendix 1) shows the operation of the database. (For the purpose of clarity the Message function and some options are omitted).

The general operating procedure for the Trainers Database is:

- Select a database from a menu of databases

- Select an operation from a menu of operations to perform on the data

- Repeat one of the above choices, or sign-off

The Trainers Database serves three functions: a source of information for and a means of communication among users, and a source of immediate safety procedures during an emergency.

Information Source

As an information source the database is divided into two areas: contents and evaluation of contents.

Contents. Conceptually, the Trainers Database may be viewed as a collection of databases, each of which (e.g., BOOKS database) is a collection of Records (specific books) identifiable by means of Elements (title, author, subject).

The user selects a database and initiates one of four operations on the contents: ADD/REMOVE (Records) or SEARCH/UPDATE (Elements).

While these operations are performed immediately upon request, the indexes reflecting these changes are not updated until sometime later. This is due to the need to interrupt service to implement the updating procedure. To minimize this interruption, entries affecting the Index (ADD, REMOVE, UPDATE) are accumulated in a separate file (Deferred Queue) and batch processed during the slack early morning hours.

An advantage of a separate file is that it offers the user a second chance to change data destined for the database. A disadvantage is that SEARCHing the index for the results of ADD/REMOVE/UPDATE operations before they are processed may yield an inaccurate statement of their availability.

- SEARCH Operation

The SEARCH operation consists of two activities:

- Selecting an Element from a menu of Elements

- Entering a system-acceptance Search Term (a list is optionally presented).

The user retrieves stored records by selecting an Element and entering a system-acceptable term. As an example, after selecting the BOOKS database and initiating the SEARCH operation on the element SUBJECT, entering the term "training" causes the SEARCH program to generate and execute the following command:

Find SUBJECT training

(Note: Adding a question mark after a term includes all characters following, thus "train?" will produce results for the words trainer, trainers, training, etc. Do not use a question mark to precede a term.)

The user reduces or increases the number of hits by using Boolean logic (ADD/OR/AND NOT), operating consecutively from left to right. As an example, the command, "Find SUBJECT training OR instruction AND methods" would provide a list of books about both training and methods as well as books about both instruction and methods. The command "Find SUBJECT training AND instruction OR methods," would provide a list of books about both training and instruction as well as books about methods. In neither example would books solely about training or solely about instruction be listed.

       (1) SEE Option

           The results of the search may be viewed before printing. A menu is presented and elements are selected concurrently (e.g., in the BOOKS database, if 1=title, 2=author, then "1 2" will produce a list consisting of the title and author of each book).

           As an example, two hits from the BOOKS database on the selection 1 2 prints out as:

              - (Title) Military Data Processing and Microcomputers
                 (Author) Ward, J.W.D. and Turner,G.N.

              - (Title) ILO Catalogue of Publications in Print
                 (Author) International Labor Office

- ADD Operation

    To add a record to the database, the user follows system prompts to feed data into an empty record. Element names are presented one at a time and the user fills in or skips an element.

    Upon completion of the filing procedures, the system automatically assigns a Record Key for identification and indexes the contents of searchable elements.

- REMOVE/UPDATE Operations

    These operations involve data already in the database. The Record Key is called for and the record is either removed entirely or modified element by element in a manner resembling the ADD operation.

    Evaluation of Contents. The user has the option of entering comments regarding an item in the database. Evaluating the contents of a database is a separate activity permitting all four operations: ADD/REMOVE/SEARCH/UPDATE. The first step in evaluating the contents of a database is to select the database containing the item to be evaluated and SEARCH for its Record Key. The second step is to select the EVALUATION Database and initiate one of the four operations. The program then prompts the user for required input.

Communication System

    Used as a means of communication, a user may send and receive messages through the MESSAGE Routines (SMSG, RMSG) to other users individually, to a specific interest group of users, or by an announcement to all users.

    Contacting an Individual User. To send a message to an individual, the user follows system prompts that request the ID of the receiver and the message.

    Contacting a Group. To send a message to a group, the user follows system prompts that call for the system-acceptable name of the special interest group and the message.

    Where conversation is desired, as opposed to leaving a note, each sender must use the Receive Message operator (rmsg), to receive a reply. In effect, (rmsg) is the visual equivalent of the "Over!" voice command of the two-way radio conversation.

Contacting All Users. Announcements to all users are made through the Database Coordinator. Usually these announcements will pertain to changes in Database operation, but it is also available for warnings of dangers affecting all users (e.g., toxic substances or unsafe equipment or practices). To avoid abuse of this capability, users follow system prompts to send such announcements to the Database Coordinator who then enters the messages into the system. The messages will appear on the screen of every user upon the sign-on.

Emergency Safety Procedures

Suggestions offered by participants have expanded the original intent of the database--capitalizing on its speed of access--by including emergency safety procedures to its original function of disseminating training information.

The Chemicals Database was introduced after a user's suggestion that if a container is leaking a chemical onto the ground, information on how to handle the contents is more quickly accessible from a computer terminal than from a manufacturer's manual where immediate access to the manual, let alone the information, is often questionable.

Additional safety databases are expected to be added to the Trainers Database as the idea gains acceptance.

COSTS FOR USING THE DATABASE

There is not charge for using the Trainers Database as it is housed in a computer owned by the University of Alberta. The user thus has access to all the computing services provided by the University of Alberta of which the Trainers Database is just one.

No advance payment of subscription fee is required to use the University's computer resources. The user is billed by the University in accordance with a Rate Schedule (in Canadian dollars) based on the amount of use of the University's computer resources ($10/month minimum).

Savings are possible for contributors of large quantities of data by making special arrangements for batch processing their tape holdings.

REFERENCES

Bellardo, T. (1981). Scientific research in on-line retrieval: A critical review. "Library Research," "3," 187-214.
Blair, J., Jr. (1982). Creating your own database. "DATABASE," "6(3)," 11-17.
Blair, J., Jr. (1982). The psychology of the human interface with a microcomputer: Machine-friendly humanware. "ON-LINE," "6(6)," 83-87.
Codd, E. (1982). Relational database: A practical foundation for productivity. "Communications of the ACM," "25(2)," 109-117.
Faibisoff, S. (1981). Is there a future for the end user in on-line bibliographic searching? "Special Libraries," "72(4)," 347-355.
Haines, J. (1982). Experiences in training end-user searchers. "ON-LINE," "6(6)," 14-23
Meadow, C. (1979). ON-LINE searching and computer programming: Some behavioral similarities (Or...why end users will eventually take over the terminal. "ON-LINE," "3(1)," 49-52.
Meyers, A. (1982). User-maintained database for trainers. "Training and Development Journal," "36(10)," 50-52.
Nickerson, R. (1969). Man-computer interaction: A challenge for human factors research. "Ergonomics," "12(4)," 501-517.

Radhakrishnan, T., Grossner, C. & Benoleil, M. (1982). Design of an interactive data retrieval system for casual users. "Information Processing & Management," "18(1)," 23-32.

Summit, R. (1967). DIALOG: An operational on-line reference retrieval system. "Proceedings" - ACM National Meeting. New York: Association for Computing Machinery, 51-56.

Swanson, R. (1982). An assessment of on-line instruction methodologies. "ON-LINE," "6(1)," 38-53.

APPENDIX 1

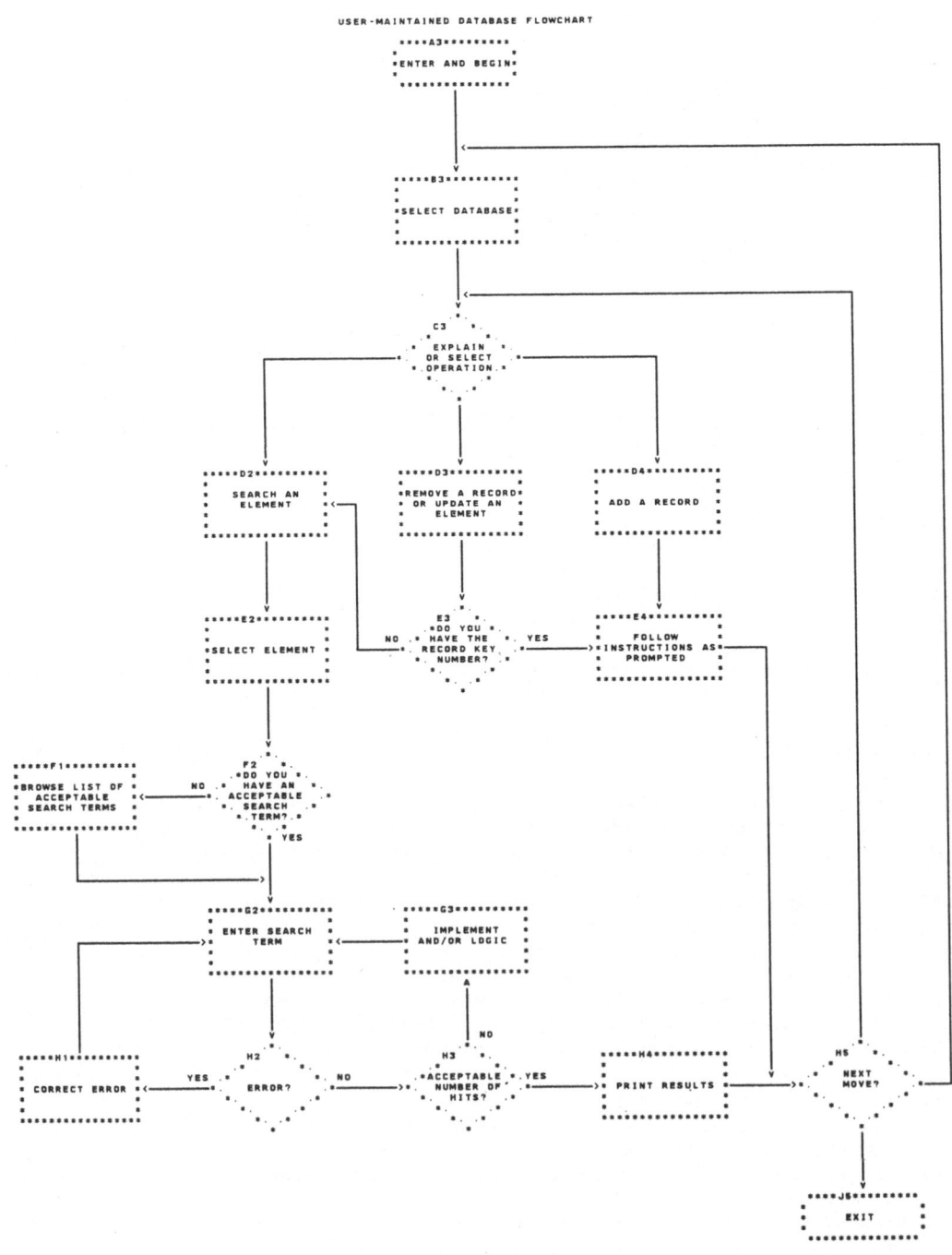

APPENDIX 2

EXPLANATION OF "HELP" SELECTION

(**BOLD**face type = User Response)

```
* 1(sel) 2(smsg) 3(rmsg) 4(stop) 5(int) H(help)
*
: Enter number preceding choice: h
*
* 1. Select database
* 2. Send message
* 3. Receive message
* 4. Leave the system
* 5. Introduction to the database
: Enter number preceding choice (If in doubt, hit BREAK):


* 1(add) 2(upd) 3(src) 4(rem) 5(see) 6(bse) 7(off) 8(sze) 9(exp) h(help)
*
: Enter number preceding choice: h
*
* 1) Add an item
* 2) Update an item (key required)
* 3) Search for items
* 4) Remove an item
* 5) Display an item
* 6) Select a different database
* 7) Signoff (To leave the system)
* 8) Display no. of items in CIJE
* 9) Describe Database CIJE
: Enter number preceding choice:


* 1(cor) 2(add) 3(alt) 4(not) 5(see) 6(opr) 7(smsg) 8(rmsg) 9(eval) 10(end) h(help)
*
: Enter number preceding choice: h
*
* Enter number preceding choice:
* 1) Begin a new search of the CIJE database
* 2) Enter additional search term (and ...)
* 3) Enter alternate search term (or ...)
* 4) Delimit the search terms (and not ...)
* 5) View results
* 6) Select a different database or
*    Add/Remove/Update/Display an item
* 7) Send message
* 8) Receive message
* 9) Evaluate an item
* 10) Exit the system (Signoff)
*
:?


* 1(add) 2(upd) 3(rem) 4(see) 5(opr) 6(off)
*
: Enter number preceding choice: h
*
* 1) Add evaluation of an item
* 2) Update evaluation
* 3) Remove an evaluation
* 4) Display an evaluation
* 5) Leave EVALUATION mode
* 6) Leave the system


* 1(rem) 2(rpt) 3(nxt) H(help)
*
:Enter number preceding choice: h
*
* 1) To REMOVE Record
* 2) ADD another record
* 3) End of ADD requests
*
  Enter number preceding choice:
```

APPENDIX 3(a)

EXAMPLE OF SEARCH OPERATION: CIJE DATABASE

(BOLDface type = User Response)

```
# sig (signon ID)
# Password?
? (Password)
# Term,Low,Internal / Teaching,Research
# Last signon was: 18:07:02
# User "ALME" signed on at 18:07:46 on Sun Nov 27/83
# so gd01:run
# $.02, $.08T
# r *spires
# 18:08:27
83/11/22 Spires user group meeting Dec. 7. SHOW NEWS for details.
-SPIRES 83.06
->) sel &gd01.protocols protocol
->) set compxeq
->) ..dispgroup
*
* 1(sel) 2(smsg) 3(rmsg) 4(stop) 5(int) H(help)
*
: Enter number preceding choice: 1
*
* 1. INFORMATION  2. PRIVATE
*
: Enter number preceding choice (If in doubt, hit BREAK): 1
*
* In SELECT Database mode
*
*  1. USERS         2. RIE           3. MEETINGS      4. MATERIALS
*  5. EVALUATION    6. ED THESIS     7. DIRECTORY     8. COURSES
*  9. CIJE         10. CHEMICALS    11. BOOKS        12. ARTICLES
*
: Enter number preceding choice (If in doubt, hit BREAK): 9
******************************************************************
*                                                                *
* Last updated with March 1983 tapes from ERIC    *
*                                                                *
******************************************************************
*
* Select OPERATION on database CIJE (Hit BREAK to exit)
*
* 1(add) 2(upd) 3(src) 4(rem) 5(see) 6(bse) 7(off) 8(sze) 9(exp) h(help)
*
: Enter number preceding choice: 3
*
* In SEARCH mode on database CIJE
*
* 1. TITLE    2. AUTHOR    3. DESCRIPTOR    4. IDENTIFIER
*
: Enter number preceding choice: 3
*
* Enter system-acceptable term for DESCRIPTOR (For list, hit ENTER key; hit
BREAK key to exit)
: (ENTER)
: Enter general term to be searched or press the ENTER KEY for a sample: (ENTER)
*
* The following are system-acceptable terms for searching DESCRIPTOR:
*
FOREIGN STUDENT ADVISERS
INFORMATION STORAGE
LOBBYING
NEUROLOGY
READING COMPREHENSION
SENTENCE DIAGRAMING
SYNTHESIS
VOLUNTARY INTEGRATION
*
* Enter DESCRIPTOR from list (hit BREAK if no term applies)
: (BREAK)
***Attn
*
* In SEARCH mode on database CIJE
*
* 1(cor) 2(add) 3(alt) 4(not) 5(see) 6(opr) 7(smsg) 8(rmsg) 9(eval) 10(end) h(help)
*
: Enter number preceding choice: 1
* 1. TITLE    2. AUTHOR    3. DESCRIPTOR    4. IDENTIFIER
```

APPENDIX 3(b)

```
*
: Enter number preceding choice: 3
*
* Enter system-acceptable term for DESCRIPTOR (For list, hit ENTER key; hit
BREAK key to exit)
: (ENTER)
: Enter general term to be searched or press the ENTER KEY for a sample: train
TRAFFIC REGULATIONS
TRAFFIC SAFETY
TRAFFIC SIGNS
TRAGEDY
TRAILS
TRAINABLE MENTALLY HANDICAPPED
TRAINEES
TRAINERS
TRAINING
TRAINING ALLOWANCES
-More? y
TRAINING LABORATORIES
TRAINING METHODS
TRAINING OBJECTIVES
TRAINING TECHNIQUES
TRANSACTIONAL ANALYSIS
TRANSFER OF TRAINING
TRANSFER POLICY
TRANSFER PROGRAMS
TRANSFER STUDENTS
TRANSFERS
-More? n
*
* Enter DESCRIPTOR from list (hit BREAK if no term applies)
: training methods
*
*************************************
* No. of records found: 563
* on the command:
FIND DESCRIPTOR training methods
*************************************
*
* In SEARCH mode on database CIJE
*
* 1(cor) 2(add) 3(alt) 4(not) 5(see) 6(opr) 7(smsg) 8(rmsg) 9(eval) 10(end) h(help)
*
: Enter number preceding choice: 2
*
* 1. TITLE     2. AUTHOR     3. DESCRIPTOR     4. IDENTIFIER
*
: Enter number preceding choice: 3
*
* Enter system-acceptable term for DESCRIPTOR (For list, hit ENTER key; hit
BREAK key to exit)
: (ENTER)
: Enter general term to be searched or press the ENTER KEY for a sample: organization
ORAL INTERPRETATION
ORAL LANGUAGE
ORAL READING
ORCHESTRAS
ORGANIC CHEMISTRY
ORGANIZATION
ORGANIZATION SIZE GROUPS
ORGANIZATIONAL CHANGE
ORGANIZATIONAL CLIMATE
ORGANIZATIONAL COMMUNICATION
-More? y
ORGANIZATIONAL DEVELOPMENT
ORGANIZATIONAL EFFECTIVENESS
ORGANIZATIONAL OBJECTIVES
ORGANIZATIONAL THEORIES
ORGANIZATIONS GROUPS
ORIENTATION
ORIENTATION MATERIALS
ORIENTEERING
ORIGINALITY
ORNAMENTAL HORTICULTURE
-More? n
*
* Enter DESCRIPTOR from list (hit BREAK if no term applies)
: organizational development
*
```

APPENDIX 3(c)

```
**************************************
* No. of records found: 2
* on the command:
FIND DESCRIPTOR training methods
AND DESCRIPTOR organizational development
**************************************
*
* In SEARCH mode on database CIJE
*
* 1(cor) 2(add) 3(alt) 4(not) 5(see) 6(opr) 7(smsg) 8(rmsg) 9(eval) 10(end) h(help)
*
: Enter number preceding choice: 5
*
*
* DISPLAY mode on Database CIJE (Hit BREAK to exit)
*
*
*     0.   All elements         1.   ACCESSION        2.   CLEAR.ACC.NUM
*     3.   ADD.DATE             4.   EJ.NUMBER        5.   MOD.DATE
*     6.   OTHER.ACC            7.   PROG.AREA        8.   TITLE
*     9.   AUTHOR              10.   INST.CODE       11.   AGENCY.CODE
*    12.   DESCRIPTOR          13.   IDENTIFIER      14.   EDRS.PRICE
*    15.   DESC.NOTE           16.   PAGE            17.   LEVEL
*    18.   ISSUE               19.   ABSTRACT        20.   REPORT.NUM
*    21.   CONTRACT.NUM        22.   GRANT.NUM       23.   BUREAU.NUM
*    24.   AVAILABILITY        25.   JOURNAL.CIT     26.   LANGUAGE
*    27.   LOCATION            28.   STATUS          29.   INST.NAME
*    30.   SPONSOR.NAME        31.   PUB.DATE.STR
*
: Enter numbers preceding choices (e.g. 1 4 3): 8 9 25 16 12 13 15 19

(TITLE)Beyond the Grid and Situationalism: A Living Systems View.
(AUTHOR)Beck, Don Edward
(JOURNAL.CIT)Training and Development Journal/ v36 n8 p76-83 Aug 1982
(DESCRIPTOR)*Leadership Styles *Management Development *Organizational
Development Training Methods
(IDENTIFIER)Living Systems *Managerial Grid *Situational Leadership
(ABSTRACT)Discusses the Managerial Grid versus Situational Leadership
approach to management development. Suggests that they need to be
supplemented by new theoretical models, called 'Living Systems.' (JOW)

*************************
(TITLE)Team Training: A Behavior Modification Approach.
(AUTHOR)Rasmussen, Ray V.
(JOURNAL.CIT)Group and Organization Studies/ v7 n1 p51-66 Mar 1982
(DESCRIPTOR)*Behavior Modification Feedback Learning Theories
Organizational Development Problem Solving Program Descriptions
*Small Group Instruction *Team Training *Training Methods
(ABSTRACT)Describes an approach to team training based on behavior
modification learning principles and describes how it differs from
other learning approaches and from common practice. While the
implications are strongest for off-site and classroom training, there
are implications for process consultation with intact teams. (Author)
*************************
* DISPLAY mode on Database CIJE (Hit BREAK to exit)
*
*
*     0.   All elements         1.   ACCESSION        2.   CLEAR.ACC.NUM
*     3.   ADD.DATE             4.   EJ.NUMBER        5.   MOD.DATE
*     6.   OTHER.ACC            7.   PROG.AREA        8.   TITLE
*     9.   AUTHOR              10.   INST.CODE       11.   AGENCY.CODE
*    12.   DESCRIPTOR          13.   IDENTIFIER      14.   EDRS.PRICE
*    15.   DESC.NOTE           16.   PAGE            17.   LEVEL
*    18.   ISSUE               19.   ABSTRACT        20.   REPORT.NUM
*    21.   CONTRACT.NUM        22.   GRANT.NUM       23.   BUREAU.NUM
*    24.   AVAILABILITY        25.   JOURNAL.CIT     26.   LANGUAGE
*    27.   LOCATION            28.   STATUS          29.   INST.NAME
*    30.   SPONSOR.NAME        31.   PUB.DATE.STR
*
: Enter numbers preceding choices (e.g. 1 4 3): (BREAK)
***Attn
*
* In SEARCH mode on database CIJE
*
* 1(cor) 2(add) 3(alt) 4(not) 5(see) 6(opr) 7(smsg) 8(rmsg) 9(eval) 10(end) h(help)
*
: Enter number preceding choice: 10
*
# 18:33:08 T=1.658 RC=0
# $1.11, $1.19T
```

APPENDIX 4

EXAMPLE OF ADD OPERATION: BOOKS DATABASE

(**BOLD**face type = User Response)

```
* In SELECT Database mode
*
*  1. USERS          2. RIE           3. MEETINGS       4. MATERIALS
*  5. EVALUATION     6. ED THESIS     7. DIRECTORY      8. COURSES
*  9. CIJE          10. CHEMICALS    11. BOOKS         12. ARTICLES
*
:Enter number preceding choice (If in doubt, hit BREAK): 11
*
* Select OPERATION on database BOOKS (Hit BREAK to exit)
*
* 1(add) 2(upd) 3(src) 4(rem) 5(see) 6(bse) 7(off) 8(sze) 9(exp) h(help)
*
:Enter number preceding choice: 1
*
*
* in ADD RECORD mode on data base BOOKS
* (Hit ENTER to bypass. Hit BREAK to exit)
*
:TITLE : Index to 16MM Educational Films (Vol I - Vol IV)
:TITLE : (ENTER)
:AUTHOR(LAST NAME, FIRST NAME) : National Information Center for Educational Media
:AUTHOR(LAST NAME, FIRST NAME) : (ENTER)
:DATE(MM/DD/YY) : 1980
:KEYWORD : reference
:KEYWORD : 16mm film
:KEYWORD : film
:KEYWORD : index
:KEYWORD : (ENTER)
:PUBLISHER : National Information Center for Educational Media (NICEM)
:COMMENTS : 7th Edition
:COMMENTS : (ENTER)
------- FORM ----
:TYPE(H-HARDCOVER, P-PAPERBACK) : P
:PRICE : unknown
------- FORM ----
:TYPE(H-HARDCOVER, P-PAPERBACK) : (ENTER)
*
* added record 35
*
* 1(rem) 2(rpt) 3(nxt) H(help)
*
:Enter number preceding choice: 3
*
* Select OPERATION on database BOOKS (Hit BREAK to exit)
*
* 1(add) 2(upd) 3(src) 4(rem) 5(see) 6(bse) 7(off) 8(sze) 9(exp) h(help)
*
:Enter number preceding choice: 7
*
# 16:54:45 T=0.571 RC=0
# $.67, $.80T
```

APPENDIX 5

EXAMPLE OF REMOVE OPERATION: DIRECTORY DATABASE

(BOLDface type = User Response)

```
* In SELECT Database mode
*
*   1. USERS        2. RIE          3. MEETINGS     4. MATERIALS
*   5. EVALUATION   6. ED THESIS    7. DIRECTORY    8. COURSES
*   9. CIJE        10. CHEMICALS   11. BOOKS       12. ARTICLES
*
: Enter number preceding choice (If in doubt, hit BREAK): 7
*
* Select OPERATION on database DIRECTORY (Hit BREAK to exit)
*
* 1(add) 2(upd) 3(src) 4(rem) 5(see) 6(bse) 7(off) 8(sze) 9(exp) h(help)
*
: Enter number preceding choice: 4
*
*
* In REMOVE mode on database DIRECTORY
*
:Enter Record Key : 19
:Do you wish to cancel this request ? (y/n) n
* record 19 has been removed
:Enter Record Key : (ENTER)
*
* Select OPERATION on database DIRECTORY (Hit BREAK to exit)
*
* 1(add) 2(upd) 3(src) 4(rem) 5(see) 6(bse) 7(off) 8(sze) 9(exp) h(help)
*
: Enter number preceding choice: 7
*
# 13:14:27 T=0.478 RC=0
# $.50, $.75T
```

APPENDIX 6

EXAMPLE OF UPDATE OPERATION: USERS DATABASE

(**BOLD**face type = User Response)

```
* In SELECT Database mode
*
*  1. USERS         2. RIE            3. MEETINGS       4. MATERIALS
*  5. EVALUATION    6. ED THESIS      7. DIRECTORY      8. COURSES
*  9. CIJE         10. CHEMICALS     11. BOOKS         12. ARTICLES
*
: Enter number preceding choice (If in doubt, hit BREAK): 1
*
* Select OPERATION on database USERS (Hit BREAK to exit)
*
* 1(add) 2(upd) 3(src) 4(rem) 5(see) 6(bse) 7(off) 8(sze) 9(exp) h(help)
*
: Enter number preceding choice: 2
*
*
* In UPDATE mode on database USERS (Hit BREAK to exit)
*
: Enter Record Key: alme
*
* 2. INTEREST
*
: Enter numbers preceding choices (e.g. 4 3): 2
RECORD KEY: ALME
(Hit ENTER to bypass element. Hit BREAK to delete element contents)
INTEREST(1) ..... computers
INTEREST(2) ..... VOCATIONAL EDUCATION
:INTEREST(1)..... (ENTER)
:INTEREST(2)..... vocational education
:INTEREST(3)..... (ENTER)
*
: Enter Record Key: (BREAK)
***Attn.
*
* Select OPERATION on database USERS (Hit BREAK to exit)
*
* 1(add) 2(upd) 3(src) 4(rem) 5(see) 6(bse) 7(off) 8(sze) 9(exp) h(help)
*
: Enter number preceding choice: 7
*
# 10:38:51 T=0.589 RC=0
# S.63, S.77T
```

APPENDIX 7

<u>ADD</u> <u>Input</u> <u>Form:</u> <u>CHEMICALS</u> <u>Database</u>

(NOTE: See: **EXAMPLE OF ADD OPERATION: CHEMICALS DATABASE**)

Chemical:

Components:

Manufacturer:

Characteristics:

Handling:

Treatment:

Comment:

Contributor:

COMPUTER-BASED INSTRUCTION IN THE DEPARTMENT OF DEFENSE: ENHANCING APPLICATION OF THE TECHNOLOGY

J. F. Funaro and N. E. Lane
*Defense Training Data and Analysis Center
  Orlando, Florida, U.S.A.
**Essex Corporation
  Orlando, Florida, U.S.A.

BACKGROUND

   The dramatic change in power, portability and affordability of small computers during the last five years has been a two-edged sword in its impact on military training. There have been compelling reasons to anticipate that these rapid advances in computational state of the art would unlock the latent potential of computer-based instruction (CBI) and finally realize the breakthroughs in training and education approaches that have been just over the horizon for the last two decades. It is true that the availability of flexible and powerful processing in small packages has materially expanded the scope of what can be accomplished with computer-based, computer-managed, computer-assisted, and intelligent computer-assisted instruction (however defined). The steady decreases in cost which have accompanied these increases in capability have also greatly broadened the classes of application for which CBI is feasible to the typical user. It is thus somewhat surprising that the applications of CBI have not grown concomitantly with the attractiveness of the technology.

   The CBI applications lag results indirectly from the same mix of positive and negative drivers associated with any technology in a rapid state of growth. The continuing revolution of capability that broadens the possibilities of CBI has at the same time brought about a proliferation of languages, architectures, authoring systems and media that inhibit the systematic development of CBI courseware. The maturity of a technology is reflected in the extent to which new applications can evolve from experience gained in previous applications so that capability can be expanded in an evolutionary way as opposed to a "dramatic leap forward." Before a "standard" or baseline technology has emerged, consumers have difficulty in resolving the claims, counterclaims, strengths and weaknesses of the different approaches, and are reluctant to make decisions without a clearer grasp of the technology. In brief, the potential new user of CBI becomes seriously confused and tends to stay out of the market until he judges the technology to have stabilized. The history of technology introduction into military systems suggests that, in the absence of some specific intervention in the technology transition process, applications will lag capability by at least one generation of technology. To date, the needed "intervention" has not occurred, and the "growing pains" associated with technology expansion have to a large extent inhibited the routine use of CBI as a solution to military training problems.

Although the military services differ in approaches toward management of training, they share a common tendency to decentralize decision making in selection of training delivery systems. In general, responsibility for configuring training packages resides with the program manager or operational activity responsible for the system or function for which training is being provided. Although this process has desirable attributes in improving accountability and in achieving best short-term use of available resources, it is also a major factor in the application gap for training technology that has slowed down appropriate use of CBI. The chronic limitations on resources available to a program manager or operational unit and the pressures for timely production of training capability have traditionally forced a reliance on "proven" training methods and an avoidance of risk involved in "gambling" on new techniques, regardless of the long-term return available from these new methods. In such an environment, the transition of technologies to applications is necessarily slow and laborious, and the need to convince each decision maker in a decentralized system of the worth of some new method can seriously delay the return realized from R & D investments. Further, when CBI is employed under such conditions, effectiveness of the technology tends to be less than expected. Montague, Wulfeck and Ellis (1983) point out the need for specific up-front attention to instructional issues and the realities of firm implementation support along with the usual focus on delivery mechanisms, and highlight the hazards of overdependence on microcomputer CBI as a cure-all for instructional problems without providing such institutionalized implementation.

The value of CBI and related techniques in improving or maintaining training effectiveness with reduced training time is well documented. Orlansky and String (1979) and Orlansky, String and Chatelier (1982) describe a review of 48 CBI applications in military settings. The typical CBI application achieved an effectiveness equal or slightly superior to conventional methods with a time savings on the order of 30 percent. Kulik, Kulik, and Cohen (1980) performed a similar synthesis of 59 studies from the college instruction domain. Their findings closely parallel those of Orlansky and String (1979). CBI made small but consistent and significant contributions to student achievement while reducing substantially the time required for instruction (about 36 percent). Montague et al. (1983) reported a comparable savings of 27 percent in time to learn material, but also reinforced the indications of Orlansky and String (1979) that the cost savings from CBI associated with reduced time have not yet been realized.

In addition to the consistent evidence of CBI effectiveness, it should be further considered that creative application of available CAI capability (particularly that using intelligent systems technology) can provide training for which conventional methods are generally considered inadequate, too risky and/or too costly. Given this unquestioned potential, it is important to look at the case of the "reluctant consumer" of CBI, to isolate factors that have prevented CBI from realizing its potential, and to determine appropriate ways to provide the "intervention" noted above. This paper describes some initiatives within the U.S. Department of Defense (DOD) to assist the services in making most effective use of CBI in military training through the establishment of a series of support systems and organizations.

CBI SUPPORT ORGANIZATIONS

A number of analyses (Pohlman [1984] for example) have looked at the issues surrounding the relatively slow rate of CBI introduction into military training. The Defense Science Board (DSB) on Training and Training Technology (1983) recommended both an acceleration of development of CBI technology and a specific focus on technology demonstration. The DSB also indicated the importance of joint-service emphasis on these problem areas. From these and other studies, three major requirements can be identified:

1. Assistance must be provided the CBI user in matching his particular needs to the available technology (a "consumers guide to CBI").

2. To the fullest extent possible, technology should be standardized across the services and common definitions developed.

3. Realistic demonstrations of CBI as a viable method of solving training problems should be developed and made widely visible throughout the potential user community.

To address these requirements, the DOD established in late 1983 a Joint Services Activity for CBI Software (JSACS). The principal goals of the JSACS are to provide for DOD activities a central system for CBI information and courseware access and to promote and encourage CBI applications on a joint-service basis. The major functions defined in the JSACS charter are (see Pohlman [1984]):

- To serve as a clearinghouse for information on characteristics of government and commercial CBI software

- To assist service users in making decisions about CBI applications

- To serve as a repository for government CBI software with configuration management and software distribution responsibilities

Since the establishment of JSACS, the organizational mechanism of implementing its functions has shifted. The JSACS was originally located with the Naval Training Equipment center in Orlando, Florida. Current plans provide for the software library functions to merge with a development and demonstration program called TRIADS (1983), with support from the Air Force Human Resources Laboratory. The data base functions will be subsumed under another DOD organization, the Defense Training Data and Analysis Center (TDAC), established in Orlando in August 1984. The TDAC is a separate DOD group responsible to the Assistant Secretary of Defense for Manpower and Force Management. It will be located with the Naval Training Equipment Center and the Army Program Manager for Training Devices.

While the TDAC has functions in service-wide training that are much broader than the specific issues of CBI, it is an important organization in supporting the enhancement of CBI applications in the services. The TDAC is in part a response to the series of specific recommendations made by the Defense Science Board (1983) for improving military training, including those previously mentioned which deal with accelerated CBI applications and greater emphasis on technology demonstration. Among the key functions of TDAC are a responsibility for defining training issues which have impact on all the services, conducting analyses of data which help to clarify the nature and dimensions of the problem, developing potential solutions, and carrying out training evaluation studies to determine solution effectiveness. Specific TDAC objectives which have direct relevance to CBI needs include the identification of new technologies that have promise for service training use, the technical support to assist application of these technologies, and the transfer of training public and international communities. An early priority of TDAC will be the development of a CBI data base and a series of surveys to define and categorize the current status of CBI technology. These efforts are discussed below.

EFFORTS IN PROGRESS

Preceding sections have discussed the problems involved in achieving the full potential of modern CBI technology and described the organizations being created within the DOD to help smooth the transition of CBI from technology to a routinely used training tool. Although the organizations involved are relatively new, several efforts are underway or in planning stages as of this writing. The principal thrusts of these efforts align with the major requirements previously outlined, specifically those of: a) assisting the user in understanding available CBI techniques and in selecting the CBI approach and methods most appropriate to his training situation, and b) providing clearly relevant demonstrations of CBI capability to overcome user reluctance to accept "unproven" technology.

Consumers Guide to CBI

The first of these thrusts is directed at overcoming the previously discussed confusion encountered by a typical CBI user when confronted by the undifferentiated mass of alternative CBI systems. It is easy to forget in the excitement of new and powerful capabilities that the typical customer for CBI is far better versed in his subject matter than in educational principles and is more likely to be looking for help in a single course or limited course sequence than to be designing a complete instructional delivery and instructional management system. Both of these applications are commonly occurring, valid uses of CBI, and both can be supported effectively with available technology.

The process, however, of determining what is appropriate, how to use it, what the hardware requirements are, and what it will cost is a challenging one even to an expert in CBI, and one on which there can be substantively different answers from different experts. It seems likely that systematic assistance for the user in decision making should considerably enhance willingness to undertake use of the technology.

Arriving at a useful and effective "consumers guide for CBI" is neither simple nor straightforward. Across the spectrum of what is generally subsumed under the categories of CAI and CMI, there are many axes or "criteria" on which available systems nor approaches can be compared. These include (but are not necessarily limited to) such considerations as the following:

- Transportability - compatibility of language, hardware dependence, special system features or communication protocols

- Scope of coverage - full system including instructional development, delivery and student management vs. selected coverage

- Student tracking, reporting and feedback characteristics - for CMI systems

- Background/characteristics of intended user - SME, training manager, analyst; knowledge expected, special training required

- Degree of system tailoring and maintenance required – off the shelf generic vs. investment in customizing applications

- Presence/absence/characteristics of authoring system – extent of support and complexity of use

- Extent of process automation – does system assist in defining objectives, course content and sequencing, media selection etc.

- Nature and completeness of user documentation

- Cost involved and dependability of cost estimation

- Hardware and physical interface requirements

- Embedding of educational principles – is theory of instruction provided by system or by user

- Proprietary vs. public domain

These criteria (and others) can be further expanded and subdivided to form a collection of categories into which, at least in theory, the bulk of CBI systems and approaches can be cataloged. It is our belief that a user needs a series of "file drawers" into which he can look to find out what he can do for a specific CBI application, combined with a way of determining which file drawer he should open. This consumer guidance should be available for both established systems and for system capabilities just emerging from R & D. Several DOD-supported efforts either underway or to be started soon will help to form the basis for the consumer's guide. A recent university grant began the process of collecting descriptive data about existing CBI software. Another recently initiated study will develop a tentative taxonomy of new CBI technology currently in developmental stages and begin the categorization process for products available in the near future. An additional study will identify already available government and commercial systems and perform a similar categorization for these existing systems, bringing together descriptive data on system characteristics.

The three studies above are all performed under the auspices of TDAC with joint service support. The crucial link among these efforts is the development of a common set of criteria on which all the systems, software, and approaches can be compared. The tentative criteria above, while indicative of the factors which must be considered, are not yet sufficiently exhaustive nor sufficiently detailed to allow for the richness or complexity of CBI technology. Further work will obviously be required to expand, refine and evaluate workability of the criteria. As with most such taxonomic efforts, the process is intensely iterative, requiring continuous "reality checks" and steady revision as new systems are discovered. It is anticipated that outcomes of these and subsequent studies will ultimately provide a comprehensive data base, along with the technical support and guidance available from TDAC and from TRIADS, should make decisions on when and how to use CBI simpler and more systematic.

Technology Demonstration

The second of the two major thrusts, demonstration of CBI technology, is proceeding principally through the mechanisms of the TRIADS program (1983) previously noted. TRIADS is a joint-service R & D effort supported by the DOD to bring together and coordinate a significant part of ongoing Service CBI development efforts. Two important functions of TRIADS concern: a) the development and documentation of a library of CBI software and courseware programs developed within the services, with a long-range goal of Ada standardization, and b) the demonstration of training capability available from new or existing TRIADS software. TRIADS is also charged with the development of functional specifications for the design and procurement of military hardware and software for CBI and with the assessment of effectiveness for CBI applications

It was noted earlier that translating the potential of CBI into real and visible impact on military training would require direct and deliberate intervention into the normally leisurely process of technology transition into training. The establishment of organizations with specific responsibilities for promoting user applications of CBI and the eventual development of detailed user guidance supported by accessible software libraries provides a beginning for that intervention.

REFERENCES

Dallman, B., Pohlman, D., Psotka, J., Wisher, R., McLachlan, J., Wulfeck, W., Ahlers, R. & Cronholm, J. (1983). TRIADS: A foundation for military computer-based instruction. "Journal of Computer-Based Instruction," "10(3&4)," 59-61.

Kulik. J., Kulik, C. & Cohen, P. (1980). Effectiveness of computer-based college teaching: A meta-analysis of findings. "Review of Educational Research," "50(4)," 525-544.

Montague, W., Wulfeck, W. & Ellis, J. (1983). Quality CBI depends on quality instructional design and quality implementation. "Journal of Computer-Based Instruction," "10(3&4)," 90-93.

Orlansky, J. & String, J., (1979). "Cost-Effectiveness of Computer-Based Instruction in Military Training." IDA Paper P-1375. Alexandria, VA: Institute for Defense Analyses.

Orlansky, J., String, J. & Chatelier, P. (1982). The cost effectiveness of military training. "Proceedings of the Fourth Interservice/Industry Training Equipment Conference," (pp. 97-109). Orlando, Florida.

Pohlman, D. (1984) The Joint-Services CBI Software Support Activity. "Proceedings of the Second Annual Air Force Conference on Technology in Training and Education," 18 (Abstract).

"Report of the Defense Science Board Summer Study Panel on Training and Training Technology," (February 1983).

TURNING EDUCATORS INTO AUTHORS: A CASE STUDY IN THE ACQUISITION OF
AUTHORING SKILLS

A. L. Droar* and A. Kennedy**

*Chichester College of Technology
Chichester, West Sussex, U.K.

**Training Technology Limited
Haslemere, Surrey, U.K.

INTRODUCTION

The need for training and retraining in all spheres of economic activity is ever more pressing. Increasingly this implies the dissemination of the skills, knowledge and experience of a small number of educators and experts to a much larger and more dispersed target audience in the most cost-effective way. Interactive Learning Technology (ILT) may be expected to have a significant role to play, yet, despite critical skill shortages in many areas, the take-up of ILT continues to be slow.

In this paper, it is suggested that the slow take-up of Interactive Learning Technology is in part due to the emphasis placed on suppliers on the "cleverness" of the underlying technology (whether Computer Based Training or Interactive Video). Whereas, experienced educators know that the critical issues are the clear definition of training to meet them. The shortage of the skills needed for these activities is a major brake on the application of Interactive Learning Technology. The provision of these skills is not offered by the suppliers nor is it particularly evident in their organizations. Nonetheless this has not prevented the suppliers from pressing the claims of Computer Based Training (and Interactive Video) and succeeding in selling systems to users. The resulting poorly utilised systems have only fueled the suspicion with which Interactive Learning Technology is viewed by many potential users.

It is argued that the provision of a high level of Instructional Systems Design and authoring skills should be a prime concern of supplier and customer alike. Technology project depends on the fruitful cooperation of vendor and client to ensure:

a. The use of well designed, user friendly and instructionally well-founded authoring systems. These systems should provide built-in support for important aspects of instructional design and present a meaningful interface to educators and trainers.

b. The willingness of the suppliers to create (and of the customer to pay for) tailored training courses which build on the customer's pre-existing capabilities (course design, presentation skills, etc.). Such a course would cover the full range of needs from front-end analysis through detailed courseware design and authoring to initial authoring case studies. Furthermore, the vendor should be prepared to follow the logic of his own sales-talk and present these courses as on-line training packages.

c. The development by the customer of a project plan which carefully integrates training on a phased basis. This would ensure that relevant Instructional Systems Design and authoring skills are acquired at the time they are needed and can be put to immediate productive use.

OVERVIEW OF THE CHICHESTER COLLEGE OF TECHNOLOGY PROJECT

The project is being jointly funded by West Sussex County Council and the European Social Fund. It uses both MicroPLATO and MicroTICCIT systems, and started in September 1984 and is expected to complete in 1986.

Its major aim is to develop a variety of computer based education and training material to assist young people of lower aptitude and motivation in their transition from school to work. The material must be in such a form as to allow users to select any subject matter which may interest them. The objective is to help them to choose an area in which either to seek employment or to take some form of vocational training at a college such as the one at Chichester.

Thus the material developed must be as interesting and creative as possible. We must catch the student's interest. If we do not succeed in this, the student will not even look at our material, and so no training can possibly take place! Consequently, there is a large element of "marketing" in the project.

Furthermore it is also hoped that some of the skills that the students learn from our courses will be of more general use, independent of whether a job is sought in that area. For example, the completion of a cheque should be of use both to a potential bank teller, and also a user of a bank's services.

To this end, the project will cover a number of curriculum areas. These are:

a. Office Skills. The traditional office skills are covered, for example, typing, filing, organising meetings, etc. Also included is the more modern use of word processing equipment.

b. Information Technology. A wide range of possible uses of Information Technology are reviewed and the meaning of "information" is discussed. In addition, an introduction on how to use computers is presented, in particular, programming in the BASIC language.

c. Money Services. This area largely concentrates on the various financial facilities available through the major banks in the UK. It also includes some of the financial processes that would be used in a small company, and gives some simple economic theory as background. As an aid to the various calculations involved, there are lessons on how to use an electronic calculator.

d. Basic Electro-Technology. An introduction to the world of electronics is presented, starting with the development of communications systems down the ages. This is then expanded into modern systems such as radio and TV. Basic ideas on circuits, their design and some of the theoretical background is also presented.

e. Car Mechanics. All of the major systems and subsystems in a car are covered, together with details of how each works. In addition, some more specialized topics are discussed e.g., the aerodynamic shape of a car body.

f. Home Maintenance. The main emphasis here is on those tasks which an ordinary house-holder would tackle rather than the do-it-yourself fanatic. Thus topics such as simple plumbing, painting and decorating, etc., are covered. Also some aspects of interior design are included.

g. Food Services. An overview of the whole range of the catering industry is presented, from serving a customer in a restaurant, through the preparation and presentation of food, to health and safety in the kitchen. Other topics include the digestive system and the need for a balanced diet.

h. Community & Health Services. A number of relatively disparate topics are covered in this area, the common factor being that they are all useful when working in the community. The subjects covered include, first aid in the home, nursery nursing, and planning the family's diet.

i. Job Seeking Skills. Most of the skills required when looking for a job are covered, including, how to decide on a career, where to look for information, how to complete an application form, what to ask at an interview, etc.

j. Building Construction. Overviews from this vaste curriculum area are included ranging from how to choose a building site, through the planning required, to the actual construction phase. In addition, there is a section on the historical development of buildings and dwellings, together with why "shelter" is a basic need of man.

k. Remedial English. Although it was originally envisaged that this topic would only be covered via "HELP" frames from other areas of the curriculum, it has been extended into an area in its own right. A number of aspects of the English language are covered including: its origin and structure, various specialised vocabularies, and puzzles and word games to enhance the usage of English.

l. Remedial Mathematics. Like the remedial English this curriculum has also been extended into an area in its own right, and covers subjects ranging from simple arithmetic operations on integers, through the use of more common units of measure, to more sophisticated examples of the practical use of mathematics.

Within each of the above areas, courseware will be produced which will enable students to sample any of the material in any order they desire. It is envisaged that this will help them to decide on which vocational areas are of particular interest. In addition, the courseware will provide more detailed training so that the student can study a particular area in greater depth if necessary.

As mentioned previously, the courseware is being developed using two computer systems:

   a. The microPLATO system supplied by Control Data Limited

   b. The microTICCIT system supplied by Training Technology Limited

Both of these systems have the capability to use interactive video, which some of the courseware developed will take advantage of.

Each curriculum area will be developed on the system which is most appropriate for that particular area. The trade-offs relate to presentation quality, use of video, the skill of the author in relation to the complexity of the authoring system, etc.

Ultimately, it is envisaged that the courseware will be able to be delivered on a small stand-alone computer, such as, for instance, an IBM Personal Computer.

THE PROJECT TEAM

The project team consists of 2 full-time members and 15 part-time members. The part-time members of the team have varying amounts of relief from their normal teaching activities within the College to enable them to work on the project. The team not only includes subject specialists in each of the curriculum areas but also experts in the presentation of graphics and on the use of video.

Team member	Proj. manage-ment	Subject matter expert	DP back-ground	Lecturing /teaching	Presen-tation skill	ISD	Progr-amming	CBT
# 1	_/			_/	_/		_/	_/	
# 2				_/	_/		_/	_/	_/
# 3		_/			_/				
# 4		_/	_/	_/			_/	_/	
# 5		_/			_/	_/			
# 6		_/			_/		_/		
# 7		_/			_/				
# 8		_/			_/			some	
# 9		_/			_/	_/		some	
# 10		_/			_/				
# 11		_/			_/				
# 12		_/			_/	_/	_/		
# 13		_/			_/				
# 14		_/			_/				
# 15					_/	_/_/			
# 16					_/	_/_/			

Figure A. Turning Educators into Authors

On the basis of the skill matrix shown in figure A, the team members can reasonably be termed educators. The Instructional Systems Design and authoring experience necessary to an author requires to be gained.

The education and training requirements of the team fall into four major areas:

a. Introduction of the project team to Computer Based Training, and the acquisition of authoring skills

b. Project planning

c. Methods and techniques

d. Courseware development on the machine

In the following sections the steps taken to meet these requirements are described.

INTRODUCTION OF PROJECT TEAM TO CBT

The initial training task for the project was to ensure that the project team felt comfortable with using the various computer equipment. In addition, they had to be introduced to the general ideas of Computer Based Training, and to the systems or systematic approach to developing training and education.

The good intentions of both the project and the suppliers notwithstanding, the pragmatics of real life played havoc with the provision of training. Suffice it to say that as regards the microTICCIT system, only three days of initial classroom training were possible. This course introduced the team to the computer equipment, and gave them an overall appreciation of CBT. However, not all of the project team was available to attend and so individual training sessions had to be conducted at our home base.

On the microPLATO system, the situation was somewhat different. One microPLATO workstation, (a PCD 110), was already installed on the College premises. It was therefore decided to use this system to provide hands-on training for the team. For this purpose simple courseware design and authoring exercises were developed. Thus, for microPLATO, no formal classroom training was initially held.

However, as one might expect, the provision of training is continuing throughout the project. To this end various short workshop sessions have been scheduled into the project plan at the points where the knowledge is needed.

As mentioned earlier, the project team members are given varying amounts of relief from their normal teaching duties to work on the project. Unfortunately, the times when people are available do not correspond very well. In fact the only time when all members of the project team can be assembled together is on a Friday afternoon. This restriction has made the planning of formal courses very difficult.

This unavailability of the team to undertake the usual instructor-led training has necessitated a self-help, learn-by-doing approach to training. The vehicle for this was a prototype course consisting of one mini lesson for each of the curriculum areas.

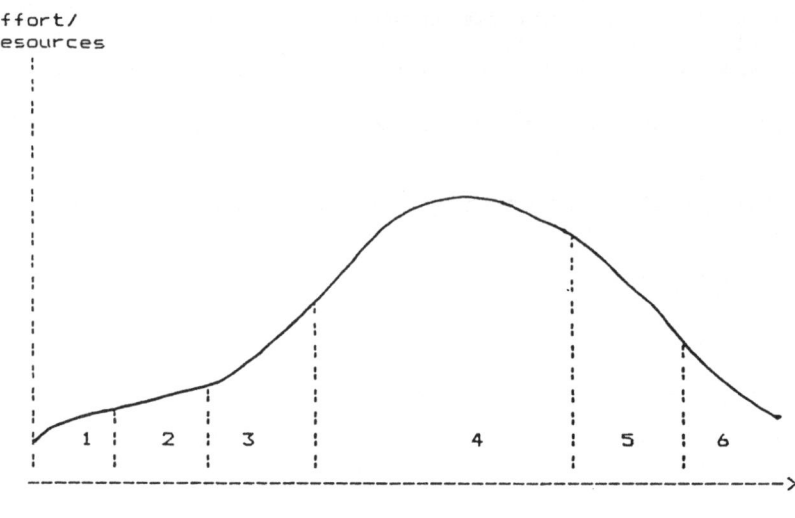

Legend:
1. Requirements gathering
2. External system design
3. Internal systems design
4. System build
5. Test phase
6. Implementation and production running

Figure B. Turning Educators into Authors

This approach enabled the project team to gain real experience of the problems of developing courseware. It also enabled any further education and training requirements to be identified. As a good prototype should, it has also been very useful in reassuring the project sponsors that all is well and it has already been used many times to demonstrate the sort of courseware to be produced on the project.

The main lesson that has been learned from this prototype exercise is that the courseware must be very carefully designed down to a low level of detail. This must be done before it is attempted to enter the material onto the system. Therefore, a procedure and a set of forms has been developed to assist the team in the design of their courseware.

PROJECT PLANNING

Part of the process of transforming educators into authors is to understand the nature of the development process. It is then necessary to work within the constraints of a management plan which defines specific activities with carefully defined inputs and outputs.

This overall plan of the project was based initially on the traditional software development life cycle (see figure B). Note from this diagram that the maximum amount of resources are normally consumed in phase 4, i.e., during the system build stage. However, one of the special problems that had to be taken into account in the planning of the Chichester project is a flat headcount for the duration of the project. This gives the resource usage the shape as shown in figure C. Within this resource profile, the actual phases or stages of the project were identified as follows:

208

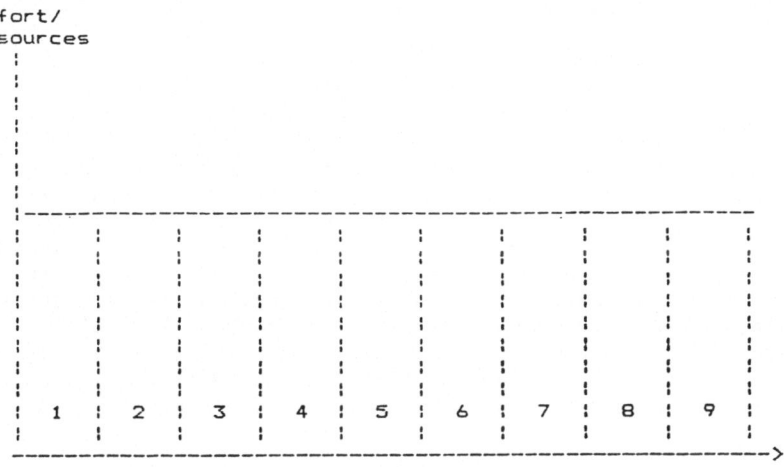

Legend:
1. Staff induction and initial training
2. Curriculum content
3. Test specifications
4. Instructional strategies and media
5-8. Detailed design and entering - a number of lessons per phase using the top down approach
9. Final project report and delivery of courseware

Figure C. Turning Educators into Authors

a. Phase 1: Staff Induction and Initial Training

   - Basic education on TICCIT and PLATO
   - Set up project management environment
   - Initial design of prototype

b. Phase 2: Curriculum Content

   - Detailed definition of curriculum areas
   - Development of learning objectives
   - Detailed design of prototype

c. Phase 3: Test Specifications

   - Overview test specifications
   - Ranking of lessons in order of development
   - Choice of system i.e., TICCIT versus PLATO
   - Entering prototype courseware

d. Phase 4: Instructional Strategies and Media

   - Detailed test specifications
   - Overview lesson designs

e. Phases 5-8: Detailed Lesson Design and Entering

   - Detailed lesson designs - using the top down approach
   - Entering test plus lessons - using the top down approach
   - Testing the lessons - using the top down approach

f. Phase 9: Final Project Report

- Final report
- Packaging of the courseware
- Final test of the completed package

At this point it is worth mentioning that the top-down design and development method is being used on the project. With this approach, a lesson is designed to the point when it is ready to be entered onto the machine. Entering this lesson onto the system then proceeds immediately. Meanwhile the next lesson work then starts on entering the second lesson. This process of alternating between detailed design and work and entering courseware onto the system then continues throughout the later phases of the project. In this way the total courseware package is slowly built up. This is in contrast to the more traditional method of completing all detailed design work before attempting to enter any material onto the system.

At the current stage of the project not enough experience has yet been gained to ascertain whether this approach will be successful. However, initial indications give every confidence.

Some of the problems that were experienced in these project planning activities are summarized as follows:

a. The content of the average courseware development model provided no basis for the development of a detailed management plan for a project of this size and complexity. Therefore is was necessary for the project to develop this detail largely from scratch. Perhaps not enough experience has yet been gained on courseware development projects for a development methodology to be sufficiently well defined and accepted.

b. Highly variable information was available with regard to estimating the various aspects of the work. Obviously, estimates can vary considerably across different organisations and different types of courseware development. However, little useful guidance was available. Thus the project was initially estimated using a development time to courseware time ratio of 50 to 1. This has already proved to be much too low. The current figure being used for planning purposes is 100:1. As the project gains more experience, actual measurements will be fed back into the estimating process, and by this means estimates should become more accurate!

c. No formal project management system existed at the College. Virtually all aspects of such a system had to be developed. In particular, the following reports and procedures had to be developed and defined:

- Definition of Phase Objectives. For each phase of the project a document is produced which defines in detail all the products to be produced during the phase. The tasks required to produce these products are then identified, and allocated to individual project team members. In addition, each task is estimated. This information is then translated into a formal plan for the phase. This document is distributed to all members of the project so that they all know what is expected of them and by when.

- Phase Summary Reports. At the end of each phase a summary report is produced which compares actual performance during the phase with that which was planned in the objectives document. This report includes a detailed analysis of all resources spent during the phase.

- Time Recording. A time recording system had to be developed. This is based on the detailed plans contained in the objectives document for the phase.

- Quality Control Procedures. This includes not only all testing of the final courseware but also the methods for ensuring the quality of the products during the development process. In particular a formal inspection process is being used on the project. All work is inspected by at least two other people before it is considered complete and accurate.

METHODS AND TECHNIQUES

Having decided in overview terms on the contents of each phase, the next stage is to define them in detail. On the Chichester project this was performed by considering each product of a phase and defining what that product should look like, and also detailing the processes by which it should be produced.

For instance, one of the first products that the project had to produce was a detailed definition of the total curriculum area(s) that were to be covered. The format and contents of the required report were defined, and communicated to the project team. In addition, the process to be used to develop the information in the report was detailed. This latter information was presented in the form of a series of relatively small tasks that needed to be accomplished to produce the final product. It also included the quality control process to be used to ensure consistency and accuracy.

To illustrate these points more fully, consider again the development of the curriculum reports. The tasks required to produce this product were defined as follows:

a. Expand on and refine as appropriate the base curriculum as contained in the original submission to the European Social Fund. Note that this submission was of a very general nature.

b. Involve a group of students (as nearest as possible in characteristics to the projected target audience) and, using brainstorming techniques, get the group to produce their ideas on what the curriculum should contain. For this type of project it was felt that as much input as possible should be gathered from members of the prospective audience.

c. From the lists produced above, group the areas of the curriculum into logical major units and subunits.

d. For each of the major units identified in c, identify the skills and knowledge required for this particular area. Repeat this process for all the subunits in the major units as necessary.

e. From d, develop and specify the learning objectives for each major unit and subunit.

    f.   Within each major unit, specify the ordering and relationship of the subunits.

    g.   Produce a draft report. Note that the format of the report was defined in detail.

    h.   Inspect the draft report.

    i.   Produce the final version of the report.

Detailed guidance on all of these tasks was produced. In addition, each task had to be estimated, and scheduled into an overall phase plan.

Note that the skills associated with these tasks are not related to any particular authoring language, but as can be seen from the skill matrix (see figure A), were required to be transferred to the project team. Again more input from the supplier would have made this job considerably easier.

The project plan supposes that the definition of the activities of each phase will have been one of the outputs from the previous phase. Thus not all of the project phases have yet been defined in detail.

This approach to project management has at least one distinct advantage. This is that the lessons from one phase can be used in the development of the plan for the next. Consequently new training and education can be easily introduced as appropriate.

COURSEWARE DEVELOPMENT ON THE MACHINE

The project has as yet limited experience in this area. However, some courseware has been developed (e.g., the prototype) and the areas where further education and training have been identified are detailed below. It is envisaged that these topics will be covered in the various workshops planned.

<u>Definition of Technical Standards and Guidelines</u>

To try to ensure some commonality of the interface between the student and the courseware, some standards and guidelines need to be developed, this would include areas such as:

    a.   Placement/colour of error messages

    b.   Common/consistent use of function keys

    c.   Good/bad practices in terms of presenting information on the screen

<u>The Use of Common Pieces of Courseware</u>

Quite a number of pieces of courseware contain the same sequence of instructions or the same type of approach is used. The examples given in the microTICCIT manuals have been of considerable use here. As the project proceeds and useful common areas/techniques are identified, then these are written up and included in the project cookbook.

<u>Production of Graphics</u>

Both the microTICCIT and microPLATO systems can produce high quality graphics. However, some methods of production are obviously better than others. The project has produced guidance and tips to help people produce the best graphics possible.

Use of Video

The project as yet has had little experience in this area, but again guidance needs to be produced on how best to use this medium.

Detailed Lesson Design Package

As with any computer system development, if you do not have a clearly defined idea of what you want to achieve then you are liable to create many problems for yourself. In order to have lessons defined in as much detail as possible before it is attempted to enter them at the machine, a package has been produced together with guidance on its use.

Entering the Courseware

Lastly, but by no means least, there comes the entering of the courseware onto the machine, and the use of the keyboard, commands, etc. This is the area that tends to be concentrated on in the current education and training offerings. Obviously effective training is required here. The project team has already received initial training plus some hands-on experience, and additional workshops on these topics are being planned throughout the project.

NEW FRONTIERS FOR COMPUTER AIDED TRAINING

G. P. Noja

Gajon Institute of Technology
Genoa, Italy

PREFACE: THE GAJON INSTITUTE OF TECHNOLOGY

The Gajon Institute of Technology, has been the leading Italian institute specializing in Electronics military training since 1949. Its most important activity is the research and development of educational technologies. Main Italian Armed Forces training centers use the Gajon training system as a "standard", while most basic courses for foreign Navies that buy Italian frigates (Lupo Class) are held at the Gajon Training Center.

Each school is provided with complete computer based hardware and customized software for courses that, from basic subjects, lead to final preparation on weapon systems, telecommunications, radar, sonar, navigation aids, avionics, data processing, automatic controls, ECM and ECCM.

Gajon also design "turn-key" training centers in electronics and related subjects.

In the NATO environment, it participates in the feasibility study of NFR-90 under training and documentation section.

In addition to Armed Forces, a minor amount of its activity is dedicated to training of State controlled, highly technological complexes, such as airlines, steel mills, communications and petro-chemical plants, where training problems have some common points with the military world.

Gajon systems are used in more than twenty countries.

The Institute occupies an entire magnificent fifteenth Century castle (national monument) surrounded by a vast park which overlooks the whole city of Genoa and the sea from its high position on the hill and is known as one of the landmarks of the city.

SUMMARY OF PRESENTATION

Starting from the consideration that in our future military environment entry skills will probably become lower and weapons more sophisticated, Gajon has developed a computer based training solution which is individual, and naturally, cost effective.

In fact, computers have been used in training for many years, but with good results for limited subjects only. The main reason for this failure seems to be the passive role of the student who is not sufficiently motivated by the simple contact with the machine.

The system Gajon introduced, combines the programmed learning method it developed for military technicians through 30 years of experience. Thus, the student himself discovers the phenomena and reaches the theory through experiences, and with the possibility offered by today's computer science, gets the advantages of both, in courses starting from basic subjects through the most advanced electronic techniques.

In a classroom equipped with Gajon systems the individual computer gives the student a procedure for the experiments he has to perform, but the student himself has to work on an especially designed desk to set the circuits and to study them, taking measurements and giving the computer his conclusions The computer can evaluate the student's answers, letting him proceed if they are correct, asking him to repeat in the opposite case, adding explanations to help him in keeping his score.

Furthermore, it controls an integrated audiovisual system based on laser videodisc which can automatically show the students films, or can remain connected with the current group of experiments he is performing.

Videodisc combines imagery, high resolution color graphics, sound and animation with the datahandling power of a computer and ease of operation of a touch-activated display screen. This technology provides nearly instant access to information in a format unmatched for completeness of content, clarity and detail, flexibility, speed and ease of use.

The instructor's function has not been cancelled, but exhalted, because through his master station he can control the complete classroom, checking student's work at any step, and helping the ones that really need his presence, without disturbing the others.

Gajon designed a system in which the student has at his disposal two instructors, the computer for the routine, and the teacher when necessary, while he can proceed at his own pace.

Experience in various countries using the Gajon system has shown tremendous interest by the students, involvement of the teacher and reduction of training time up to 50% according to traditional systems.

LIMITS OF COMPUTER BASED APPROACH TO THE TRAINING OF MILITARY TECHNICIANS

Talking about Computer Aided Instruction could seem obvious today, as this kind of machine is more and more influencing our way of life.

As a matter of fact the effort to apply computers to this important field started long ago, probably with Computer Science itself, but if we look deeply inside the results, we can see that these results are encouraging only when limited subjects are involved.

It is not easy to resume in a few words the reasons for this partial failure (which someone can call a partial success), but we think that it was mainly caused by an original vice, still uncancelled: the unlimited trust in the computer as in a sort of magic box, which is able by itself to solve any problem, without taking into account that the learning process is the result of a lot of elements, and that it is not realistic to expect to reproduce this process simply by putting a student in front of a machine.

In this way we can explain the fact that good results have been achieved when, for example, what we call "the student" was a previously trained technician whose aim was to get some particular specialization in his field.

In this case it is possible to get results due to the capacity of the computer to sort information and to show them to this particular student, due to its speed in evaluating his answers and to change accordingly its teaching strategy, together with the limited extent of the subject.

But let us consider another case. Just to keep close to my company's experience, and to my own, too, let us take a student who knows nothing about electronics, and who is supposed to become a technician able to maintain the sophisticated circuits of a Fire Control System.

Even if from a theoretical point of view we can imagine a computer able to manage the enormous quantity of information necessary to achieve this goal, we have to face at least two problems. The first one is the cost of such equipment, which must be able not only to store this amount of information, but also to identify and correct a number of possible mistakes, which is very big due to the vastness of the subject itself.

If, as we mentioned above, it is relatively easy to implement a program to teach a technician how to use a new component or a new piece of equipment, it could be more difficult for a computer to eliminate student's doubts about Ohm's Law, and in no other field as in computer business the difficulty of this problem is increasing the final price.

But the second point is even more important. To maintain and to repair electronic equipment, a technician need more than theoretical knowledge.

What he knows about electronics must be integrated by his ability to use it to solve practical problems; this means to be able to use measuring instruments, to correlate different phenomena and, last but not least, to use his own hands.

Moreover, if the technician we are talking about is a military one, the difficulty of his duty is increased not only by the complexity of the equipment he has to cope with, but very often by the particular conditions he is working in, which force him to solve the problems in a time as short as possible.

To reach this target he needs what we resume in a single word: experience.

But Armed Forces, who need this kind of skilled technicians, are seldom in the condition to prepare them, due, for example, to service reasons which often compel to more experienced people to different positions, but mostly because of the lack of time which is at disposal for training, together with the necessity to send people to their final jobs as soon as possible.

A NEW COMPUTER APPROACH

<u>The Computer as "an Element" of the Training System</u>

These problems cannot find a satisfactory solution in traditional training methods, neither can a computer do it by itself.

However, it can be done in an easy way using a computer as a component, no longer as "the component", of a training system including elements which a computer can coordinate and control in a proper way.

Before starting the analysis of the Computer Aided Training System we are introducing, it is better at this point to take a step backwards, because the system is the result of an evolution taking years, and to understand it completely it is useful, perhaps necessary, to take a look at the intermediate levels of this evolution, which are strictly interconnected with the development of the company which implemented it.

The Experimental Programmed Learning System for Military Technicians and Computer Improvements

The Gajon Institute of Technology, established in 1949 and since the very beginning involved in military technicians training, realized the necessity of studying a new training methodology to solve the problems of preparing skilled manpower at the satisfactory level in a shorter time, and, if possible, at a lower cost.

A basic point is the following one: the student has to participate in the learning process in an active way.

This active behavior can be resumed in two aspects:

1) The student has to reach the fixed level of knowledge working according to his learning rate.

2) The student himself must be considered an interesting teaching resource, both from the self teaching point of view and as a useful help for the real teacher.

On the other hand, the continuous increase of scientific knowledge to be assimilated pushes the students to accelerate their learning rate; but unfortunately, very often the learning rate is slower than the transmission of knowledge.

Deep changes in the methodology are therefore necessary to improve teaching productivity.

Another problem is the growing of the scholastic population; the increase of knowledge in quantity and quality is not balanced by a proportional increase in number and preparation of teachers.

To solve the problem, we have to work towards two directions: a better use of the teacher as didactic means and the realization of an individualized autonomous teaching.

These considerations together with the study carried on learning process, suggested to adopt a "learner centered" method.

The Gajon answer is a learning philosophy different from the traditional one: through a direct experimentation the student is pushed to observe and to analyze phenomena in order to reach the conclusions by himself.

On the contrary, the normal training method is composed of theoretical lessons and subsequent experiments to apply and test the studied concepts.

With the Gajon system the student is brought to discover by himself the laws regulating the phenomena following the same way of the scientists; it is evident that in such a way the student will understand completely the laws and will be able to apply them without forgetting them.

The teacher's task is exalted as he has not only to dictate formulae but he must amplify and deepen the concepts and, above all, help the student to develop his own capacity of observation, synthesis and reasoning, the real bases of knowledge.

The results we have been getting for twenty years employing our special programmed learning method have been satisfactory. However, in the educational field you cannot expect to have reached the top, and that is even more true for an Institute engaged in the training of electronic military technicians.

On the other hand, we realized that there were some problems due to the particular market we were working in: very often, the instructors we prepared in our Center in Genoa, after two or three years had to leave their schools for other destinations because of changes in their careers and it was not easy to replace them.

In our training philosophy, the equipment is important, but even more important is the method to use them, and this is something that only instructors prepared by us know; in our services additional training for several groups of instructors is included, but it seldom happens for various reasons connected to the rigidity of military organizations.

Therefore, we started trying to add something to the system to make it easier for the new instructor to follow our training method.

The solution of the problem could not have been a simple manual, but it had to be something alive and able to guide the instructor step by step keeping him close to the right procedure.

But we were also looking for something so flexible as to let the experienced instructor modify the medium itself according to its philosophy, once he got complete control on the system.

We discovered that a properly designed computer could give a positive solution to our investigations.

Of course, the possibility offered by the computer added to the system to avoid problems connected to the change of instructors has not been the sole reason why we took that decision.

As a matter of fact, the computer aided training is a logical improvement of an experimental programmed learning system as the one we developed; it adds to the system several advantages:

- It makes it easier to have a wider possibility of ramifications, with a consequent increase of self-adapting capability and personalization of the course itself.

- The information can be automatically stored and managed.

- Through special algorithms, the computer can satisfy requests which ask for elaboration (like execution of mathematical operations).

- With some restrictions, answers freely expressed can be accepted and evaluated.

- It is possible to generate files of data, having a fast access to use or to correct them. This is an important condition to have the necessary feedback in the program: the changes which experience may suggest are not so easy to be done if the training means is a manual or a teaching machine.

- Taking into account the previous curriculum (preliminary test results, previous answer, etc.) automatically stored in the memory, it is possible to adapt the sequence of the course to students' characteristics.

Due to the modularity of our programs and to step by step procedure of our course it did not seem difficult to modify them slightly to transfer them in a computer memory.

Moreover, we wanted to take the advantages offered by the development of audiovisual aids, as well. Our instructor should have had the possibility to manage a complete audiovisual set, integrated in the classroom, including CCTV system, videoslides, VCR, while an interactive laser videodisc should have been automatically operated by the computer at the proper moment of the lesson.

Taking into account all these requisites we had to make a first important choice: an intelligent terminal for each student connected to a main computer managing the complete classroom or the whole school, or an individual microcomputer?

We preferred the second possibility, for the following reasons:

- More economical

- More flexible

- Most important, in case of system failure, only one student would have been affected, and not the entire classroom.

We could not find on the market a microcomputer matching all our requirements, so we designed our own; we solved a lot of technical problems, but we think that the results can be defined satisfactory.

THE TRAINING DEVICE

To reach these targets a new training medium had to be designed. In a classroom equipped with our computerized training we have two different types of desk: a number of Student Desks (from 1 to 20) and a Master Desk for the Instructor, connected with multiple lines to each student.

The Student Station: An Open System

The heart of the system is the Gajon desk for training in basic electricity, electronics and advanced techniques.

It is a unique "space - age" stainless steel design, complete "open end" computer based electronics laboratory with an integrated system of circuit assembling, circuit feeding, instrumentation, electronic components, computer with touch screen, keyboard, printer, interactive videodisc player, and bidirectional audio, video and computer lines connected to the Master.

The whole system makes it possible to produce any kind of electronic circuit including complex and professional types.

Most training systems employ pre-assembled block circuits which become obsolete because of the fast evolution of electronics.

On the contrary, the Gajon desk is an open-end system as it allows the greatest liberty in assembling every kind of electronic circuit, also the most complex ones, employing standard or special components.

On the desk even a complete video set or a radar bearing generator can be assembled.

The Basic Desk can perform programs of Basic Electricity, Basic Electronics, Basic Digital Electronics, Basic Communications.

There are also many additional kits for training in advanced techniques such as: electrical machines, servosystems, automatic controls, telecommunications, videotechnique, antennae, microwaves, radar, sonar, digital techniques, computers. These kits are additional components which fit perfectly on the basic desk system.

This equipment practically covers the entire field of electronics but in case of particular requirements, other additional materials can be provided, due to the complete flexibility and standardization of the system, enabling the school to follow any desired program.

These things are the best guarantee that the Gajon system will never become obsolete, saving investments.

Circuits Assembling The desk provides a work surface which allows the assembling of very complex circuits without soldering, using transistors, integrated circuits, microprocessors and any kind of other components (even tubes, if necessary).

The work surface is composed by movable plates which may be taken out with the assembled circuits, leaving the surface free for other students, for multi turn utilization.

Circuits Feeding The desk power supplies give all the voltage values necessary to make the circuits work through an automatic feeding line integrated in the work surface.

All the power supplies are electronically protected against short circuits; an acoustic alarm indicates overcurrent conditions and a control panel shows the overloaded power supply. A digital system continuously scans power supply cards and a coded system warns immediately on the failure of each card which can be substituted in seconds by the instructor.

Instrumentation A low profile and long turret is provided to keep about 30 analog and digital measuring instrument and signal generators instruments are modular plug-in types and range from the educational modules to the state of the art industrial standard 6 channels delayed oscilloscope to keep trainees with the realism of their job.

Electronic Components Common and special components are supplied according to courses to be performed; all components are mounted on standard bases with inscription of type and value. Connections are made with special elements.

The Desk is provided with a storage trolley for components and instrument modules when not used.

Computer Section Central unit: 16 Bit CPU, 256 K central memory, 10

M Bite hard disk, graphics processor, 640 x 400 pixels color resolution, laser videodisc controller, text/graphics overlay on videodisc imagery, touch screen interface, external control line to master station.

    <u>Keyboard</u> Alphanumeric keyboard ASC11 encoded cursor, control and special function keys.

    <u>Monitor</u> 12" high resolution color monitor, 80 columns by 25 lines, 640 x 400 color pixels, 0.31 mm. dot pitch; touch activated screen.

    <u>Printer</u> Ink-jet; replaceable 12 dots head, 150 cps, extremely silent, friction and tractor feed, single pages or normal telex paper.

    <u>Videodisc Player</u> Laser videodisc, 54.000 images for each disk side, single frame fast access, segments, dual languages; in alternative OMDR laser videodisc, recordable, 22.000 images.

<u>Bidirectional Lines:</u>

- Audio. Direct and private communication between student and instructor; headset with microphone.

- Video. Reception of video images from Master or pick up by Master of student image.

- Computer. Computer request of help from student; master permission at any necessary step.

<u>The Instructor Station: A Complete Control of Classroom Activity</u>

    The instructor station (master), which has the same size as the student desks, is equipped with a sophisticated system which allows complete control of the classroom, through three channels: bidirectional video/channel, to send video images coming from video camera, overhead projector videocassette player or videodisc, or to transfer student video image to instructor; computer progress control channel, which allows complete control over progress of the student.

    Controls are individual, group and overall.

    Instructor station, is also equipped with same student computer and peripherals; furthermore, it is a lesson production center, where anyone with no knowledge of computer programming, is able to modify Gajon lessons, prepare his own lessons and transfer them immediately to students.

    On the front panel, there are all digital interfacing with the student Desks and a 9" monitor used by the teacher to preview audiovisual programs.

    On the surface there are 4 keyboards, printer, and a transparent crystal used as an overhead projector thanks to the CCTV camera placed on top of the crystal.

    Slides are projected on the same crystal from the slide projector placed underneath, allowing the pick-up from the CCTV camera.

    In the trolley beside the desk are mounted the videodisc and the video cassette recorder and a storage area is provided for videocassettes, transparencies and slides cartridges.

The Desk includes:

- front panel with all controls
- 12" CRT video graphic alphanumeric display
- 9" CRT monitor
- alphanumeric keyboard
- electronic symbols graphic keyboard
- special functions keyboard
- numeric keyboard for graphics production
- computer and interfacing facilities
- audio/video intercom
- CCTV camera
- slide projector
- video cassette recorder
- laser videodisc
- printer

Monitors and computer are plug-in modules, allowing quick substitutions in case of breakdown.

The computer is provided with an autodiagnosis board to reduce trouble-shooting time.

There are some differences between the student's computer and the teacher's one.

Additional keyboard and software control functions allow the teacher to generate special graphic characters, to prepare lessons and to dump them on disk.

A very interesting feature offered by our master computer is the possibility for the teacher to modify the standard programs we supply together with the system, or to write brand new programs even if he is not a computer programmer.

To make it possible we developed an authoring language and to solve the problems usually connected to graphic programs , we designed a special graphic keyboard.

To each key of the last a graphic electronic symbol or a part of a symbol are corresponding in the computer memory.

If the teacher needs an electronic symbol to draw a circuit on the screen, what he has to do is simply press the key corresponding to it.

If the symbol he needs is composite, it means composed by several parts on different keys, he can press a special sequence key corresponding to that symbol and automatically the computer will collect the single parts to draw the complete symbol.

Two symbols correspond to each key; the choice is made by pressing one of the two function keys, the yellow or the green one.

Naturally the Instructor can modify the graphics characters at his desire; 126 different graphics are available for each single lesson.

<u>The Portable System</u>

The system is available as standard size for fixed installations, or portable, with miniature master and laboratories, which can be installed in a few minutes, through a small and flexible 16 line cable, which from the Master Station provides student laboratories with AC line, audio, video and computer channels.

One outlet is sufficient in the classroom to feed from the Master all student laboratories. A typical classroom contains Instructor station and from ten to twenty student sets.

This solution has been envisaged whenever, special school changes or immediate need is an important factor. A small van for transportation of an entire classroom, and a long table or a series of tables measuring no more than 5 meters by 1.6 meters total are sufficient to have a 12 student plus one master set-up.

While the operating system of the portable classroom is nearly the same as the fixed model, some differences must be found in the student station:

- Circuits Assembling. Reduced supplies; electronic protection but no digital scanning on cards available.

- Instrumentation. Fixed miniature instruments provide basic range of necessary measurements: 4 trace oscilloscope, voltmeter, ammeter, V.O.M., digital meter, frequency meter, digital reading, function generator, digital reading RF generator, clock generator.

- Electronic Components. Fit directly into the breadboards and are stored inside the cover.

- Computer Section. Same as fixed model with 9" CRT, or lower grade computer for reduced performance (CBM SX-64 has been used successfully).

- Videodisc Player. Same as fixed model.

- Bidirectional Lines. Same as fixed model, except for computer line, which does not exist in case of lower grade computer.

As far as the Master is concerned, there are no major changes, if not in the dimension and the absence of the video slide projector.

Both Master and Student Stations measure a minimum 70 x 40 x 25 cm., are foldable and have handles for easy transportation. Weight is 30 Kg. each.

THE GAJON COMPUTER BASED SYSTEM AT WORK

The philosophy of the training method is unchanged: the student has to work on the desk, making his own practical experiences and reaching the laws which regulate the phenomena correlating his observations and the measures he can take.

At any step the student is guided by his own computer.

In fact, as we mentioned above, each student desk is provided with processor with all peripherals.

The instructions for the student and the graphical representation of the circuit he has to assemble appear on the screen controlled by the computer.

This special display can be used as a graphic terminal for the computer and also as a normal video screen for the audiovisual aids, with text and graphics overlay on videoimages.

Through the keyboard and touch screen the student gives the data to the computer about the measurements he has done on the circuit, answering the questions the computer asks him.

In the student computer memory the complete sequence of the experiments has been stored together with the numerical results of the experiments; the student must perform them according to the instructions received from the computer.

A program makes the comparison between students' results and the right ones in a range of approximation.

If the student's answer is correct, through the display the computer shows him the next experiments to be performed; in the opposite case it asks the student to check again the circuit and to set it up in the correct way.

If the results remain incorrect, automatically the computer sends the student additional information to perform the lesson correctly. If the answers are still wrong, the computer will call the teacher through the computer line.

At the same time the computers keep the score of the student, which will be a part of his curriculum.

To complete the subject the student is studying, the computer automatically shows him short films or slides on the display, through the videodisc.

The computer system is controlled by the master desk.

At any moment the instructor can copy on his screen what is appearing on the student's one and vice versa; he can also verify the individual score or the score of the complete class to check the general progress.

In such a way, the teacher may also give his judgement about the student's progress if it cannot be resumed by a simple numeric answer.

As the lesson goes on, everything the student writes is printed on paper automatically, so that at the end of the course each student will have his personalized manual.

The student proceeds at his own pace, according to his learning capability. The proceeding of the course is the best available, because it has been prepared by the Gajon specialized instructors, starting from entry level up to the requested target.

In this way each student has an instructor at his own disposal, the computer. Teacher's function is not cancelled, but exalted, because him aim will be to help the student where the computer, as a machine, cannot succeed without being bothered by routine explanations; it will not be necessary to keep the marks of each student, because this is done by the computer.

The time the teacher can use to perform new research has been increased and he can modify the program whenever it is needed.

In fact, as we mentioned above, he can change the programs in the computer memory by simply typing the new lesson on the keyboard, even if he does not know anything about computer programming, due to the special microprogrammed keyboard he has got at his disposal.

THE AUTHORING LANGUAGE

Most important for the above purpose, Gajon developed its own authoring language which permits the composition in "real time" of any lesson, including graphics, questions, answers, student score, video control, master call and any other necessity.

In fact, we felt that there was no sufficient advantage for a military school in utilizing a computer based system, if the same school could not have the possibility of eventually producing its own programs, utilizing its "non programmer" instructors.

The consideration we made was simple: usually programmers do not know how to teach and teachers do not know how to program; so the choice was compulsory: the programming language had to be simple enough to be used by any person and powerful enough to allow a true transfer of knowledge from instructor to student.

Such a language was not available, so we had to design it and, as far as we know, it is the only language available today, which allows a person to type any lesson using the computer like a normal typewriter, thus composing lessons in "real time", but adding all features of a full interaction.

To achieve this goal, first of all we had to determine a standard for the development of a lesson of electronics; using our experience we chose a format of 8 video pages. Then we divided each page from 1 to 9 windows, for a total of 72 windows, which were to be treated separately, containing text, fixed and moving graphics, completely interacting step by step with student answers, with continuous student evaluation, final lesson marking and control of images coming from videodisc player, this also interacting with student answers.

In electronics lessons detailed graphics are a "must", so we added to the ASC11 keyboard an additional one, containing 63 keys with a shift key, which produces 126 very high resolution, (256.000 pixels), electronic symbols for each lesson. As the graphics symbols are loaded for each lesson and are not necessarily equals, we have 126 x n lesson symbols (practically we use more than 500 electronic symbols, that are permanently stored in the memory).

Moreover, we added a special numeric pad, which addresses directly locations of memory and produces graphics symbols at desire, simply filling data in a single or composite matrix.

At the end, we added a function keyboard, which facilitates instructor operations.

Let's now suppose we wanted to compose a lesson, say the multivibrator. We push a key marked "lesson"; the computer is transformed into a word processor, which also processes graphics.

We choose any window we want among the 72 at disposal in 8 pages and start writing the title, then we draw the electronic circuit with the electronic symbols keyboard, then we follow by typing components and instruments that should be used, procedure for the assembling of the circuit and execution of the lesson and for each of these points we have the space for the student to write his own observations and conclusions.

In doing so, we immediately see exactly what the student will see and we can appreciate the complete transfer of knowledge. When we have finished, we imagine what difficulties the student might encounter during this particular lesson; then accordingly, we fill a number of windows with additional help, e.g. flowing of the current super imposed to the circuit, additional questions to drive the student to the right conclusion, additional explanations, etc.

Again, we can see in practical terms, what will be real help to the student, composing them immediately, as the instructor thinks of them.

Every time we finish a window, we push the key "end" and everything is transferred to memory.

When we have finished all necessary windows, we write on a line some extremely simple commands that establish the action and interaction of the computer for a procedure, which takes care of all student answers, evaluated one by one and determine the branching to any one of the 72 windows, or even modify current windows, adding sentences, moving graphics or inserting video stills or segments from the video disc.

If 8 video pages are not sufficient for a single lesson, we can add 4 or 8 additional pages, or a branching can be made to other lessons.

A complete typical lesson does not take more than one hour to be fully programmed by any teacher, including graphics composition.

Typical time for an instructor to learn to use the full authoring language is 2 days (without having any previous programming experience.

SERVICE

The Gajon Institute provides some services which has enabled the school to operate with the maximum efficiency through the years.

Preparation of Programs

Specific programs are prepared exactly according to school requirements, both in basic and advanced training. All the programs are based on programmed learning according to the Gajon system.

Teacher Training

Teachers are invited to participate in special courses of pedagogy in Gajon Institute in Genoa or on customer site. Aim of these courses is to make teachers aware of the Gajon programmed learning of all the possibilities of the Gajon equipment. Courses last from one week to months.

Maintenance Technicians Training

This course is designed up to third level maintenance on Gajon equipment and lasts two weeks. With this, the school becomes completely independent.

Long Term Consultant Service

This special service lasts ten years and enables the school to request the preparation of new programs according to its new requirements.

Long Term Guarantee

The Gajon equipment is guaranteed for the period of ten years against

defects of construction and quality of materials. This means that the
school can easily make a financial plan without taking into account unknown
future expenses.

SYSTEM DATA

Tests Performed

Among the various tests performed, one is of particular significance.

The Air Force wanted to evaluate Gajon computer based system. To have
a right base for comparison, in June '82 they divided a course of 20
students into two groups of ten. The course was on Digital Techniques.

10 Students followed the course in the traditional way and 10 others
used the Gajon computerized system.

The examining commission was the same and so was the starting date, the
mixture of trainees and the number of hours per week.

Results were the following:

- Time Taken: Traditional: 8 Weeks
  Gajon   : 5 Weeks

- Theory Output Level: Traditional: Good
  Gajon   : Good

- Application Output Level: Traditional: Low
  Gajon   : Extremely Good

This test does not need any comment.

Typical Performance

One of the main points has been the reduction of training time, up to
50% in comparison to the traditional course. As an example, a course of
1100 hours has been reduced to 660 and another of 1330 reduced to 540,
these courses, aimed at maintenance technicians starting with 8th grade,
included Basic Electricity, Basic Electronic, Telecommunications, Antennae
and Servosystems. Practically speaking, a two year course has been reduced
to one year.

Second point, there is no longer a need of separate instructors for
theory, mathematics and laboratory because everything is done in the same
classroom by a single instructor, if necessary with one assistant.

Normally classes have a duration of three hours a day, which allows the
execution of 2, 3 or even 4 turns a day. Due to the modularity of the
system, each of these turns can perform different subjects, without
disturbing the composition of the classroom. If necessary the same
classroom can perform several different programs (e.g. Basic Electronics,
Microprocessors and Radar) at the same time.

Student Attitude

One of the negative points regarding computer based training, is the
fact that if programs are not well developed or not interactive enough, the
student, after an initial curiosity, loses most of his interest.

With the Gajon system, reality proves the contrary; typical computer automatic request for help from teacher does not exceed 20%. It has often occurred than when a student had a 10 minute interval between his 50 minute periods, he rarely used this facility.

As a matter of fact, it is almost a problem to kick them out of the classroom at the end of the lesson!

The greatest surprise was when a complete classroom, though having the right to a one day rest after an injection, asked to spend their time in a Gajon classroom.

Instructor Attitude

Initially instructors are quite doubtful and intimidated by the system, both because of the apparent complexity of managing the Master Desk, and because there is a remarkable difference between explaining theoretical phenomena on the blackboard and following real experimentation with each student.

However, after the first week, instructors realize that most students are proceeding at their own pace and it is quite pleasant to control by video every single position just sitting at the Master, informed by the computer on student progress and communicating through a private line with students who need help.

Consequently a new feeling arises; the security of having control over the classroom; and more a continuous check on students through the computer leaves him free of the worry of continuous interrogations and personal tests.

However, this does not mean that his work has been reduced; on the contrary he must prepare himself very well for each lesson, because when a student needs his help it may be a difficult intervention on a circuit trouble shooting or a theoretical explanation. For this purpose, the instructor may preview at fast speed with his computer the contents of the lesson and theory, which is usually given through videodisc and videocassette player.

Cost/Effectiveness

A typical complete 15 Student Desks and Master Desk has a value of half a million US dollars. Considering the fact that a classroom is guaranteed for 10 years, we may obtain a cost of 50.000 dollars per year.

In a classroom one can rotate from 2 to 4 turns per day, meaning 30 to 60 students per year; dividing 50.000 dollars by 30/60 students we obtain a cost per student variable from 1.666 to 833.

Considering that the system reduces training time by 50%, there is no minimum doubt that the year which has been saved, costs much more than 1.666 dollars in the worst case.

There are very simple calculations, which do not take into consideration additional parameters, but whatever parameter or expense is added, one fact is evident: saving of money and reduction of time.

And all this without taking into account the superior preparation of a student who, at the end of his course, will have performed several hundreds of experiments and measurements and will consequently manage industrial type instruments and circuits with ease.

THE DEVELOPMENT AND TEST OF A HAND-HELD COMPUTERIZED TRAINING AID

R. A. Wisher

U.S. Army Research Institute
Alexandria, Virginia, U.S.A.

INTRODUCTION

Advances in semiconductor technology are making possible the development of hand-held training aids that can accompany a soldier in a variety of living and working areas. Such training aids can package, to large measure, many of the known advantages of computer-based training (CBT) into a more convenient delivery medium. When scaled down to such a size, the opportunities for CBT use increase dramatically. In a recent Army study (Francis & Levey, 1982), for example, ten hand-held computers were reviewed for their potential as low-cost training devices. The study concluded that these hand-held computers are capable of performing important training tasks. The purpose of this chapter is to describe the development of a device that is dedicated to training applications, present evidence for its training effectiveness in a field setting, and discuss planned changes in its design and capabilities.

The condensation of increased computational capability on a decreased physical area is the cornerstone of microprocessor technology. The development of new integration techniques that involve the compacting of thousands and even millions of circuit elements on a single piece of silicon will lead to shrinking system sizes, expanding address spaces, increasing speeds, and falling prices. This trend towards greater speed, higher density, and lower costs will extend to many product areas. The result will be that for a given level of product performance, costs will be reduced. For training applications, the implications of this trend are twofold: (1) advances will be made in miniaturizing training aids and devices to dimensions suitable for personal use by soldiers; and (2) faster computation and larger memories will enable advances in artificial intelligence to drive the cost-effective design of the smart training systems of the future. The focus of this chapter is the first implication.

Microcomputers and Training

Whatever else a microcomputer may be good for, it is first and foremost a rather powerful computer. It is a general tool designed to satisfy the needs of businesses, laboratories, homes, and schools. The desktop microcomputer, because it is a general tool, is equipped with capabilities that are beyond the need of a training-only application. For example, keyboards are needed if one is to enter text as a response in an instructional routine. In many CBT applications, however, responses are often limited to a small set of keys, such as a four-item multiple choice or yes or no answers. In these cases, the response-limited aspect of CBT renders the standard keyboard an unnecessary feature of an instructional delivery medium. Arguments can also be made against the cathode ray tube, the standard 24 x 80 character display area, and other hardware features standard on a microcomputer. They are of debatable need for a training-only application. Instructional design issues have not driven the engineering development of instructional technology products, with the exception of large scale simulators and training devices. The issue here is not whether these features can be used for training, but rather do they need to be applied and should their costs be amortized by a potentially large training market?

The microcomputer has served well in validating the efficacy of training by means of electronic delivery. Its availability and decreasing cost are instrumental factors in its growing presence in the classroom. But therein lies the problem. The still rather bulky dimensions of the microcomputer and its power requirements tie it to a classroom or institutional setting. In view of the changing technology, this physical limitation will be removed, and personal-use learning aids will emerge. Until the technology is housed in a form that is as available and portable as a book, its full potential as a training aid will not be realized.

With this forecast for technology in mind, the U.S. Army Research Institute (ARI) sought to develop, in incremental phases, a hand-held computerized device dedicated to training. The purpose of the initial phase was to demonstrate a training concept, validate its effectiveness, and then programmatically engineer a prototype that would enable training technology to be made available to soldiers outside the classroom. In September, 1981, ARI awarded a contract for the development of such a device to the Franklin Research Center. One intent of the contract was to have instructional concerns drive the hardware design. Although hand-held electronic learning aids, such as Texas Instrument's "Speak and Spell," have been developed, they lack relevance to military training needs, and they are not designed to withstand a level of environmental impact typical of military training environments. A military-specific training aid was needed.

HARDWARE DESCRIPTION

The initial device developed by the Franklin Research Center is referred to as the Hand-Held Tutor, or simply the Tutor. Housed in a 23 cm x 28 cm x 4 cm rugged plastic casing, the Tutor technology was built around a familiar and useful instructional medium -- the book. An indented molding retained a 12 cm x 12 cm booklet that contained graphics, instructional text, and test questions that would be used in conjunction with Tutor prompts and feedback. (See Figure 1.)

The Tutor hardware consisted of the following main items:

- 8-bit central processing unit
- 32k bytes of read only memory
- Voice synthesis processor
- 32 character liquid crystal display
- 18 key dome-type membrane keyboard
- Nickel-cadmium battery pack
- Printed circuit board with supporting electronics

The total weight of the Tutor device, including batteries but excluding the booklet, was 1.9 kg.

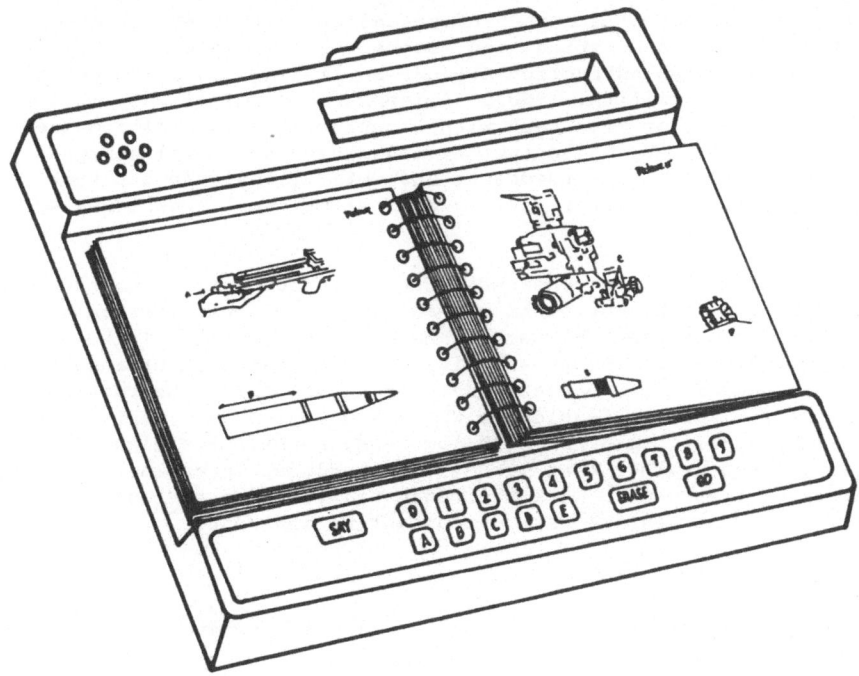

Figure 1. Original Hand-Held Tutor

INSTRUCTIONAL OVERVIEW

Job-related technical vocabulary was selected as the initial training task to be incorporated on the Tutor. Soldiers must know the terminology related to their military occupational specialties in order to comprehend training and field manuals, and to communicate effectively in the classroom and on the job. Vocabulary acquisition is especially difficult for low-literate soldiers, those reading below a sixth grade level. In addition to addressing this training program, technical vocabulary emerged as a good application because there was an ample research literature for computer-based approaches to training vocabulary (Block, 1982). This would force the incorporation of more sophisticated learning algorithms into hardware of hand-held dimensions.

The vocabulary for cannon crewman was selected for the initial field test. Cannon crewman operate field artillery pieces, and regularly deal with words, such as trunnion, lunette, and equilibrator, that are not found in civilian life. Based on frequency counts in training manuals and ratings of importance by instructors, 124 words or short phrases were selected for incorporation into the Tutor.

A decision was made not to seek the single best method for teaching vocabulary, but rather incorporate a number of instructional algorithms into the hand-held device. An important aspect of the Tutor design was the recognized advantages of reserving part of the instructional delivery for a textbook, which was attached to the device. In a sense, the technology would be built around the textbook. Although considered a traditional medium, the textbook continues to serve as an effective, stable instructional system (Rothkopf, 1976). It remains the most widely used, and most familiar, medium in the schoolhouse. Books can condense a large amount of printed and pictorial information. Typographical techniques allow the development of a number of visual stimuli which influence the reader's attention, perception, and memory. For example, the keyword method of vocabulary instruction depends on linking visual images of a word with its meaning (Griffith, 1980). A learner can selectively move through a book, jump ahead, or move back without entering a specialized query code through a keyboard. By balancing the advantages of a well-designed textbook with the control, feedback, and motivational aspects that technology offers, a greater variety of instructional techniques was made possible.

This was important in considering the intended user. Constant use of a single technique might not sustain a soldier's interest over an extended period, whereas a variety of techniques would be more likely to do so. Furthermore, there was the possibility of a trait-treatment interaction, which would diminish the effectiveness of a particular instructional technique for a subset of soldiers who measured low on a particular trait (REF). For example, soldiers with low reading abilities might learn better if more pictures, rather than words, were included in an instructional technique, or treatment. With the range of aptitudes currently present in the military, this feature was of substantial interest.

Instructional Techniques

Three relatively independent but mutually supportive instructional techniques were developed:

(1) A pretest and explanation sequence

(2) Word War - a drill and practice sequence

(3) Picture Battle - matching spoken word to a picture

Pretest and Explanation. The cannon crewman vocabulary was divided into groups of words with related meanings or describing a related set of functions. For example, words used in descriptions of ammunition formed one group such as detonate, fuze setter, and superquick; words that described parts of the cannon, such as muzzle, bore, and tube, formed a different group. These functional groups served as the basis for segmenting the instruction into 25 separate units.

Each unit pretest consisted of multiple-choice questions with 4 or 5 answer options for each question. The questions and answers appeared in the book, and the soldier responded by pushing the appropriate response key on the Tutor. Upon completion of the pretest questions, the soldier was given voiced feedback as the number of correct answers. This number also appeared in the display area. An option to review each individual question was available, with corrective feedback provided for incorrect answers. Research (Rothkopf, 1966) has demonstrated testing to serve as a facilitator to learning, so the pretest was intended to provide a direct instructional benefit.

The explanations for each question with supporting illustrations were presented in the book. The text provided basic definitions for the word with supporting contextual materials. The general approach was to embed the definition in a context that was meaningful to the soldier. Research has demonstrated imagery stimulated by pictures to be an effective instructional technique (Gagne & White, 1978), so pictures were used throughout the text. The keyword teaching method mentioned earlier was also used. A significant technological feature of the explanations segment is the capability to have designated words that appear in the text pronounced by the voice synthesizer.

Word War. This drill and practice technique consisted of groups of ten words and their definitions. The word groups were formed from a combination of several units including the words from the current unit together with words from the immediately preceding unit. A brief definition would appear on the display area. Afterwards, three vocabulary words would appear sequentially in the display area, and be simultaneously voiced. The soldiers task was to select the word that corresponded to the definition. Corrective feedback would occur through the voice synthesizer.

The word war used an increasing ratio review in which an item that was answered incorrectly would be presented again after an interceding item, a 2-later review, and then again after three items have been presented, a 4-later review. Research has demonstrated the increasing ratio review to be superior to conventional drill and practice (Siegel & DiBello, 1980), where missed items are not repeated until the end of the list. The technique reportedly promotes the transfer of the definition from short term to long term memory.

Picture Battle. The soldier views a picture with various parts labelled A through E. After the device pronounces one of the parts, the soldier's task is to identify that part with the appropriate keystroke. A gaming feature was built into this exercise. A special character, shaped as an arrow or projectile, appears on either end of the display area. For each correct answer, the arrow moves four spaces towards a target on the right side of the display area; for an incorrect answer, the "enemy" arrow moves six spaces toward a target on the left side of the display area. The object of the game is simply to destroy the enemy target before the enemy destroys you. Hitting the enemy target is accomplished by a sound effect akin to an artillery shell exploding. The intention was to create an intrinsic motivator for learning in a job context.

FIELD EVALUATION

The purpose of the field evaluation was to: (1) determine whether hand-held training aids would be used profitably by soldiers during the field training exercises; and (2) compare the training effectiveness of hand-held training aids to the training effectiveness of traditional, workbook and pencil methods of instructional delivery. Data collected in the classroom indicated that the Tutor was an effective trainer, in that it increased a trainee's ability to match correctly technical vocabulary items with their definitions. Its real test and ultimate payoff would be determined by its effectiveness in a field environment.

An agreement was made between ARI and the U.S. Army 197th Field Artillery Brigade (the New Hampshire Army National Guard) to evaluate the Tutor during their annual training exercise, held at Fort Drum, New York in May, 1984.

Participants

Ninety (90) soldiers participated in the evaluation. These soldiers were divided into three groups, between 29 and 31 per group:

(1) Technology Group - used the Tutor throughout.

(2) Workbook Group   - a workbook and pencil rendition of the content of the Tutor.

(3) Control Group   - no intervention. Pre- and post tests only.

Each group was attached to a different company of two battalions within the brigade. The groups were physically isolated from each other, and there was no knowledge within groups that other groups were participating in a field evaluation.

Evaluation Method

Pre and post test, a multiple choice format for the 92 vocabulary items available for instruction, were administered by traditional paper and pencil methods. These 92 items were covered in the 20 units of instruction covered in the evaluation. For the Technology and Workbook groups, the pretest was administered immediately prior to the first opportunity to learn from either the Tutor or the workbook. This pretest and initial training time, about 90 minutes, was set aside by the company commanders for purposes of the field evaluation. Otherwise, each group was to find time during lull periods, equipment downtime, adverse weather, breaks, etc., to complete the 20 units of instruction chosen for the evaluation.

The post test was administered on the same day that the participant completed the instruction, or at the end of the 72-hour evaluation period, whichever came first. Evaluation monitors were available to administer the pre- and post tests, and to monitor the initial training period. Throughout the evaluation period, the demands of the field training exercise, of course, took precedence over the evaluation of the training aids. Indeed, the opportunities and inclination to train concurrently on the Tutor while meeting the demands of the field training were of vital interest to the intention of the evaluation. In general, each soldier was entrusted with the responsibility to complete the instructional program according to his opportunities.

The Technology and Workbook group had access to their respective training methods over a 72-hour period. The workbook group actually had increased access, since some of the Tutors were returned during evening encampment for battery recharging, mostly as a precautionary measure against power loss during daytime training opportunities. Nevertheless, each group had ample opportunity to complete the approximately five hours of training.

Results

There were two aspects to the evaluation. First, would soldiers make profitable use of technology-based training aids concurrent with field training, and second, how do such training aids compare to traditional, workbook methods in terms of training effectiveness?

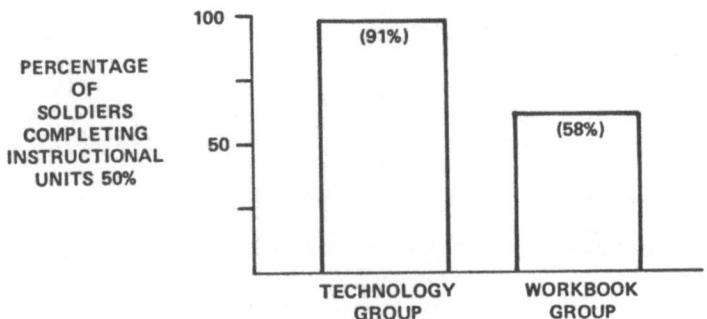

Figure 2. Rate of Completing Instructional Units

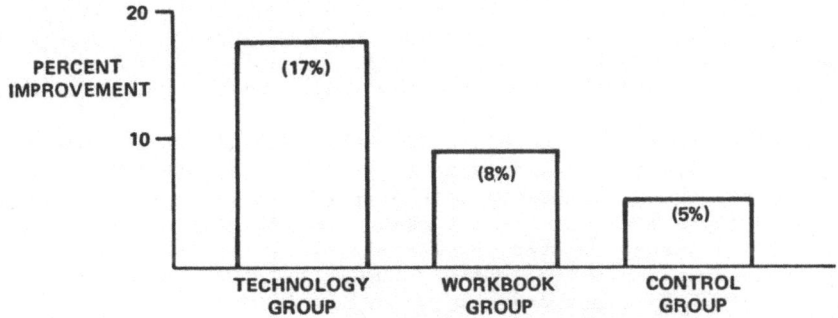

Figure 3. Improvement in Word Knowledge

With respect to the first question, the Technology group did remarkably better than the workbook group: 91% of those in the Technology group completed all 20 units, versus only 58% of the Workbook group. (See Figure 2.)

With respect to the second question, the dependent variable was the difference between pre- and post test scores. Again, the Technology group excelled, with nearly a 2:1 improvement over the Workbook group (p <.06, sign test). The fact that the Control group, which was given a pretest and, 72 hours later, a post test, exhibited no statistically significant difference from the Workbook group (p >.1, sign test) indicated no instructional efficacy of the workbook method. (See Figure 3.)

Discussion

The field evaluation demonstrated that soldiers were able to make profitable use of a hand-held training aid concurrent with the demands of a field training exercise. Moreover, the training effectiveness of the technology-based aid was superior to the effectiveness of traditional, booklet forms of instruction. The soldiers participating in the evaluation had been exposed to the vocabulary items during previous military occupational specialty training for cannon crewman (MOS 13B). It is likely, but not empirically known, that the training effectiveness of the Tutor as demonstrated in the field evaluation would have been higher if the participants had been less familiar with the terminology at the outset of the evaluation. Of course, the same statement can be said for the workbook group.

The 2:1 training effectiveness advantage of the technology, when multiplied by the nearly 2:1 advantage in completion rate, translates into a powerful overall demonstration of the efficacy of hand-held training aids in field training exercises.

PLANNED CHANGES

The Tutor is undergoing electronic and instructional modifications that will lead to the engineering of the CHIP, or Computerized Hand-Held Instructional Prototype. CHIP, then, is a next-generation Tutor. It is also a joint, U.S. military service effort to build an interoperable training aid that can be used by all branches of the U.S. military.

Retaining many features of the predecessor Tutor technology, the CHIP will include a 2 by 40 character display area (1 by 32 in the Tutor), improved electronics and power circuitry (50 hours between battery recharge versus 10 hours in the Tutor), an automatic data collection feature that will maintain individual student information (none in the Tutor), and a data communication capability that will allow transfer of that information. A more durable, unified body will house these improvements.

Current plans call for the delivery of 400 CHIPs in the summer of 1986, with field evaluation for each service to begin the following autumn. Large scale procurement of the CHIP training aid will, of course, hinge on the success of these evaluations, a compelling cost-effectiveness training evaluation, and a strong interest by operational users in determining how a hand-held training aid can best satisfy their training needs that are currently fulfilled by classroom methods.

REFERENCES

Block, K. (1982). "The instructional design implications of some vocabulary learning strategies observed under two methods of CAI." Manuscript, University of Pittsburgh, Learning Research and Development Center, Pittsburgh, PA.

Francis, L. D., & Levey, G. W. (1982, May). "An evaluation of the feasibility of using hand-held computers for training" (TDI-TR-82-2 Final Report). Ft. Monroe, VA: U.S. Army Training and Doctrine Command.

Gagne, R., & White, R. (1978). Memory structures and learning outcomes. "Review of Educational Research," "48," 187-222.

Griffith, D. (1980). "The keyword method of vocabulary acquisition: An experimental evaluation" (Technical Report ARI-439). Alexandria, VA: U.S. Army Research Institute.

Rothkopf, E. Z. (1966). Learning from written instructive materials: An exploration of the control of inspection behavior by test-like events. "Army Educational Research Journal," "3," 241-250.

Rothkopf, E. Z. (1976). Writing to teach and reading to learn: A perspective on the psychology of written instruction. In N. L. Gage (Ed.), "The psychology of teaching methods" (pp. 91-129). Chicago: The National Society for the Study of Education.

Siegel, M., & DiBello, L. (1980, April). "Optimization of computerized drills: An instructional approach." Paper presented at the annual meeting of the American Educational Research Association.

CONSIDERATION OF INSTRUCTION AND TRAINING IN HUMAN OPERATOR MODELS

J. Marguin

Société d'Etudes et Conseils AERO
Paris, France

> "Man is such a complex machine
> that it is impossible at first
> to understand and consequently
> to define him."
>
> Le Mettrie (1748)

INTRODUCTION

   Mathematical models play a growing role in the conception of new systems. Weapon systems are not an exception to this evolution.

   Today, a relatively important number of human activities can be represented by mathematical models in conditions of acceptable realism.

   These models are no longer interesting from their biomechanical aspects alone, but also take into consideration the physiological aspects and notions of the mental load of operators and crew.

   The domain of privileged application of these models is the assistance to the conception of new systems. In fact, it permits, before any realization, to foresee the operational performances of a system under project, taking into consideration the qualities and limitations of the operators who will work time.

   After a brief reminder of the main categories of methods of modeling of human activities, we will examine the main parameters and hypotheses taken into consideration.

   This analysis will result in verifying that the factors connected with instruction and training are practically nonexistent in present models.

INTEREST OF AN ASSISTANCE MODEL IN THE CONCEPTION OF THE INSTRUCTION FIELD

   The cost analyses show that in modern weapon systems, for example a warship, the education expenses represent from 7 to 10% of personnel cost.

This percentage should not be underestimated.

It is therefore important to try to reduce these costs while at the same time improving education.

In order to do this, adequate models should represent a precious assistant.

Another way to reduce education costs is evidently to automate as much as possible, and even robotize the systems.

In fact, if one represents instruction costs versus the complexity of the system one will get the "bell-shaped" curve shown in Figure 1.

Present systems are still mainly situated in the climbing section of the curve. Now the problem of improving education arises and will continue to arise in coming years.

Besides, the nature of education has evolved in relation to the complexity of systems: in fact, automatization starts with the most repetitive tasks in which superior faculties of human intelligence are not particularly necessary. The present tendency is to privilege the faculties of making decisions and of adaptation which are the most difficult to automate.

The tendency to intellectualize tasks makes problems of mental load more and more crucial. At the same time it does not facilitate the task of the modeler, who would logically analyze in detail the processes of human learning, which are not in his field of competence.

In the meantime, this effort of modeling would give some first stages of conception:

- To determine the best economical compromise within the degree of automation of the system and the level of education and training of the operators

- To adapt instruction more efficiently according to needs

- To select human operators more efficiently

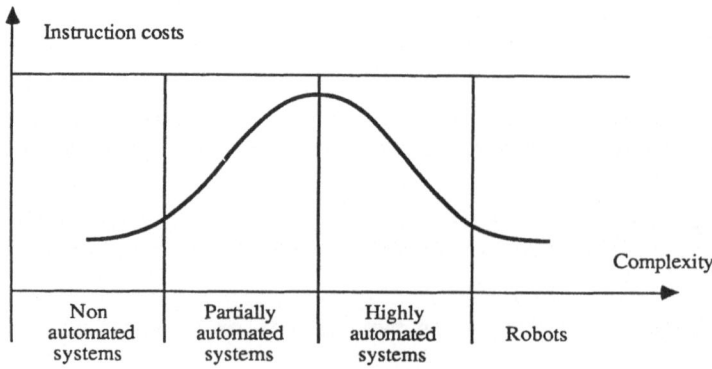

Figure 1

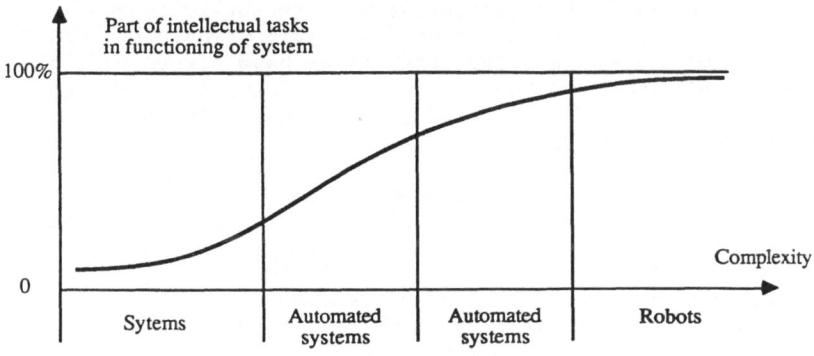

Figure 2

MATHEMATICAL MODELS OF THE HUMAN OPERATOR

For the past fifteen years mathematical models have been used more and more in the conception of systems. In the first phase of studying feasibility and definition of a future system, they are very precious for comparing concurrent technical solutions, for searching for the best compromises and evaluating the concepts.

In the later phases of development, they often avoid trials and building of mockups thus gaining in time and cost.

The prime difficulty of mathematical models is obviously the search for the best compromise within the complexity of the models and accuracy in representing reality.

Usually two types of models can be distinguished:

- Explicative models

- Phenomenological models

Explicative models aim at representing as accurately as possible the mechanisms and actual internal processes of the system. They are therefore primarily realistic, but use an enormous amount of complicated data and are difficult to evaluate. One therefore often tends to use the phenomenological approach still called the "black box" or "the grey box". This approach allows minimum hypotheses on the internal functioning of the system, but tries to represent its "external" behavior as well as possible. This type of model generally simplifies reality considerably, but insofar as it is validated through experiments, it can be used under certain restrictive hypotheses, which must be set out clearly ("domain of validity" of the model).

The advantage of this approach is the relative ease of identification of parameters of the model and the restricted number of necessary data. On the other hand, the domain of validity may be reduced and must be perfectly understood.

In the domain of technical models of the systems, the two approaches are utilized readily and with great profit. Recently progress of technical models has made it necessary to consider the presence of human operators who are an integral part of the complex systems (man "in the loop").

Thus, during the past ten years an activity has been created for mathematical models of human operators. In this domain it is obviously the phenomenological approach which predominates. Strangely enough, it was initiated and led by engineers starting from basic principles laid down by doctors and psychologists. However, the latter have always remained hostile towards this work and have occasionally criticized it vigorously, not realizing that in the domain which concerns us, only the operative value of the model is important.

A detailed analysis of present weapon systems in operation in the Armed Forces has enabled us to draw up ten functions or categories of tasks in which the human operator participates, they are:

- Detection, surveillance, and observation
- Recognition, classification, and identification
- Pursuit, guidance, and aiming
- Communication, transfer of data
- Exploitation of data, making decisions
- Driving, piloting a platform
- Regulating, verification, control, and test
- Filing, putting into memory, registering
- Mobility, displacement of human operator
- Muscular transport

In all of these functions, the effect of modeling is especially based upon visual functions (detection, recognition, identification) and the neuromuscular and biomechanical functions of administering and piloting.

Three approaches have been explored:

- Theory of servomechanism and of optimal control

- Analysis of task diagrams

- Artificial intelligence (algorithmic approach and expert systems)

<u>Modeling through Theory of Subjection and Optimal Command</u>

These models deal specially with the psychomotor activities of operators.

They have been developed and applied in order to represent pursuit tasks and piloting on a reduced number of parameters.

Chronologically, it is the theory of linear servomechanism which was first applied (frequential approach of McRuer & Krendel (1984)). A typical diagram of this model is seen in Figure 3.

The method has been extended and perfected through introducing more recent techniques of optimal control (temporal approach of Kleinman, Baron & Levison (1970)).

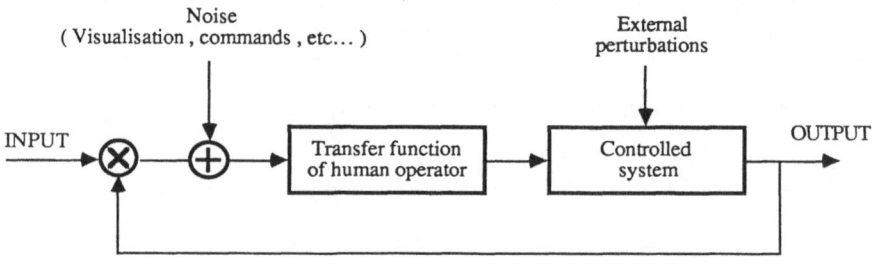

Figure 3

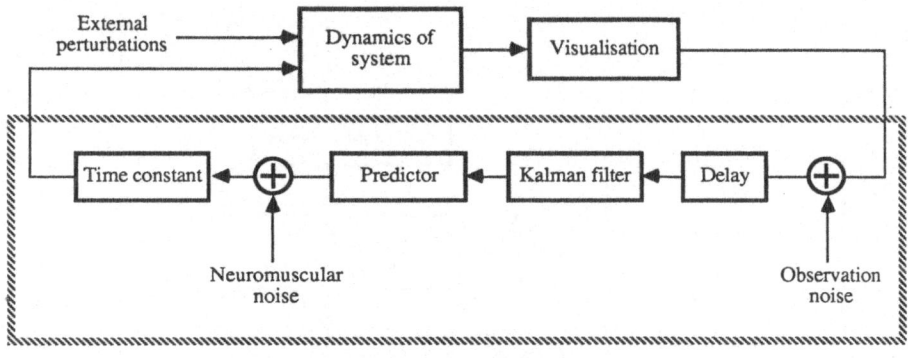

MODEL OF HUMAN OPERATOR

Figure 4

However, this approach is limited to linear phenomena and rarely takes into consideration the facilities of exceptional adaptation of the human operator. Moreover, it supposes that the operator optimises a criterion of root-mean-square deviation, but that is left to be proven.

These models are very useful in foreseeing the performances of the man-machine system in very specific conditions and in an environment with very little disturbance.

Analysis of Task Diagrams

A complex task performed by one or more operators together can be subdivided into a combination of elementary tasks in the form of a diagram. A diagram can emphasize the elementary duration of a task and at the same time the conditions of priority to be respected. This diagram can be treated by a classical method of planification (i.e., PERT).

This method was successfully applied to the task analysis of a project of a combat helicopter (AERO, 1984).

Moreover, the Aerospace Medical Research Laboratory has developed a language to describe human tasks (SAINT = Systems Analysis of Integrated Networks of Tasks; cf. Wortman et al. (1978), Laughery (1984)).

The applications of this methodology are in rapid extension.

Artificial Intelligence

The main disadvantages of the previous approaches is that it does not consider the decision processes which characterize the Human Operator.

The present tendency is therefore to use techniques of artificial intelligence.

Two approaches have been developed:

- An algorithmic approach based upon a branching of decisions

- A nonalgorithmic approach based upon the logic of propositions and expert systems

The algorithmic approach was especially developed in France by Wanner and Soulatges for the simulation of air-transportation piloting (MIOCHE model from ONERA).

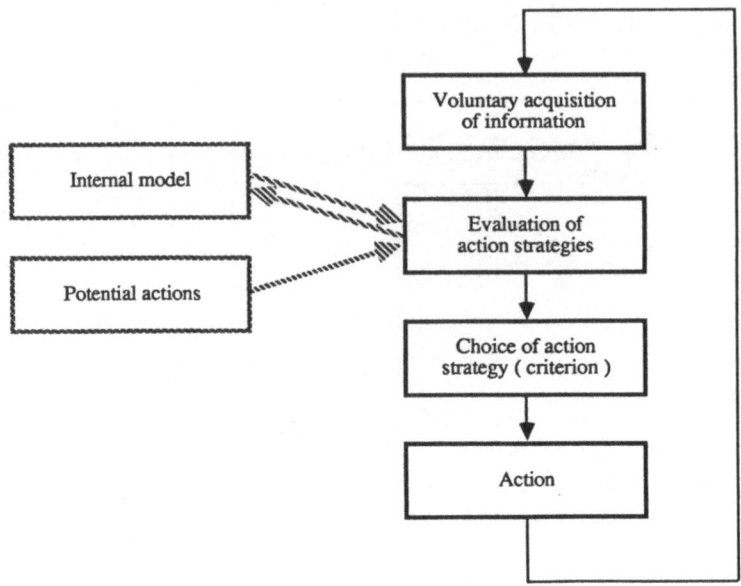

Figure 5

The general procedure is specified in Figure 5.

One should assume that the information - mainly visual - is voluntarily and sequentially acquired. The sequence to acquisition is simulated by a Markovian process, whereby the matrix of transition derives from oculometric measures.

In reference to an "internal model" of the system that is piloted and following a list of potential action strategies in his memory, the operator evaluates the strategies and chooses one by following a criterion, which may vary (minimax, minimum risk, etc.). The action is executed, the system reacts and the process is repeated.

As one can see, this approach is potentially interesting for introducing formation and instruction by modifying the internal model and the strategy list.

In the nonalgorithmic approach (or nonprocedural), one no longer makes a hypothesis regarding the process of making a decision. One just exploits a principle of "production rules" which up the knowledge of experts.

An "inference engine" systematically applies these logical rules starting from information acquired through the senses (facts data base) in order to reach a conclusion. The production rules data base can be the result of a learning process and the facts data base of a sequential or nonsequential acquisition process.

The diagram of this process is seen in Figure 6.

This approach has the advantage of making as few presuppositions as possible about the human operator, but on the other hand needs preliminary expertise which can be very difficult.

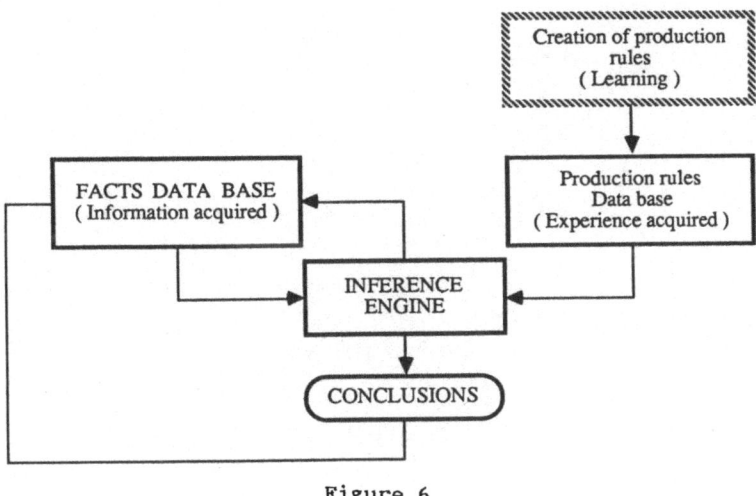

Figure 6

MAIN HYPOTHESIS OF OPERATOR MODELS

The approaches of the modelizing described above are usually based upon three fundamental hypotheses:

- Sequential or nonsequential processing of information ("one channel hypothesis")

- Existence of "internal model"

- "Optimal" character of performance of operator (existence of "criterion" of optimisation)

Sequential Treatment of Information

Many authors agree that the acquisition of information needs a voluntary act on behalf of the operator, except in certain particular cases, when an intensity threshold has been surpassed (intense alarm, for example).

The information would thus reach the "human processor" in the form of temporary sequences. Senders has even proven that the operator proceeds with a visual pattern very similar to the theory of Shannon (cf. Moray (1976)).

Consequently it was easy to suppose that the human operator carries out a sequential information pattern when distinguishing between conscious performance and reflex performance. More precisely, one generally admits that the "operator process" functions in the time sharing in order to deal with reflex information (cf. Wanner (1981)).

Johannsen (1979) sums up this hypothesis with a very clear comparison:

"The conscious planification might be comparable to the execution of an 'interpreted program' while the unconscious planification comparable to the execution of a 'compiled program'."

This purely operative comparison with the functioning of a computer has allowed certain authors to build work load models and to calculate the duration of tasks. These models, confronted with reality, seem to confirm directly the hypothesis of the "one channel hypothesis."(cf. Card (1979)).

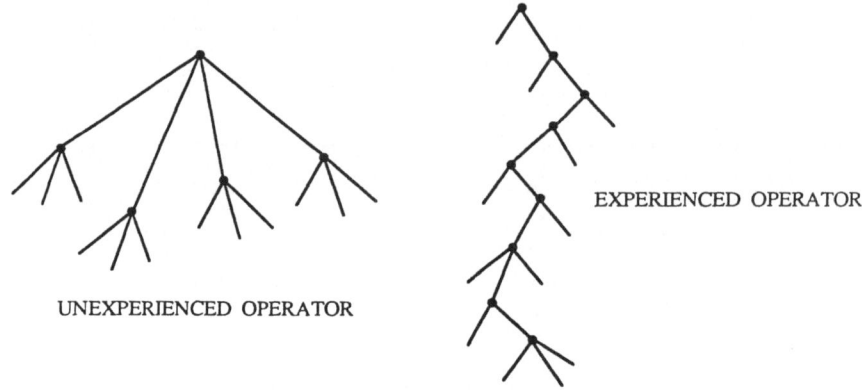

Figure 7

Existence of an "Internal Model"

The studies of psychologists on the relations between memory and work have brought forth the notion of an "operational memory" defined by Bisseret (1970) as a "temporary memory of actual data organized and structured by the work process" (cf. also Speradio (1975)). This notion leads to the frequently used concept of an "internal model" which would be an interiorized representation of the behavior of the "machine". According to Velshuyzen and Stassen (1977) the internal model is made up of knowledge on:

- Machine to be driven (structures, parameters, etc.)
- External disturbances and their effects
- Task to be completed

Soulatges (1976) and Jacacinski (1978), who have applied themselves to the identification of the internal model in relatively simple tasks, have proven that this representation can only have a very distant relation to the actual functioning of the machine.

Optimisation of a Criterion

Linear models suppose that the human operator aims at minimizing a root-mean-square deviation. This criterion leads to simple algorithms, but one has never proven that the human operator had such behaviour.

On the other hand, the branching algorithmic method authorizes a wider choice of criteria. Finally, the approach through expert system, no longer makes a hypothesis of optimality.

HOW TO CONSIDER INSTRUCTION?

We have seen how advantageous it would be to be able to modelize the effect of formation and instruction. However, the present models rapidly described in the section on artificial intelligence do not consider parameters of instruction.

It is clear that linear methods of optimal command are limited in this case, as it would be necessary to correspond to each level of instruction a transfer function or different algorithmic command. It seems difficult to envisage such procedure.

In the method of representation through task diagrams, the instruction level runs through the duration of the elementary tasks. In order to consider it, it would be necessary to define experimental protocols to measure the duration of the elementary tasks for different instruction levels. This procedure is imaginable, but certainly difficult to carry out. The methodological procedure could be the following:

- Numbering of elementary task types in the frame of a certain problem

- Definition of experimental protocols:

    - Choice of a pattern of subjects

    - Measure of duration of tasks during the learning phase isolated tasks or tasks placed in a sequence, etc.

    - Statistical analysis of results to emphasize the influence of learning, variability among individuals, etc.

The methods of artificial intelligence can also be used for determining instruction factors.

In an expert system, for example, the instruction level is directly linked to vastness of the knowledge database (the production rules database). There again the experimental protocols could be elaborated.

In the branching algorithmic method elaborated by Wanner and Soulatges, instruction takes place at two levels:

- Adequacy of internal model

- Characteristics of decision phases

According to Wanner during the course of instruction and training the human operator progressively builds the behavior model of the machine. One should therefore imagine the identification procedures of these models. This pattern would also have the advantage of allowing research of simpler and more efficient models in order to recommend them to the instructors.

According to Kalsbeek (1974) the mental load is bound to the number of decisions to be taken.

For a given task, learning therefore involves a reduction of the mental load. That is translated directly into the structure of decision branching.

An inexperienced operator will explore a large number of ways which will give no results. The experienced operator, on the contrary, for the same work load, will make long term forecasts (cf. Soulatges (1974)).

CONCLUSIONS

Today's models of human operators could mostly consider parameters of instruction. Ways of research have been indicated which could allow one to reach this aim. All of these methods require a better knowledge of human learning processes.

A lot of work is still to be done. This must be a common endeavour of pluridisciplinary groups consisting of specialized systems engineers and psychologists who are interested in the practical application of their knowledge to the domain of technique.

REFERENCES

AERO. "Etude methodologique de la modelisation de l'operateur humain" (Contract No. 77/992). Paris.

AERO (1984, April). "Etude ergonomique du tir air-air helicopter" (Final Report, Contract No. 82/85030). Paris.

Bisseret, A. (1970). Memoire operationnelle et structure du travail. "Bulletin de Psychology," "24(5-6)," 280-294.

Card, S.K. (1981). The model for making engineering calculations of human performance. "Proceedings of the Human Factors Society," "25th," 301-305.

Jacacinski, R.J. (1978). Describing the human operator's internal model of a dynamic system. "Human Factors," "20(4)," 425-433.

Johannsen, G., & Rouse, W.B. (1979). Mathematical concepts for modeling human behavior in complex man-machine systems. "Human Factors, "21(6)," 733-747.

Kalsbeek, J.W.H. (1974). "Prevention of excessive mental load and how can the industrial engineer and the ergonomist cooperate." Conference of European Federation of Productivity Services, Berlin.

Kleinman, D.L., Baron, S., & Levison, W.H. (1970). An optimal control model of human response, Parts I and II. "Automatica," "6," 357-369, 371-383.

Laughery, K.R. (1984). Human operator modeling: A new technology for addressing human factors during design. "NAECON '84 Proceedings," 857-865.

McRuer, D.T., & Krendel, E.S. (1984, January). Mathematical models of human pilot behavior. "Agardograph," "188."

Moray, N. (1976, March). Attention, control and sampling behaviour. "International Symposium on Monitoring Behavior and Supervisory Control" (pp. 160-182).

Soulatges, D. (1974). Theory des questionnaires: modelisation de la charge mentale d'un pilot. "Onera - NT," "230," 31.

Sulatges, D. (1976, November). Prise en compte de certains facteurs ergonomiques lors de la modelisation du comportement du pilot. "Colloque BIOMECA II" (pp. IV-1-IW-8). Toulouse.

Speradio, J.C. (1975). Complements a l'etude de la memoire operationnelle: Deux experiences sur des controllers de navigation aerienne. "Le Travail Humain," "38(1)," 41-62.

Velshuyzen, W., & Stassen, H.G. (1977). The internal model concept: An application to modeling human control of large ships. "Human Factors," "19(4)," 367-380.

Wanner, J.C. (1981). Le facteur humain dans la conduite des grands systemes. "Le Progres Technique," "21," 35-43.

Wortman, D.B.. (1978, July). "Using SAINT: A user oriented manual" (Report AMRL-TR-77-61). Aerospace Medical Research Laboratory.

COMPUTER-ASSISTED PROGRAMMED CASES: A LEARNING METHOD FOR IMPROVING THE UNDERSTANDING OF PERSONS

L. Van den Brande

Free University of Brussels
Brussels, Belgium

In several professions (i.e. army officers, psychologists, educationalists, forensic experts, members of the police force, nurses and others) it is part of the job to be a person with high psychological and interpersonal skills; one has to have an accurate interpersonal perception and a high degree of psychological insight. Assessing the accuracy of psychological insight and interpersonal perception has long been a troublesome area in psychology. The same holds for the training of such skills.

All the processes that play a role in 'getting to know a person' such as person impression, person perception, image-building, person judgement, prediction and person description can be encompassed by the term 'psychological insight'. Psychological insight refers to the individual's ability to understand the personal characteristics and motivational processes of people (Greenspan, 1981). A review of the literature based on a computer-search revealed: (a) that there is no adequate and acceptable taxonomy of the constructs 'social and psychological insight' available (in other words a lack of conceptualization), and (b) that there are no adequate techniques to measure psychological insight (in other words a lack of operationalization.)

The concept of psychological insight has a broad and confusing variety of possible meanings. The only attempt known by me and therefore used is the taxonomy of social awareness by Greenspan .

The term 'social awareness' may be defined as the individual's ability to understand people, social events and the processes involved in regulating social events. In the taxonomy of Greenspan, social awareness (or social intelligence) is divided into three component abilities: (1) social sensitivity as the individual's ability to label accurately the meaning of a social object or event, at a given moment in time, (2) social insight as the individual's ability to understand the processes underlying social events and to make evaluative judgements about such events and (3) social communication as the individual's ability to understand how to intervene effectively in interpersonal situations and influence successfully the behaviors of others. For a broader discussion of the abilities social sensitivity and social communication see Greenspan (1981).

The second major component of awareness (social insight) is divided

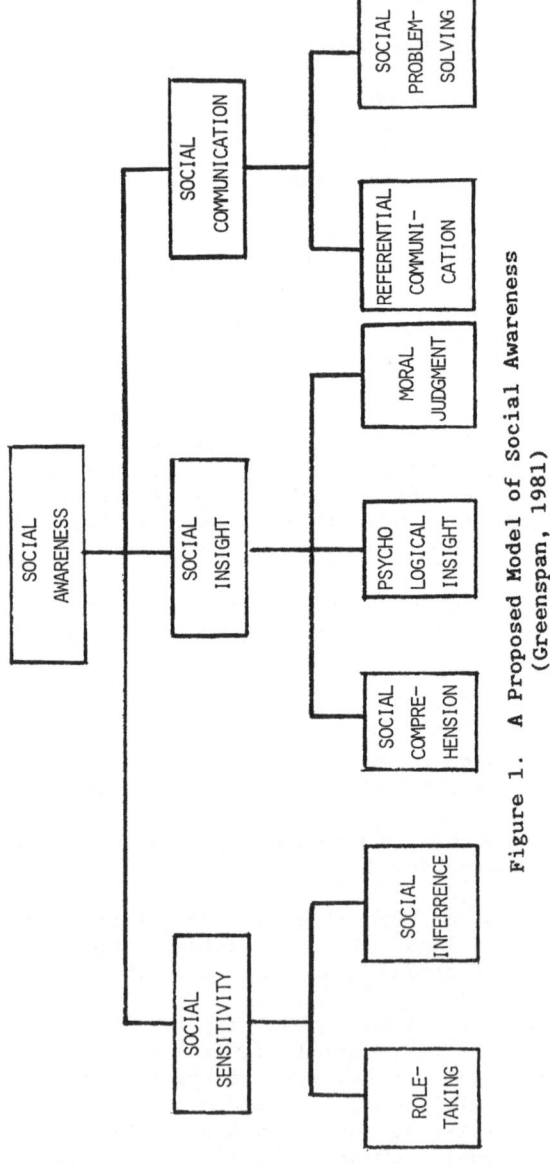

Figure 1. A Proposed Model of Social Awareness (Greenspan, 1981)

into three constructs: 'social comprehension', 'psychological insight' and 'moral judgement'. The term social comprehension refers to understanding of social institutions and processes. The term psychological insight refers to the understanding of people, how they differ from each other (person perception), and why they behave the way they do (person prediction). The term moral judgement refers to the ability to think about social rules and about ethical matters.

In all three of these constructs the emphasis is upon the ability to generalize about interpersonal behavior and events, rather than the ability (as in social sensitivity) to phenomenologically respond to a concrete social event. Such concrete events can be used, however, in assessing social insight. It is just that the question being asked is different. Instead of being asked to show a surface understanding of the event (what is happening?), the person is being asked: why is it happening and what is its significance in a broader scheme of things? For more details of these constructs see Greenspan, 1981.

The main reason for the lack of an adequate operationalization of 'psychological insight' is that most of psychological insight tests don't deal with a 'genuine situation with real persons' (Thorndike, 1920). Most of the psychological insight measures have been modeled after traditional tests (mostly intelligence tests) which are primarily composed of items that are abstract, decontextualized and have little or nothing to do with one's actual competence in real-life social situations. Studies in the accuracy of interpersonal perception used to set subjects the 'guess the quantity of a trait' task (McHenry, 1968). In the 'guess the quantity of a trait' task, subjects are given a list of personality traits and they are required to state the quantities in which these are possessed by certain stimulus persons. Often a comparison is then made between the subject's judgement and the stimulus person's view of himself. In the 'guess what he would write' task a stimulus person is required to fill in a personality inventory and it is the task of subjects after meeting him or seeing him on film to fill in the same personality tests as he thinks the stimulus person did. But these interpersonal judgements which as the subject one asked to make in the laboratory are not similar to those he is used to making in everyday life.

In complex problem tasks like the task 'getting to know and judge accurate a person' are the actors an active element in a complex network of active and passive elements (Dorner et. al., 1984). The reality wherein the actors act is:

(1) Complex: there is a lot of information available.

(2) Intransparent: a lot of necessary information is not available.

(3) Self dynamic (eigendynamisch): the situation and the other persons are active and autonomous (selbstbewegend).

There has been in recent cognitive psychology and problem solving psychology research on problems of a whole other kind: the problems are very simple, transparent and static (for instance the prisoner's dilemma). As a consequence, most of psychological research is totally inadequate for the analysis and the understanding of complex problems and especially complex social problems.

As Ford and Tisak (1983) clearly stated, a measurement approach is needed in which the behavioral effectiveness criterion for defining psychological insight is translated into precise, relevant and practical operationalizations of the construct which retain at least some of the richness and meaning of real-life social interactions. So what is needed in order to study psychological insight is a task that deals with the behavior of real persons and which have a biography. In others words, a 'what he would do' task. The technique of the programmed cases refers to such a task.

Not only assessing the accuracy of psychological insight has long been a troublesome area in psychology, but the same holds for the training of such skills.

ESSENTIAL FEATURES OF PROGRAMMED CASES

Programmed Cases is a method constructed by Dailey (1971) and further developed by J.P. De Waele (1971) with the purpose of improving one's ability to predict behavior and increasing one's understanding of other people.

The method of Programmed Cases can be defined as an application of methods of programmed instruction to the study of simple cases (life histories). A Programmed Case is a biography of an individual divided into time-segments, called episodes. The case is presented one event or episode at a time to the subject and the subject is required to forecast the next or following behavior. Each episode consists of two data: (1) situational data and (2) five possible reactions, behaviors, attitudes of the person upon the situation. For example:

Situational Data:

> During his military service he gains the confidence of his lieutenant because he is the only married man and already has two children. He becomes the confidant, shows himself to be very discrete and is appointed as telefonist. This gives him the opportunity to render some services concerning love affairs to his lieutenant. At the end of his military service, the lieutenant becomes interested in the future of X. As X has no fixed goals, the lieutenant advises him to apply for a job with the police. What will X do?

Five Different Reactions:

(1) He does not accept the lieutenant's offer and returns to his former employer.

(2) He prefers to stay in the army.

(3) He applies for a position in the police force and is accepted.

(4) He starts taking a course in electronics.

(5) He applies for a job as an electrician in the city services.

While an information of an event is always real, there is one and only one real reaction of the person. The task of the subject consists in predicting the really happened behavior of the described person on the basis of the given information. Then the subject is informed as to which of the five reactions did in fact occur.

It is assumed that informing the subject of the truth of each forecast permits him to accumulate information about the person and that accuracy of forecast in a case indicated the subject's understanding of the case.

CONSTRUCTION OF PROGRAMMED CASES

To construct a programmed biography, the investigator uses single-case data collected in an intensive and idiographic study. De Waele in his article about the Brussels Method (1976) stated that for a systematic personality assessment the convergent use of four approaches is required:

(1) The autobiography is the first step which must enable the person to give his definitions of his present and past situations and his self and other conceptions within his own time perspective.

(2) Direct observation of behavioral patterns in various institutional or social settings.

(3) The social inquiry.

(4) Experimentally contrived problem and conflict situation.

These four sources of data are characterized by the fact that they are homogenious because (a) they have to do with common every day behavior and situations and (b) belonging to a world of meanings shared by the person and by the investigator they are accessible to both, and expressible in the same ordinary language.

For these reasons, the data obtained lead to accounts (justifications, argumentations, commentaries) whose correctness and authenticity can be checked by negotiating them with the focal person and various informants. They can also be verified independently by field study as well as the use of documentary evidence.

However, to be coordinated with each other, these four sources of data must be linked to a common frame of reference and must, at least as far as 'first order constructs' are concerned, be integrated within the more or less unified system of cognitive structures manifested by the person. In order to reach these two objectives, a technique called the Biographical Inventory is used by De Waele (1979). This is a systematically organized collection of open questions, questionnaires and ratings which (a) are to be used by the investigators and by the investigated person alike, (b) are systematically linked up with the four sources of data mentioned above, (c) are so organized that multiple cross-references and comparisons are made possible, (d) once they have been analyzed, become the starting point for detailed interviews oriented towards situational and interactional structures and (e) allow for comparisons with other sources of information.

The reconstruction of a biography according to the Brussels Method of De Waele, which forms the basis of each programmed biography is the result of a very intensive and idiographic research and conceived a cooperative achievement between a team which ideally consists of about half a dozen people, each bringing to the task a different professional background such as sociologist, psychiatrist or psychologist, and the participant whose biography is to be generated.

This life-history material is then divided into the smallest possible behavior units, called episodes, that are still significant. Under an episode we understand a behavioral event occuring at a particular time and place, in response to a particular situation, to include overt behavior, words and gestures which indicate the feelings and probable motives of the person.

For each episode the case-writer prepares then four distractors: four plausible but fictitious reactions of the person to the given situation.

Before the subject or student predicts the first episode of a childhood event and proceeds the life history in chronological order, he is given some more information about the social and familial background of the case person or participant. The aim for each programmed biography is getting to know the person. In order to control the plausibility of the distractors, the participant predicts his own life-history and criticizes the four distractors.

Until now nine programmed cases have been constructed and predicted by several students in the paper and pencil form: 3 cases of fifty episodes and 6 cases of twenty episodes. For more details about these cases see De Waele (1971) and Van den Brande (1984).

It is also possible to construct a computerized form of a programmed biography. It will be argued below that computerized programmed biography have several advantages both for research and educational purposes.

ON-LINE COMPUTER ADMINISTERING OF PROGRAMMED CASES

Within the frame of a research project at the Free University of

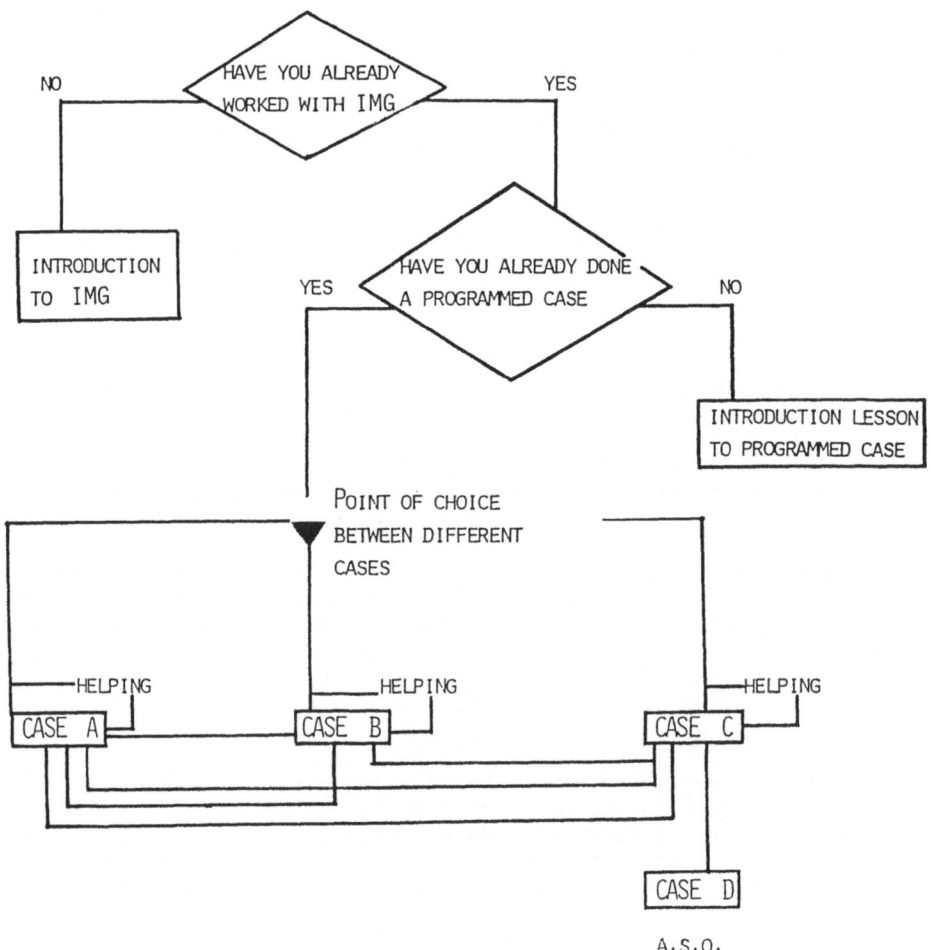

Figure 2. Macro Flowchart

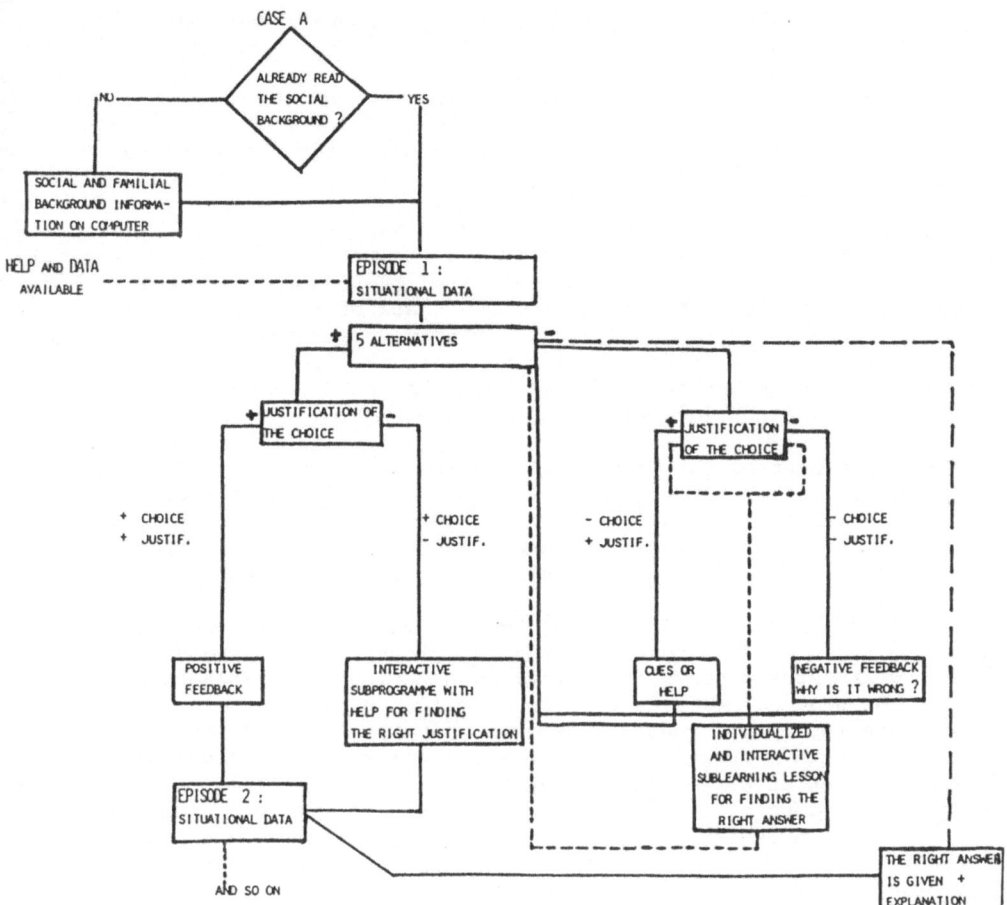

Figure 3. Micro Flowchart

Brussels (Department of Personality Psychology and Department of Education), several cases were designed and programmed by means of an author system: the Instruction Modulator Generator system (IMG). A macro and micro outline of programmed cases on IMG are shown in Figures 2 and 3.

The IMG system is an interactive computer network designed by IBM for computer-based instruction for noncomputer specialists like educationalists or psychologists, so no computer background is needed. The IMG system has been especially designed to facilitate the two major aspects of computer based education: Computer Managed Instruction (CMI) and Computer Assisted Instruction (CAI):

(1) Computer Managed Instruction. The software for CMI on the IMG system allows testing of students, routing of students to appropriate lessons and recordkeeping routines that keep track of the lessons the student has completed.

(2) Computer Assisted Instruction: The actual lessons used for CAI or for CA research on IBM are constructed using the IMG system. This system is particularly powerful for:

  Displaying textual and graphical material

- Inputting and judging students responses and controlled branching through the program

A programmed cases courseware is started by two introduction lessons, one to the system IMG and one to the method of P.C. Then the students are routed to appropriate cases, depending upon the interests, background, study of the student, and others.

The micro outline shows the structure of one single episode. First of all the subject reads the situational data and tries to predict the really happened behavior of the described person on the basis of the given information. At the left you can see the track of the student when his choice was right. He is asked for a justification. When the choice and the justification are right, he is given positive feedback. But when his justification is wrong, he is routed to an interactive subprogram with help for finding the right justification.

The right part of the outline is the track of a student who has made a wrong choice. After a second mistrial, he is routed to an individualized and interactive sublearning lesson for finding the right answer depending on the answers on the episodes before. So the feedback is different for each person. After a third mistrial, he is given the right answer.

The most important advantage of CPC composed to paper and pencil administering are the interactive and individualized responses. The student works at his own pace. After each choice and justification of that choice, the student receives feedback namely cues, suggestions or exercises to do it better. This feedback depends upon the followed route of the students through a programmed case. Besides interactive and individualized responses, sophisticated graphic capabilities ranging from line drawings to animation are possible. Also microfiche facility available which involves the backscreen projection of images into the terminal, e.g. of a problem and conflict situation and interaction is possible among terminals for predicting programmed cases in group.

So the advantages of CPC compared to paper and pencil administering are: (1) automatic collection of student data by storing student records, responses and scores, (2) control of presented information and randomization of potential variables such as order of presentation, (3) routing of students to appropriate lessons and recordkeeping routines that keep track of the lessons the student has completed, (4) interactive responses, (5) individualization: the student works at his own pace, (6) product and process evaluation, (7) sophisticated graphic capabilities ranging from line drawings to animation are possible, and (8) also microfiche facility available which involves the backscreen projection of image into the terminal, e.g. of a problem and conflict situation and interaction is possible among terminals for predicting programmed cases in group.

PROGRAMMED CASES AS A RESEARCH INSTRUMENT AND A TRAINING METHOD

Programmed Cases and Computer-Assisted Programmed Cases can be used both as a research instrument for studying psychological assessment, psychological insight and the methodology of single case study, and as an educational tool for psychologists, educationalists and other social scientists with the aim of improving their ability to predict behavior and to understand persons.

Several experimental studies conducted at the Free University of Brussels revealed: (1) evidence that the understanding of other people or the ability to predict behavior increased during a series of cases, and (2) evidence that a learning pattern was discernable within the individual cases. The first findings indicated that subjects were 'generalizing' the results of what they were learning.

The principal aim of that ongoing research is substituting clinical experience by the development of a courseware of Computer Assisted Programmed Cases to be used in the training of army officers, psychologists, educationalists and forensic experts.

Therefore an optimalization of the method as an educational instrument is a primary condition. The series of experiments treated here were related to the following four topics:

(1) Psychometric research: difficulty level, error analysis, item discrimination or validity, item reliability

(2) Learning within the scope of a case: does the subject 'learn' another person in the sense of making increasingly accurate predictions of the other person's behavior as he receives increasing amounts of information about that person. To test the learning within the scope of cases, one may compare the prediction score of all subjects at successive points within the cases. The method used was a correlation between the first fourth (Q1) and the difference between the first fourth and the fourth fourth (Q1-Q4). An experimental investigation (Thewissen, 1967, involving n=29 subjects) making detailed analysis of three cases (AB, D and X) revealed that the Programmed Case Method did in fact result in measurable improvement in the ability of the subjects to make accurate predictions.

(3) Learning between cases: Is there a generalization of this prediction skill of subject from one person to the next? To test for generalization of the skill from case to case, the prediction scores of all subjects at successive points during the series of cases were compared (n = 29) (Sloore, 1967). The correlations between the cases are relatively high, when we take into account that the cases are very different in content.

Case AB $r = + 0.64$
Cast D $r = + 0.49$
Case X $r = + 0.87$

Figure 4. Correlation Between Q1 and (Q1-Q4) (n=29)

Case	first choice	s	sum of trials	s	%
AB (52 episodes)	27.34	8.22	90.76	19.09	52.57
D (56 episodes)	31.69	9.44	93.96	21.32	56.59
X (56 episodes)	34.48	9.38	89.24	18.40	61.57

Figure 5

	r	
AB (1) - Dr (2)	+ .73	(p = 0.001)
AB (1) - X (3)	+ .64	(p = 0.001)
DR (2) - X (3)	+ .77	(p = 0.001)

Figure 6. Correlations Between the Cases

	cognitive complexity (n=29)	ego identity (n=29)	examens in (n=29)		
				MATH.	MATH.
AB+D+X	+ 0.05 (ns)	− 0.11 (ns)			
AB	+ 0.03 (ns)	− 0.05 (ns)	+0.02 (ns)	0.00(ns)	0.27(ns)
D	+ 0.11 (ns)	− 0.16 (ns)	−0.11 (ns)	−0.21(ns)	−0.01(ns)
X	− 0.00 (ns)	− 0.06 (ns)	−0.13 (ns)	−0.27(ns)	0.00(ns)

	Vocabulary	Cattell (n=80)
AB+D+X	−	− .12 (ns)
AB	−0.13 (ns)	− .25 (ns)
D	−0.15 (ns)	− .15 (ns)
X	−0.19 (ns)	+ .01 (ns)

Figure 7.

(4) No significant correlation was found between programmed cases and cognitive complexity (REP-test), ego identity of Kelly test, exams, vocabulary test and intelligence (Cattell).

However, these results can be criticized on several points and further research is necessary. It can already be concluded that subjects do 'learn another person' if the data are programmed as in this experiment and that there is a measurable degree of generalization of this skill to other cases. The implication for education is that something may, indeed be learned from the case method.

The second line of research was gaining new insights in the field of conceptualization and judgement of persons.

Four steps showed to be essential in predicting Programmed Biographies:

(1) Noting the significant. Significant statements are:

- the ones about the events most likely to influence the future behavior and attitudes of the individual

- the ones that show an action of an attitude that may be characteristic of the individual

(2) Interpreting the data by questions like "What is this person trying to do?", "What kind of approach does he take in trying to do it?"

(3) Forming the image: an observer must construct a mental image of an individual so that he will be able to tell why that person acts as he does.

(4) Comparing episodes with the image.

However, further research involving these four steps is necessary in order to answer following questions below:

(1) What should a subject predicting a programmed biography discover? Or an analysis of the tasks of each case.

(2) How is a good performer solving these tasks? Is he using more data and argumentations to claim an alternative? Is he predicting as he moves along a programmed case following a growing

abstraction level? Is he using 'naive' personality theories and if so which one is useful?

(3) How can bad performers be thought to predict more accurate programmed biographies? Research has shown that initial lessons for using adequately the four steps and feedback at several stages, helping the subjects to argumentate their choices and better conceptualize the person, increase the accuracy of prediction with 25%.

On these results, three IMG Programmed Biographies were designed and programmed with a lot of feedback and sublearning programs. In ongoing research (n+40) the hypothesis is tested that subjects perform better on Computer Assisted Programmed Cases than on the paper-and-pencil version.

CONCLUSION

By way of conclusion, it can be stated that a series of Programmed Biographies and Computerized Programmed Biographies constitute an adequate training in the clinical study of an individual case (clinical didactics).

It should be noted that: (1) also psychopathological data can be inserted in Programmed Cases. This would allow to incorporate a training of the DSM III diagnostic categories in a study of whole single persons; and (2) not only biographies but all processual psychological data (i.e., action psychological data) can be the subject of the programmed instruction method.

REFERENCES

De Waele, J. (1971). "La method des cas programs." Bruxelles: Dessart.
De Waele, J., & Harre, R. (1976). The Personality of Individuals. In R. Harre (Ed.), "Personality." Oxford: Basil Blackwell.
De Waele, J. & Harre, R. (1979). Autobiography as a psychological method. In Ginsburg, J. (Ed.), "Emerging Strategies in a social-psychological research." Wiley.
Dorner, D. et al. (1983). "Lohhausen: Vom Umgang mit Unbestimmtheit und Komplexitat." Bern: Verlag Hans Huber.
Ford, E. & Tisak, M. (1983). A further Search for Social Intelligence. "Journal of Educational Psychology," "75(2)," 196-206.
Greenspan, S. (1981). Defining Childhood Social Competence: A Proposed working model. "Advances in Special Education," "3," 1-39.
McHenry, R. (1968). New Methods of Assessing the Accuracy of Interpersonal Perception. "Journal for the Theory of Social Behavior," "1(2)," 109-119.
Sloore, H. (1967). "De conceptualisatie van personen en de gedragsbeoordelingen in geprogrammeerde gevallen." Unpublished thesis. Free University of Brussels.
Thewissen, P. (1969). "Geprogrammeerde gevallen." Unpublished thesis. Free University of Brussels.
Thorndike, E. (1920). Intelligence and its use. "Harper's Magazine," "140," 227-235.
Van den Brande, L. (1984). Computer Assisted Programmed Cases. Poster presented at the First European Conference on Personality Psychology. Bielefeld.

ELECTRONIC DELIVERY OF JOB PERFORMANCE AIDS[1]

W. E. Hartung

U.S. Army Research Institute
Alexandria, Virginia, U.S.A.

INTRODUCTION

   Booher (1978) summarized several studies which demonstrated that when maintenance technicians, with only a minimum of training and experience, use a Job Performance Aid (JPA) their performance meets or exceeds that of technicians with much higher levels of training and experience. Further, when highly skilled technicians use JPAs they make fewer mistakes (Foley, 1973). However, when these research results were applied to technical manuals, the expected improvements were not forthcoming.

   Schurman, Porsche, Garbin & Joyce (1982) report on a field study of the performance of maintenance technicians in fifty Army units. These units performed organizational level maintenance on wheeled and tracked vehicles. They found that of all the maintenance tasks observed only 23% were performed without error. Part of the reason for this poor performance was the fact that the technical manuals were often missing, dirty, out of date, or inaccessible. Also, some technicians ignored the technical manuals completely and relied on their own past experiences. When these technicians encountered a problem they could not understand or with which they had no experience, they relied on their more experienced companions.

   In another study of similar units (Dressel & Shields, 1979), of Line Replaceable Units (LRUs), which were removed in the process of maintenance, were traced back through the depot repair facility. When these LRUs were tested at the depot, it was found that 40% of them did not need repair and should not have been removed.

   Maintenance performed in this manner results in costly losses, both in terms of wasted manpower resources and in terms of the unnecessary replacement of parts. When the readiness of the US Armed forces is a primary objective of maintenance, such a waste of resources cannot be tolerated.

---

[1] This chapter draws heavily on material from a paper by Hartung and O'Neil (1985). Additional comments and discussion are solely the responsibility of the author.

TECHNICAL MANUALS

A technical manual is designed to be the sole source of technical information for the maintenance technician. When field research found that JPAs offered significant gains in the quality of maintenance being performed, it was decided to structure technical manuals in this format.

When these "new look" technical manuals were being created, the authors discovered that branching, which is necessary in all troubleshooting procedures, made the manuals impossibly large. Cross referencing was introduced to reduce the volume of paper. However, cross referencing causes the user to jump from section to section in one volume and often requires reference to several manuals. It is not unusual for one troubleshooting task to require access to three or more manuals. For example in the M-1 Abrams tank technical manuals, which follow a simplified block flow type of design (MIL SPEC 63038), a simple procedure to troubleshoot and repair the Thermal Imaging System entails over twenty-five references in five different volumes.

Obviously, technicians find such procedures difficult, even frustrating to follow. In addition, even with extensive cross referencing, the volume of paper required to print all these procedures is enormous; the procedures themselves are difficult to write; and, they are difficult to keep up-to-date because it takes so long to write, print, and deliver new pages.

The result is that instead of promoting better maintenance, the current system of delivering maintenance information is achieving just the opposite. The technician is alienated by the bulk and complexity of the paper-based technical manuals and job aids and feels punished by a system which is purported to be supportive. Kern (1985) has discussed this phenomenon in some detail.

In this whole process, the user was not consulted. The assumption was made that the findings from the research on JPAs would be sustained when implemented on a large scale. It is this assumption which has been proven to be false.

A NEW PROPOSAL

The opportunity for a radical shift away from page oriented, paper-based maintenance information is provided by increases in the speed and capacity of micro-processors, and memory devices, and decreases in the size and power requirements of display devices. The increase in speed and capacity of micro-processors permits the real-time processing and display of information from a large and complex database in less than one second. The increase in speed and capacity of memory devices permits the storage and high speed retrieval of vast amounts of data which, if stored on paper, would occupy several volumes. The shift in display technologies from cathode ray tubes to high resolution flat panels permits the development of a hand-held delivery device.

The PEAM (Personal Electronic Aid for Maintenance) program is aimed at applying these technological advancements to the problems of delivering JPAs for Organizational Level maintenance on military systems. PEAM is a Joint Service Research Development effort directed from the Office of the Under Secretary of Defense for Research and Engineering.

PEAM PROGRAM OBJECTIVES

Primary Objective

The primary objective of the PEAM program is to demonstrate that the efficiency and effectiveness of the maintenance performed by military personnel on all types of military equipment can be improved by replacing paper manuals with an electronic Job Aid. This primary objective is supported by three sub-goals.

The principal sub-goal of this program is to design and build a system which will satisfy the information seeking needs of expert, less-than-expert, and novice technicians. This sub-goal is based on research reported by Kern and Hayes (1983) and Kern (1985) which indicates that the technician performing the work have immediate and easy access to accurate information.

Another major sub-goal of the PEAM program is to insure that the material which is presented to the technician is easy to understand. The importance of this sub-goal is driven by the prevalence, within the Services, of technicians with poor reading skills and the penchant for the engineers who write the technical manuals to write for engineers. Achievement of this sub-goal requires careful control of syntax and vocabulary. Both a controlled vocabulary and a limited, standardized syntax have a significant positive impact on the intelligibility of technical text (Joyce, Chenzoff, Mulligan and Mallory, 1973). Further, there are good explanations of what is required to produce a good JPA (e.g., Smillie, 1985).

The third and, in light of the previously quoted research, the most crucial sub-goal is to build a system which will be attractive enough to the mechanic that he or she will use it. The critical nature of this sub-goal is clearly pointed out by the findings of the field research reported above.

Secondary Objective

The secondary objective of the PEAM program is to reduce the enormous burden of training which presently exists. Accomplishing this objective is supported by the sub-goals stated above. However, the impact that the use of PEAM might have on training has not been documented. Further, there are powerful arguments over what should be taught and what should not be taught.

On the one hand there are those who advocate that technicians should be taught all they need to know to maintain, troubleshoot and repair the equipment for which they are responsible. This doctrine leads to training programs in which the student is taught not only the basic skills and elementary knowledge of the principles underlying the system which they are to maintain, but the detailed procedures they are to use in maintaining the equipment.

The purpose of raising these issues is to point out that there is no body of research upon which one can draw to arrive at a definite conclusion. Further, there appears to be no present desire to perform the needed research, as it would require bridging two areas which have not yet been joined. Hopefully, the advent of devices such as PEAM may stimulate this needed research.

ASSUMPTIONS

Assumptions Supporting Primary Objectives

Whether or not PEAM succeeds in what it proposes to do rests on two assumptions:

1) Technicians of all skill levels are willing to use an electronic device, which delivers a hierarchically organized JPA, as their primary source of technical information.

2) The research on JPAs is valid even when it is applied to a large set of tasks, e.g., organizational level maintenance of the Fire Control System of the M-1 Tank Turrett. This includes the assumptions that technicians are willing to follow step-by-step instructions for the performance of both simple and complex tasks to insure accuracy of their work; and that in doing this they will perform in a more efficient and effective manner.

Assumptions Supporting Secondary Objective

The potential impact of this program on training is dependent on other assumptions:

1) When provided accurate detailed information which is comprehensive and comprehensible, mechanics will gain an understanding of the topology (Kieras, 1985) of a system as a product of repeatedly performing specific task sequences. A corollary of this assumption can be stated as: Those who wish to learn, will learn.

2) Given the above assumption, the next assumption is that by delivering detailed step-by-step procedural information to the technician, there will be no need for training of specific procedures on specific equipment.

3) Given the second assumption, it follows that the majority of training which technicians receive should be on basics (e.g., mechanical, electrical, and hydraulic systems) and the basic skills required to use the tools of the trade.

SYSTEM DESIGN

Much is known about and much has been published on JPAs. The problem addressed in the PEAM program is not how to build a better JPA, but how to put it into an electronic device for delivery to users with widely different levels of experience. In other words, what is the best form of and format for an electronic JPA; and, most importantly, how should this device and its information be configured so that the technician will want to use it and, in using it, will perform more effectively and efficiently.

In formulating the system design, many issues were raised for which there was insufficient data upon which to base a decision. The design analysis is documented in the Final Report of the exploratory development study (Texas Instruments & XYZYX Information, 1981). In this study, the above mentioned objectives were kept in mind as the technologically possible alternative designs were reviewed. Out of this process came a list of essential functional characteristics.

Design for a Database

Designing the database in a hierarchical fashion was seen as the best means of satisfying the wide range of experience and expertise of the technicians who are the potential users. A wide range of experience implies a wide spectrum of needs for technical information. At one end of this spectrum of needs are those of the highly skilled and experienced technician who requires a minimum amount of data on routine tasks and more information on seldom performed but important tasks. At the other end of this spectrum are the needs of the novice technician to have detailed information including graphic illustrations with single step-by-step instructions for most tasks.

The hierarchy of the PEAM database is based on level of detail. The highest levels contain menus of symptoms. Each succeeding level down the hierarchy would progressively expand, in detail, each element until, at the highest level of detail, there is a single graphic with a single instruction.

Design for an Authoring System

As has been noted above, designing the content of JPAs for optimum effect on unskilled and low reading ability readers has been discussed in detail by other authors (e.g., Smillie, 1985). However, the ability to achieve close control over the production of massive amounts of JPA materials is still in its infancy.

The PEAM program addresses the problem of creating the form and content of the JPA by placing the burden of responsibility for control on an "intelligent" authoring system. This authoring system is designed to control the size of the vocabulary used and the variety of syntax employed in the construction of sentences for the JPA. This control is exercised by the software system under the guidance of one Technical Writer. The authors are Subject Matter Experts (SMEs) with little or no writing experience. These SMEs perform the task of writing the detailed instructions by selecting both syntax and vocabulary from menus.

Design for the Delivery Device

The functional characteristics for the design of the delivery device are aimed at making it as attractive as possible to the user.

1) It should be self-contained (i.e., function without any external communication or power link).

2) It should be as small and light as is technically possible; at a minimum it must be hand portable.

3) It should provide simultaneous text and graphics whose quality is equal to paper based technical manuals.

4) It should be easy to use (e.g., cross reference should be transparent), and should not require any typing skills (i.e., minimize keyed inputs).

5) The information should be accessible at any one of several levels of detail, at the option of the user.

6) It should be rugged and able to function at whatever time and place organizational level maintenance must be performed.

Each of these characteristics was specified on the basis of general knowledge and not specific research findings. Their validity will be one of the principal questions to be addressed in the field tests of the PEAM system.

ENGINEERING DESIGN

Overall Design of Delivery Device

In the present design, the delivery device consists of two removable components packaged in a large briefcase. These removable components are: a Man Machine Interface (MMI); and a Mass Memory Unit (MMU).

The MMI, which is connected to the carrying case by a cable, contains a 5 x 7 inch Thin Film ElectroLuminescent (TFEL) display screen, eight membrane type keys, a speaker, volume control, and a plug for a headset with a microphone. The MMU contains CMOS memory chips for storage of up to one megabyte of digital data and the batteries which are required to sustain them.

Integral to the carrying case are the electronic components and resident software which are required to: a) perform an initial internal check out procedure and other housekeeping functions, b) access the MMU, c) display the graphics and data on the MMI and d) perform the voice input and output functions. Two types of power cords which can be used to connect the case to a variety of power sources including a portable battery pack are stored in the cover of the case together with a light-weight headset with a boom mike.

Display

Specification of the display size and resolution were based on the best guesses of the design team and were constrained by the limits of technology. For, to achieve a hand-held device which conforms to military specifications, requires that the device weigh 10 pounds or less. The number of display devices which are capable of conforming to this requirement are few in number.

At the time of the design freeze, the TFEL flat panel display was clearly the best choice in terms of power consumption, resolution and viewing characteristics. Nevertheless, it consumes fully three fourths of the power required by the entire PEAM device and recent tests indicate that the luminance is less than originally forecast. Supplying power to this display results in greater size, weight, and cost than are desirable.

Mass Memory

The sizing of the mass memory started with an analysis of a broad selection of technical manuals for aircraft, shipboard and ground vehicle systems. The design team also judged that, at a minimum, the user should have access to all information for an entire major subsystem, such as the M-1 tank turret. The combination of these two inputs resulted in a tentative requirement for 1 million bytes of storage in the MMU.

The design choice for the memory chip used in the mass memory was the 64 Kbit (8K x 8) read-write Static CMOS (Complementary Metal Oxide Silicon). This was chosen to minimize long term power requirements, maximize speed of data retrieval, and minimize time required to load in data. These chips are placed directly on ceramic leadless chip carriers. This design specification will change in response to changes in the availability and cost of solid state memory chips.

Voice Input and Output

The original design specification did not identify voice Input and Output (I/O). However, because this technology was rapidly emerging and offered significant advantages, it was included in the system specification.

Speech synthesis was chosen for three reasons. First, it provides another means of circumventing problems caused by the limited reading ability of some technicians. Secondly, it makes it possible to deliver instructions to the user while he or she is looking at the task at hand. What quality of speech is required, is an unanswered question. Third, the design team thought that a device which is capable of speaking is one which a technician would be more likely to carry and use.

The capacity to recognize spoken commands was included in the design so that the technician can direct the flow of information without having to remove his or her hands from the task. The fact that this technology is presently limited to speaker dependent voice recognition can be seen as either a gain or a loss. It is a gain, if it is desirable to identify each technician. It is a loss to the extent that the requirement to enroll tends to make the technician avoid using it.

User Controls

The specifications for the means by which the user makes inputs to the system and controls the outputs of the system were created out of general experience rather than specific experimental research data. The design goal was to make the control of the system as simple and easy as possible. A specific goal was to avoid any requirement for a full keyboard, a large key pad, or a key pad which included number keys. In the present design, the system is controlled by pressing one of eight keys or by speaking one of eight commands. Eight keys were selected because this was about the absolute minimum number to achieve all required actions.

In operation, the screen contains either a menu, a list of procedural steps, or a single drawing with one procedural step. When there is a menu or more than one instruction on the screen, the cursor, in the shape of an arrow, is moved up or down the list by pressing NEXT or LAST. If the user is at the greatest level of detail and only a single drawing with one instruction is on the screen, pressing NEXT or LAST will present the next or last instruction and the associated graphic.

To obtain more information on one procedural step, the user presses SELECT. (This is equivalent to traversing the hierarchical data structure from the roots toward the leaves.) To return to a previous menu or level of detail the user presses BACKUP. (This is equivalent to traversing the tree from the leaves to the roots.)

YES and NO keys are for responding to direct questions. These questions might occur from a system function (e.g., "Do you wish to resume?") or they would occur in a troubleshooting routine (e.g., "Is the fault light still on?").

The last two keys are special use keys. MENU selects a master menu from which the user can branch to other menus or take other actions. SPEAK causes the device to speak the line of text at which the arrow is pointing.

DESIGN OF PEAM AUTHORING SYSTEM

The design of the authoring system incorporates the field tested and proven concepts of paper-based job aids into a hierarchical, highly structured software system which creates a digital database. The authoring system permits non-writer technicians to create easy to read text, with a minimum of human supervision. Their creative activity is tightly

controlled by the software system which places limits on the size of the
vocabulary and the variety of sentence structures.

The software design concept underlying this authoring system is a
hierarchical database development and management system called KMS
(Knowledge Management System) (Akscyn, 1984). This system permits a single
highly trained technical writer to oversee and tightly control the
distributed production of a database. Several technicians, each at their
own computer-terminal/work station, may simultaneously operate on different
modules of the same database. The technicians are led through the creation
of the text material by extension use of menus. The authoring system
tracks the production of their individual work and monitors the
construction of the entire database. As each unit of information is
created by a technician, the system creates the links which tie it to other
steps and procedures in the database. The result is a highly
interconnected set of nodes in a hierarchically organized database. Each
node contains a series of procedural steps or a single instruction and
graphic. Each node is linked to other nodes within the structure so that
the flow of information to the technician depends upon the outcome of a
test or the choice of the user.

The product of this authoring system is a digital database which
conforms to the requirements of the PEAM delivery system. Also, the design
of the authoring system and the database permits rapid updating and
electronic transfer of this updated information directly to the field units
where the delivery devices can be loaded. This technology is in dramatic
contrast to the current method of updating paper based technical manuals.

EVALUATION AND TEST

The present design of PEAM represents one engineering solution to
satisfy the objectives which were established for the program. What still
is unknown is whether or not this design approach satisfies the military
requirements. This is the question which must be answered prior to making
a decision to buy a system which can be fielded. The bottom line is: "Do
maintenance technicians use PEAM by choice and does using it improve their
effectiveness?"

The answer to this bottom line question is influenced by the answers to
other question such as: "Does a hierarchical database satisfy the full
range of the skill spectrum?" and "Does voice I/O provide a gain sufficient
to justify its cost and complexity?" A more general questions is: "What
elements in the present design of PEAM should be changed to make it more
rugged and more attractive and easy to use in the field environment?"

To gather data to answer these and other questions, the Army is
conducting an evaluation and test of the PEAM device. The prototype
devices will be used by technicians to perform Organizational Level
maintenance on the Fire Control System of the M1 tank turret and its
subsystems. This system was chosen because it encompasses a broad spectrum
of technologies and is serviced by one technician with the MOS of 45E.

FUTURE PLANS

The field tests described above are the start of a longer range
examination of the issues involved with delivering information to a
technician at the site of the task and on an as needed basis. Further, it
is only the beginning of what will be required if a decision is to be made
regarding a change in the present philosophy of training maintenance
technicians.

Many questions still remain to be answered. Is it a possible and realistic goal to reduce the amount of training that technicians receive and provide them instead with an electronic storehouse of knowledge which they can use to perform their tasks; and, given this electronic storehouse of knowledge, will technicians begin to learn more about the specific functioning of the equipment and the principles which underlie its operation? Research must be performed to determine if such a concept can be realized in practice. The center of this issue is the question: "What should be taught in a classroom environment and what should be learned through hands-on experience?"

REFERENCES

Akscyn, R., (1984, January). "Knowledge Management System: An Introduction," TR #152. Pittsburgh, PA: Information Technologies.

Booher, H. R. (1978, July). "Job performance aids: Research and technology state-of-the-art." (NPRDC TR 78-26) NPRDC. San Diego, CA. (NTIS No. AD A057562)

Dressel, J. D., & Shields, J. L. (1979, April). "Organizational Maintenance Performance," (RPR 79-8) U.S. Army Research Institute, Alexandria, VA.

Foley, J. P., Jr. (1973, November). "Description and results of the Air Force research and development program for the improvement of maintenance efficiency" (AFHRL-TR-72-72). AFHRL, Brooks, AFB, TX. (NTIS No. AD 771 000).

Hartung, W. E. & O'Neil, H. F., Jr. (1985). Personnel electronic aid for maintenance (PEAM), "Proceedings of the NATO Symposium on Computer Based Instructions in Military Environments."

Johnson, R. D., Thomas, D. L. & Martin, D. J. (1977, June). "User acceptance and usability of the C-141 Job quite technical order system" (AFHRL-TR-77-31). AFHRL, Wright-Patterson Air Force Base, OH. (NTIS No. AD A044 001).

Joyce, R. P., Chenzoff, A. P., Mulligan, J. F., & Mallory, W. J., (1973, December). "Fully proceduralized job performance aids (Vol. I); Draft military specifications for organizational level and intermediate maintenance." (AFHRL TR 73-43[1]). AFHRL. (NITS No. AD 775702).

Kern, R. P. (1985, April). Modeling users and their use of technical manuals. In T.M. Duffy & R. Waller (Eds.), "Designing Usable Test." Academic Press.

Kern, R. P. & Hayes, J. F. (1983, November). "Research findings to aid supervisors and trainers in improving maintenance performance" (ARI RP 83-14). (NTIS No. AD A144655). U.S. Army Research Institute, Alexandria VA.

Kieras, D. E. (1985, June). An Augmented Computerized Readability System: Final Report, FR-85/ONR-22.

Orlansky, J., & String, J. (1981, August). "The Performance of Maintenance Technicians on the Job." (IDA Paper P-1597), Institute for Defense Analysis, Arlington, VA (NTIS AD A104347).

Schurman, D. L., Porsche, A. J., Garbin, C. P. & Joyce, R. P. (1982). "Guidelines: Assessing use of information sources and quality of performance at the work site." (ARI Research Note 82-7), U.S. Army Research Institute, Alexandria, VA. (NTIS No. AD A 125366).

Smillie, R. J. (1985). Design strategies for job performance aids. In T. M. Duffy and R. Waller (Eds.) "Designing Usable Text." Academic Press.

Texas Instruments, Inc & XYZYX Information, Corp. (1981, August). PEAM Final Report (Prepared for NTEC & PM TRADE, Contract No 61337-80-C-0134) Lewisville, TX.

VIDEO GAME TECHNOLOGY AND TRAINING RESEARCH

C. Heaton

Army Personnel Research Establishment
Farnborough, Hants, U.K.

INTRODUCTION

Two projects are currently being carried out at the Army Personnel Research Establishment (APRE) to research and apply microcomputer and video games technology to some aspects of military training and selection. This paper discusses the area in general and is based on an APRE publication [Heaton & Segal, in press]. The original aim of the work was to take advantage of the available technology in order to produce portable and cheap Microprocessor Controlled Video Simulators (MCVS) for training, that could be used by Army units and schools to support more traditional training methods. However, after an initial consideration this aim appeared to be a very modest one and the wider implications of using MCVSs as a means of extending personnel training and testing in other areas were considered. In this context the development and application of new technologies was seen as an exciting area of applied research.

A paper entitled 'Video games: A New Behavioral Technology' was presented at the August 1980 meeting of 'The Technical Cooperation Panel' (TTCP) Sub Group U 'Behavioural Sciences'. The paper extolled the virtues of using video games as behavioral tests and training devices for several reasons. These games involve many skills; playing them repeatedly constitutes so many trials of practice. They are wonderfully self-motivating and most video games are highly speeded. This feature accounts for much of their appeal. In fact their being so fast may permit them to tap aspects of human functioning that were not accessible when dealing with essentially mechanical tasks. Three possible uses of such games were suggested: performance testing, predictive testing, and as training aids.

The paper concludes that "the new games are not adequately understood as so many additions to an existing arsenal of behavioural techniques and devices; potentially, they represent a new foundation for behavioural technology". There is no doubt that the technology that is currently used to produce video games, can be used to produce inexpensive, compact, Microprocessor Controlled Video Simulators which will have great potential as vehicles for both behavioural research and training applications. When discussing MCVSs in this paper, I am referring to devices that have high task fidelity but probably a low degree of realism in the engineering and scene content sense (Miller, 1954). The video screen is used to present

information relevant to the task or skill in a symbolic visual form that
will enable a student to construct cognitive representations of the task or
skill structures. These structures are functionally similar to the
cognitive representations formed in carrying out the real task (Goett, Post
& Miller, 1980). To meet this aim, it is important that a simulator
environment is established that encourages purposeful information gathering
behaviour, as would occur in the real world. A simulator presented as a
video game can set the scene for highly motivated activity, might be
expected to fulfill this requirement.

VIDEO GAME TECHNOLOGY

Video game technology is a generic term for the combination of hardware
devices and software techniques used to produce video games. There is
unfortunately no logical way, apart from their different applications, of
distinguishing between the concept of a video game and say the task
presented by a sophisticated computer-graphics flight simulator. The
distinction is largely founded in the capabilities for a given equipment
cost, and in the commercial viability for recreational applications. With
the increasing power and decreasing costs of computing and especially
computer-graphics, it is likely that tomorrow's video game technology will
be similar to much of today's flight simulator technology.

Therefore, it is necessary to adopt a pragmatic approach in defining
the current limits of video game technology. Video game technology is at
present broadly characterised by machines that possess the following
features:

a. They are capable of presenting a task in the form of a game using
    animated synthetic video images, usually with sound effects.

b. The player's goal can usually be obtained by manipulating objects
    on the screen using real time controls.

c. The machines are inexpensive not more than two thousand pounds,
    and often considerably less.

d. Devices are generally small, self-contained, portable, and robust.

These features were originally characteristic of video game machines
that consisted mainly of dedicated logic circuitry in the form of
integrated microelectronic circuits dedicated to one type of game. With
the introduction of the microprocessor in the mid 1970s, the situation
changed dramatically as video game technology shifted to using general
purpose microprocessors. For the first time it became possible to specify
a game in software only, thus allowing the use of a single system for a
wide variety of games (Op Het Veld, 1978).

Though general purpose microprocessors are more flexible than dedicated
hardware, they are slower. Major processing bottlenecks occur particularly
in the generation of visual and sound displays, thus the trend is to
consign these functions to their own specialised hardware. Consequently,
current video game systems are based on general purpose microprocessors
with varying degrees of specialised hardware support, usually in the form
of 'Graphics Display Processors' and 'Sound Generators'. Further
developments are likely to be due to a combination of increasing power and
more sophisticated specialised support hardware. This perhaps is
reminiscent of flight simulators and other serious applications of
computer-graphics. There are a number of different ways in which
commercial video games are currently implemented:

a. Arcade Video Game. Behind the attractive front panel there is usually a single printed circuit board containing a dedicated microprocessor that drives a specially designed video display processor for moving shapes around on the screen. Other special parts on the board produce sound and special visual effects. The board is dedicated to run on sophisticated game only. Theoretically this game could be changed by reprogramming some of the memory chips on the board, but in practice most games use their own special effects chips so that the whole machine is replaced rather than reprogrammed.

b. Semiprogrammable Video Game Players. At present these are usually programmable either by a magnetic tape cartridge or by a cartridge containing plug-in memory chips. They contain a microprocessor driving a single chip video display processor and accepting inputs from games' controllers such as joysticks. These machines only play off-the-shelf games supplied by the manufacturers.

c. Fully Programmable Video Game Computers. These video game machines are essentially the same as video game players, but with facilities, such as a keyboard, that enable one to write one's own computer programs. It is difficult if not impossible to write games of a similar standard to those supplied by the manufacturers of the machines, whose games are written on larger machines with special development software tools.

d. Personal Computers with Video. These are general purpose microcomputers with facilities that enable one to write one's own games. These games are usually written in a high level language such as Basic. Video games thus produced are not as good as those written in a faster low level language. Many machines have video output hardware that is not particularly suited to video games. This means that manufacturer written games may be faster than those written on the machine itself, but may not be as effective for a given application.

The basic hardware for all these machines is similar; the controls are joysticks, push buttons, etc., and in the case of the more general purpose machines a keyboard may be added. None of the machines available are configured for the behavioural scientist interested in their use for training or selection. The exact hardware configuration is largely determined by market forces, which is heavily dependent on the nuances of the recreational market place. However, many video game machines are cheap, readily available, and provide an apparently sophisticated game capability. In view of this, psychologists and other traditionally nontechnical behavioural scientists and those interested in training, may be tempted to make use of off-the-shelf games, rather than to configure their own equipment. This approach may indeed be useful for investigating some behavioral aspects of video gaming in a recreational context. However, currently available video games and equipment suffer from at least three major drawbacks when applied to training and testing situations:

a. The games are often designed around the limitations imposed by the hardware/software configuration. This produces, to some extent, only an illusion of considerable sophistication. If one tries to reverse the process, that is to use a given configuration to produce a particular game, then problems very soon arise.

b. The hardware itself is designed for recreational rather than scientific purposes. Consequently the types of controls that can be connected are very limited; there may be no facilities for event timing, data recording, or voice output etc.

c. The software can afford to be highly sophisticated in commercial video games, as they are distributed in commercial quantities for which it is relatively easy to recover the development costs. This contrasts with the smaller quantities that would be used in most training, testing and research applications.

There is therefore a requirement for MCVS systems configured to meet the practical needs of training and research. This could be achieved fairly easily and cheaply from a hardware point of view by the following methods:

a. Adapting a suitable personal microcomputer by adding appropriate peripheral boards to provide a complete MCVS/software development system

b. Constructing an MCVS by utilising one of the standardised microcomputer bus systems and plugging together the required hardware modules. The software is produced on a separate development system and is then transferred to permanent memory which resides in the end-user target system.

The exact choice of hardware will depend on such factors as, the extent to which reprogramming is required in the field, the physical robustness required (which might exclude the use of relatively fragile magnetic memory equipment), the required sophistication of input controls and audiovisual outputs and, of course, cost constraints. The choice of hardware will also often depend on whether the machine is going to be used for research or in the field by an end-user. However, if the application of MCVSs is to become a practical reality, a necessary philosophy is that the results of research obtained on the hardware system should be directly transferable to devices that meet all the operational requirements for use in the field. One of the attractions of microprocessor-based systems is that the research tool and end-user device may essentially be the same machine. The main differences are likely to be that the research device will have expensive memory disk peripherals, a keyboard and all the equipment associated with the development of software. The field version will be stripped down to a minimum configuration, housed in a suitably robust container.

A somewhat more difficult issue than the choice of hardware for MCVS applications and research, is the development of suitable software. With the advent of really cheap powerful hardware, the effort required to provide and maintain reliable software is often overlooked. Many projects have failed as a result, often leaving the whole technology damned in the eyes of the injured parties. The general acceptance of MCVSs for routine training and selection, may depend very much on the facility with which software can be produced and maintained.

Without discussing in depth the attributes and advantages of various computer languages, the following general guidelines for developing software for MCVSs are offered for acceptance:

a. A structured, modular, high level language (eg PASCAL) should be used to develop all the speed insensitive parts of the program.

b. A macro-assembly language, linked to high level language procedure calls, should be used to implement the speed dependent parts of the system.

c. The software should be produced as self-contained functional modules that can be transported to other programs, perhaps by means of a library.

It is now widely accepted that modular software is the key to cost-effective programming for most all computer applications. It is clear that the production of sufficiently cheap software to drive MCVSs for individual training and testing applications will rely quite heavily on a modular approach. Once a software module has been designed and written, the objective would be to use it as a component in a 'software machine' in a similar manner to the way in which parts are used to construct mechanical devices.

If MCVS applications are to be cost-effective, there must be a clear understanding of the kinds of general functions that might be assembled into reusable software modules. There are likely to be a number of functions which are common to a particular training or selection area. For example, most types of weapon system training and selection would require a moving target function, a method of scoring hits and misses and perhaps a function that would return information regarding procedural errors that a trainee makes when operating the system.

Some modules, such as peripheral drivers or a video object 'explode' routine, will be technical in nature, while others, particularly those to do with the user environment, will depend more on their design on a knowledge of human behaviour. For example, a module which controls the speed of movement of objects on the screen in accordance with a tracking difficulty criterion attached to each object would accept various parameters such as control law order, video screen control law damping, no control system lag, and so on. In this way, the findings of behavioral research can be used to define the kinds of software modules available to the MCVS technologist, and to impose restrictions on software functions to keep them within the limitations of the behavioral theories.

Although software portability can be achieved within an individual video game hardware system, portability between systems may be both more difficult and in some ways less essential for MCVSs than it is for other computer systems (Blandford, 1982). MCVSs will be dependent on specialised peripherals, such as video display processors, which uniquely dictate the kinds of displays which are possible. Consequently, the rationale behind much of the software will be dependent on a particular piece of hardware. However, the cost of hardware is generally so small that it is more cost-effective to purchase the appropriate peripheral than to attempt to adapt the software, and it is in this sense that intersystem software portability may be less important than in other areas.

MICRO PROCESSOR-CONTROLLED VIDEO SIMULATION AND COMPUTER-ASSISTED LEARNING

It is perhaps understandable if many psychologists and behavioural scientists are sceptical about the introduction of a new computer training methodology, especially where the achievements of Computer Assisted Learning (CAL) are used as a yardstick. The amount of material that has been published by psychologists and other specialists about the bright future of CAL is vast and yet its implementation has been limited, confined on the whole to educational or other establishments with an intrinsic interest in the problems of implementing CAL and organizations such as banks or computer system manufacturers possessing huge computer resources with spare computer capacity.

The stumbling block of CAL has been the practical problems of its implementation rather than its theoretical basis. The optimistic forecast of the universal computer in every home and school, has not yet been realised thus the hardware has not been available in the quantities expected.

With the advent of cheap extremely powerful microcomputers and the appearance of local networks, resource sharing and the rapid deployment of small computer systems, the hardware problems of CAL may soon be overcome (Alty, 1982). However, software production will still be a major problem. The difficulty lies in justifying the expense of the enormous manpower effort required to analyse and program even a small knowledge domain into a suitable computer with all the testing, assessment, and feedback facilities implied by CAL, especially when resources are stretched for maintaining traditional training methods.

The types of training and testing problems for which MCVSs can be used are liable to be less affected by this resource allocation problem. The application area will generally require the mapping of relatively small amounts of knowledge into the training or testing device, especially where part-task skills are concerned. In the case of skills training the devices are likely to have intensive use, because many repetitions are usually required to practise a skill. Testing applications will generally be subject to a large throughput of personnel perhaps over a long period of time. In either case the cost/benefit ratio is liable to be better than for CAL which will usually be concerned with imparting a much broader range of knowledge. MCVS applications might include:

a. Real time skills training - controls coordination, task scheduling, procedural learning, tracking tasks (especially where these are part-task)

b. Real time skills testing - both performance and predictive

c. Standardised ability testing - including intelligence, personality, decision making

d. As a research tool - investigating, for example, the effects of stress on performance, task scheduling, and factors influencing decision making

As Nawrocki and Winter (1983) suggest, the post hoc selection of a video game to support instruction is likely to be far less effective than the development of a game specifically designed as part of a coordinated instructional package. They propose a classification of games in terms of their characteristics and predicted learning transfer in different skills areas. Such a classification, based on the objective results of task analyses transfer experiments, and validation of existing devices should ensure that intrinsically motivating devices can be appropriately incorporated into a training programme.

RESEARCH ISSUES

The use of small simulators, based largely on video game technology, as tools for examining human behaviour, is a new area that has almost no history of research. Some research questions are particularly important in the military context where much of the value of MCVSs will stem from their ability to simulate the movement and interaction of objects on the battlefield. A characteristic of current video game technology is the very simple representation used for physical objects and their movements, that is they may have little visual reality or fidelity. Other features are also highly stylised, for example, the environment (cockpit, or gun turret) may have little fidelity in the engineering sense. In a game these factors are of little importance and the lack of realism does not necessarily detract from the "psychological reality" of the game. However, when put to more serious use, more needs to be known about the psycho-perceptual constraints and the limitations which might need to be imposed on applications.

Miller (1954) states that, "At least from the standpoint of economy the development of training devices should rest on psychological simulation rather than engineering simulation. Therefore to the extent that engineering simulation is a matter of selection and of degree, the selection of variables should be based on psychological considerations as to what will maximise the validity of training". In other words, the device should be constrained by the task, rather than engineered to replicate real-life equipment (Dallman, Pieper & Richardson, 1983). In this respect it is rather surprising that the literature on visual simulation and visual perception contributes remarkably little to the process of visual information acquisition as applied to real world, purposeful behaviour (Hennessy, Sullivan & Cooles, 1980). A second area of interest is in the use of MCVSs for performance and ability testing. The use of a range of commercially produced video game has already been investigated (Kennedy, Bittner, Harbeson & Marshall, 1982; Jones, Kennedy & Bittner, 1981). Until recently the most popular video games were of the 'track and destroy' variety, such as Space Invaders. This is now a trend towards games which possess a greater scheduling component, such as those which involve the 'closure' concept. In these games one's movements must be scheduled to either avoid being trapped or to trap or enclose others. Closure games generally require a series of rapid choices to be made, with performance being dependent on spatial and temporal judgements as distinct from motor skills. This sort of task might prove useful for testing personnel for jobs, that have a large task scheduling component. This type of game might also prove effective in investigating the effects of stress on some aspects of decision making, an important issue in military psychology.

Where MCVSs are used in a training context, it will be particularly useful to discover any general factors that might help to sustain motivation, for example, the role of challenge, curiosity and fantasy (Nawrocki & Winter, 1983). Although well known psychological techniques may help in this respect, such as operating a partial reinforcement schedule, other motivators are certain to be found. Video game sound effects are a well known example, where their absence considerably decreases the attraction and continued motivation to play the games. In an experiment by the manufacturers of "space invaders" the sound beat which increased in tempo as the game progresses was removed. The revenue captured by the machine was considerably reduced, even though most of the sounds, guns firing and invaders being destroyed, remained.

The justification for research into MCVSs and video game technology by nonacademic organizations must to a large extent depend on there being a strong indication that potential users are willing to commit themselves to the new technology. APRE's own initial research efforts into MCVSs found an early practical outlet in training aids required by the Royal Armoured Corp to supplement their more complex team training systems.

A PART-TASK GUNNERY TRAINING AID

An experimental part-task training device was developed, to enable tank gunners to practise some of the basic procedural and coordination skills required to operate the Chieftain Improved Fire Control System (IFCS) controls. The Chieftain IFCS is a semiautomatic weapon control system designed to optimise line-of-sight engagements on moving targets. The gunner operates this weapon system via two main controls, a right-hand thumb operated joystick that controls the movement of the main armament,

and a left-hand multifunction handle that contains switches that effect
various system functions. Trainees experience difficulty in coordinating
the operation of the left and right hand controllers while following the
correct procedures and tracking the target. The experimental trainer was
designed to enable trainees to practise and acquire this skill.

The training task was presented as a video game whereby the trainee was
required to destroy a schematic moving target to obtain points. This was
done by following the correct drill with his weapon system controllers.
The relationship between the gunner's control inputs and the information
presented on the video screen was similar to the real tank. The trainee
could experiment with the training aid, building up a picture of how the
controls influence the functioning of the weapon system. Unlike the real
tank however, any errors made by the trainee during the procedure were
immediately indicated and the run was terminated.

Both the difference in the number of procedural errors and hits were
significant ($p<0.01$ and $p<0.02$ respectively). We may conclude that PTT
training has had a real impact. These figures, although effective
statistically, do not adequately reflect the extent of the qualitative
difference between the two subgroups that were observed from the video
recordings of GTS runs. The PTT trained subgroup was seen to perform with
much smoother tracking and a much more confident approach. The fact that
both subgroups have produced the same number of tracking errors is probably
due to a tendency for proper tracking to precipitate more procedural
errors. As tracking errors were classified as such only when there were no
procedural errors, some tracking errors will be masked by procedural errors.

The experimental system was designed to be as flexible as possible so
that suggestions and criticisms put forward by military users could be
immediately tested and incorporated as design modifications. This is
inherently possible with training aids based on microcomputer technology
which, with its dependence on general purpose processors, is heavily
software based. It is particularly significant that the great flexibility
provided by a 'software machine' approach allows one to 'bootstrap' the
design; initial versions can be used to provide information to guide more
advanced versions of the design.

The IFCS part-task trainer has since been transferred from its current
hardware environment into an operational package to be used for further
trials and demonstrations. The new environment, although stripped to a
minimum configuration of microprocessors, the Motorola 6809, which is
particularly suited to high level modular programming. This processor is
coupled to a high-powered, yet cheap, graphics display processor which has
been developed by Texas Instruments specially to support video gaming and
educational requirements. The facilities provided by this hardware have
enabled the game value of the IFCS part-task trainer to be considerably
enhanced.

THE BATTLEFIELD ENGAGEMENT SIMULATOR AND TRAINER (BEST)

A large component of military skill is essentially concerned with the
manipulation of objects in space on the basis of information which is
visually acquired from the scene. This applies particularly to the
acquisition of targets by gunners, target allocation by commander, and to a
lesser extent, to the deployment of men, vehicles, and weapons. Training
in these skills is difficult as field exercises are expensive and often
dangerous. Because ammunition is costly and dangerous, the circumstances
in which it can be used for training are extremely limited. It is also
expensive and time consuming to use real vehicles for routine military

training. Furthermore, mock battles and other pre-arranged training scenarios do not exhibit many of the characteristics which may be important for training visual acquisition combat skills. Where training is difficult research is even more problematic. Pratically, it is not possible to generate many of the scenarios that would be of interest, or to instrument these on training grounds to obtain the necessary data.

As the running costs of the real equipment increase, the use of simulators is becoming more attractive, especially for routine training. Simulators also offer more controlled environments for research. However, simulators that provide a suitable visual environment for practising combat skills are available only at great cost. A major problem for visual acquisition type simulators lies both in providing and manipulating the required features in the visual scene. A particular difficulty is in providing targets that exhibit characteristics that are realistically challenging to combat skills. For research, targets should possess features that will encourage subjects to practise strategies that they would, and for training purposes should, employ in actual combat. Targets should take evasive action, disappear and appear from behind objects, conform to certain terrain structures, and change apparent size and shape as they rise and fall with the terrain surface. They should cluster together, move apart, turn, stop, start, accelerate, and of course, return fire. Almost all military training targets are deficient in the majority of these features. Most simulated moving targets merely traverse a scene at constant speed. These criticisms then apply to both range targets and targets currently supplied with many simulators, including the Chieftain IFCS GTS, although some improvements to both are envisaged.

It is possible to generate a suitable display for a visual acquisition type combat trainer by making use of very powerful computer graphics techniques. There are however several problems:

   a. The simulator display technology would be as complex and hence as expensive and bulky as the most sophisticated flight simulator displays.

   b. The display would still fall below the visual complexity of the real scene. Perceptual cues vital to many combat tasks might still be missing.

The expense alone would almost certainly destroy the viability of this type of simulator.

There is a possible alternative in providing a simpler computer display which contains the perceptual cues necessary for part-task rather than whole task, skills training. This is consequently much less expensive. Part-task training simulators will more often be concerned with the psychological equivalence of the simulation to the real task, rather than 'engineering' realism per se. However, a clearer understanding of the task components is generally required than for whole task simulators. A detailed task analysis is usually required to identify the critical components that affect performance. Once these have been isolated, a number of options must usually be considered regarding which task components to train independently, whether to train them as a general skill rather than a task specific function, and so on, depending on the task. Although the technical complexity of part-task simulators over whole task simulators may be reduced, the psychological basis has to be firmer, which will add to development costs (particularly those associated with technical expertise). Current microprocessor technology pushed to its limits should be able to meet the less stringent criteria of a part-task simulator display. A display based on advanced microprocessor technology can faithfully simulate the changing geometrical consequences of the movement of objects in the world, but can only effect a rather schematic visual representation of the scene. Nevertheless, a stylised scene can be very convincing, if the display can provide a consistent subset of important psycho-perceptual cues. The human perceptual function tends to compensate for missing perceptual details by interpreting images according to the expectations of previous experience (Gibson, 1980; Neisser, 1976). It therefore seems likely that training the essential components of many visual acquisition military skills may be feasible, even though many of the more subtle cues in a visual scene may not be available. This type of training may be especially relevant where these skills are concerned with the functional significance of objects rather than their fine details.

A device has been developed by APRE to investigate the training impact of providing different combinations of psycho-perceptual cues developed by advanced microprocessor graphics display technology, and to determine what constraints a display containing stylised objects will place upon training applications. The device, called the 'Battlefield Engagement Simulator and Trainer (BEST)' will also be used to investigate strategic engagement skills in target acquisition and allocation, as well as acting as a model for a future battlefield engagement trainer.

The BEST is conceptually an extension of the most sophisticated arcade video game machines. The video display screen acts essentially like a moveable window into a three dimensional world of objects and terrain. The observer, who is operating the window, can move through the world and interact with the objects within it in various ways. The objects may be, for example, tanks, missiles, trees, houses, or any other previously defined components of the world. The point of observation is itself represented by a previously defined object, perhaps a tank or a helicopter. The objects, including the observer's vehicle, can interact with other objects and terrain in the world, for example, colliding with other objects and precipitating various predefined consequences.

The device itself, which is expected to cost in the region of £25,000 (at present prices for a production version), consists of a specialised high speed graphics display processor (GDP) linked to a data base containing the world object descriptions. The GDP is associated with a powerful 16 bit microprocessor (a Motorola 68000) that passes and receives information from the GDP and controls the overall operation of the device. Many types of controls may be connected to the machine's flexible input/output facility, which also contains a sound generator. The video output is compatible with a RGB monitor and has a resolution of 512 x 416 pixels. Three-dimensional objects may be generated with faces each of a different colour if required. The edges of these faces may be etched in different colours to emphasis an object's shape. The maximum number of complexity of objects is governed only by the influence this has on the animation rate of the simulation and the screen resolution. The more complex an object, the more time it will take to draw and hence the animation rate will be reduced accordingly.

The relationship between animation rate and scene complexity undoubtedly has important and general consequences for the effectiveness of skills training. This is an example of the kind of psycho perceptual unknown that can be thrown up by the technology itself, and for which it would be worthwhile attempting to provide some general guidelines. Typically the real time animation rate of the BEST is in the region of between ten to twenty five frames per second with no appreciable delay between frames. This specification produces a flicker-free animation.

Since its initial conception, several facilities of particular

importance in a research role, have been added. The most significant of
these is the ability to define and follow terrain. It will be possible to
incorporate different terrain models and investigate fidelity features of
the display produced. In addition the BEST has the facility to connect
several simulators together. Individual vehicles in the same 3-dimensional
world can then be controlled from their own consoles, with a view of the
world depending on their particular vantage point. This facility is
expected to be useful for investigating and training target allocation
strategies, where a commander designating targets must take into account
the different fields of view of vehicles under his command and their
relationship to the targets. If required, targets themselves can be under
human control and can therefore operate the tactics of the opposing force.
The main features of the device are outlined in an APRE Memorandum
currently being drafted.

The BEST is currently at a stage where the major design problems have
been overcome and the single simulator prototype has been built. Initial
experimental work is planned for 1984, although demonstrations of some of
the machine's capabilities have already taken place. Some current flight
simulators can produce comparable or superior displays, but the BEST is
revolutionary in terms of cost, size, and the kind of military scenarios
for which it has been optimised.

CONCLUSION

The military systems being used by the Army are becoming increasingly
complex in two ways:

a. Weapons systems such as tanks are being increasingly loaded with
    new equipment.

b. The equipment itself is becoming increasingly 'clever', under
    computer control.

This has several consequences for the personnel operating these
systems. The workload on operators and especially commanders is increasing
due to both the sheer diversity of equipment, with corresponding checks and
status information that must be processed, and to the increased number of
military options made available. Furthermore, computer controlled systems
often require the operator to translate external events into information
that can be understood by the machine, by making a sequence of responses
that are often complicated, counter-intuitive, and which therefore require
much practice. Furthermore, these responses must often be highly speeded
to accord with the response time of the system. The learning environment
provided by small video simulators of the type discussed, would seem to be
excellently suited to practising the essential drills and skills to operate
many of these systems.

The logistics of supplying high technology for training purposes are
somewhat different from the Army from other Services, for example the Royal
Navy can make use of large shipboard computer resources. The availability
of highly portable, robust training aids as opposed to a large fixed
installation is particularly important to an Army which has to be able to
maintain training in the field.

Increasing complexity is also rejected in the cost of equipment for
both field use and training. By reducing complexity of training aids (by
adopting a low fidelity part-task approach) the costs of training equipment
may be greatly reduced, without necessarily reducing training
effectiveness. However, in order to ensure that training is not degraded

as a result of the introduction of such devices, fidelity issues must be taken into account early in the design of equipment and sufficient consideration must be given to the design of the overall training package, and the possibility that each tank squadron possess its own training device, which can be transported with the squadron to wherever it happens to be stationed. This would apply generally to the application of cheap, portable training aids in various Arms and Corps.

As with most video games, the subjects' continued interest in the game was enhanced by vision and sound effect. A competitive element was introduced by using a 'role of honour' feature found in many arcade games, whereby the high scoring trainee could eliminate a competitor and enter his own initials and score into a list of prominently displayed top scores.

The most common errors were determined by carrying out a task analysis of the basic engagement against a moving target for both the large turret based simulator and earlier versions of the part-task trainer. These errors fell into three main categories, procedural errors, timing errors, and tracking errors, each error being flagged up by its own error message.

Two important questions were raised early in the design: is a diagrammatic, nonrealisitic display suitable; and is there a need for accurate weapon system controls and control law? The first question was easily answered as the difficulties experienced by trainees operating the system are not so much in acquiring visual information, but in scheduling their operation of the gun controls according to the required procedure. It was held therefore that a stylised display would be suitable providing it could supply the relevant information in a clear fashion. The second question was more difficult to answer. Provision of the actual controls and control law could expect to maximise the transfer of training and improve the face validity and hence acceptability of the device. On the other hand an attempt to provide these would complicate the training device and considerably increase its expense. It is conceivable, that provided the controls and control law are functionally equivalent to the real thing and effect a similar information processing load, then an accurate simulation of the controls may be unnecessary for acceptable transfer of training.

In that event, the current training device is a combination of the real IFCS controls, and a control law of the same order as on the real tank which is subjectively acceptable to experienced gunners. In fact, the schematic display was accepted almost without question and the fifteen experienced IFCS gunnery instructors who were approached, clearly stated that they did not believe the device required a more complicated display or control law.

Initial trials have indicated that the trainer produces a significant transfer of training from the PTT to the large Gunnery Training Simulator (GTS). A group of 10 gunners who were IFCS naive, was split in half, each half being balanced for initial ability, as judged by a preliminary instructional session on the PTT. One half was given further training on the PTT and a comparison of performance on the GTS was made between the half that was given extra training and the half that had no extra PTT training. The performance of each man on each GTS was categorised as either a miss due to procedural error, a miss due to a tracking error, or a hit.

The following results were obtained:

	Percentage Procedural Errors	Percentage Tracking Errors	Percentage Hits
PTT Trained	27	29	44
Not PTT Trained	61	29	10

REFERENCES

Alty, J. L. (1982). The Impact of Microtechnology. A case for reassessing the roles of computers in learning. "Comput. & Educ.," "6," 1-5.

Blandford, C. (1982). CAL Software Design for Transferability. "Comput. & Educ.," "6," 165-174.

Dallman, B. E., Pieper, W. J. & Richardson, J. J. (1983). A Graphics Simulation System - Task Emulation Not Equipment Modelling. "Journal of Computer-based Instruction," "10," 70-72.

Gibson, J. J. (1979). "The ecological approach to visual perception." Boston, MA: Houghton Mifflin Company.

Goett, J. M., Post, T. J. & Miller, G. G. (1980). "Maintenance training and simulator development utilising imagery techniques" (AHFRL-TR-80-3). Air Force Human Resources Laboratory, Technical Training Division.

Heaton & Segal (in press). "Training by microprocessor-controlled video simulation" (APRE Memorandum, draft No. 82N). Army Personnel Research Establishment Farnborough, Hants.

Hennessy, R. T., Sullivan, D. J. & Cooles, H. D. (1980). "Critical research issues and visual system requirements for a V/STOL Training Research Simulator," (NAUTRAEQUIPCEN 78-C-0076-1). Orlando, Florida: Naval Equipment Center.

Jones, M. B., Kennedy, R. S. & Bittner, A. C., Jr. (1981). A video game for performance testing. "American Journal of Psychology," "94," 143-152.

Kennedy, R. S., Bittner, A. C., Jr., Harbeson, M. & Marshall, B. J. (1982). Television Computer Games: A 'New Look' in performance testing. Aviat. Space and Env. Med.

Miller, R. B. (1954). "Psychological considerations in the design of training equipment," (WADC Tech Report 54-563, AD-71 202). Wright-Patterson AFB, O4: Wright Air Development Centre, Aero Medical Laboratory.

Nawrocki, L. H. & Winner, J. L., (1983). Video Games Instructional Potential Potential and Classification. "Journal of Computer Based Instruction," "10," 80-82.

Neisser, U. (1976). "Cognitive Psychology." New York, Appleton-Century-Crofts.

Op Het Veld, S. J. (1978). "Microprocessor-controlled video game electronic components and applications," "1(1)."

The Technical Cooperation Panel (1980). "Video games: A new behavioural technology." (TTCP point papers). Cambridge, England.

EXPERIENCE-CONSOLIDATION SYSTEMS: A SKETCH OF A THEORY OF COMPUTER-BASED INSTRUCTION IN ILL-STRUCTURED DOMAINS

R. J. Spiro

University of Illinois at Urbana-Champaign
Champaign, Illinois, U.S.A.

Experience-Consolidation Systems are microcomputer software intended primarily as training devices. In particular, their purpose is to "telescope" some aspects of the process by which practical field experience leads to the acquisition of judgemental expertise. In situations where rules, general principles or statistical models are insufficient, some other way of thinking is required for correct performance, one that is more appropriate and impressionistic. In the inexact language of everyday usage, that mode of thought is commonly referred to as "intuition." It is what allows people to think for themselves when explicit guidelines are lacking. Intuitive judgements are required when complex, overlapping patterns of rules and past behavior must be analyzed and weighed. This pattern information and the intuitive process that utilize it are built up over the years from experience with large numbers of richly textured cases. Experience-Consolidation Systems aim to shorten the time required for experience to accumulate, so that acquisition intervals can be measured in hours and days instead of years.

It is impossible to merely hand over knowledge of this kind using traditional technologies of schooling (lectures, textbooks, conventional educational software). These means of instruction depend on the presentation of rules and general principles. The problem is that the real world will not cooperate in this tendency towards "artificial neatening" of subject matter. The world is messy, partially irregular, entangled. Experience-Consolidation Systems acknowledge this characteristic of real situations and make it the heart of their training philosophy. [Experience-Consolidation Systems resemble simulations in many of their aims. However, the two approaches differ fundamentally from each other, as will become clear during the course of this paper, with the differences summarized at the conclusion.]

In other words, Experience-Consolidation Systems teach what cannot be conventionally taught, what has traditionally been left to the vagaries of "experience in the field". They make the user familiar with the intertwined, mutually influencing patterns inherent in individual cases by presenting rich case information in a psychologically convenient way made possible by advances in cognitive theory and by the power and flexibility of the computer. They teach the contexts that determine when rules will work and when they will not. They make it easier to decide what you should do when there are no rules prescribing what to do. They help you to think for yourself.

UNDERLYING PRINCIPLES

The theoretical and methodological breakthroughs that make this telescoping of experience possible are very extensive and technical. Given the purposes of this paper and limitations of time and space, we will just sketch the general outline of our approach and the theory that underlies it, with much of the detail and complexity omitted. [More complete written accounts are forthcoming shortly and will be available from the author.]

We begin with the premise that there are two kinds of knowledge. One kind is well-structured and is amenable to the formulation of widely applicable, general principles for correct behavior. It is in these well-structured knowledge domains that educational practice has had the most success and that cognitive psychology and artificial intelligence have made the greatest advances.

The other kind of knowledge is relatively ill-structured, and has some of the following characteristics. It is difficult to identify a single set of properties or attributes found in all cases (examples, situations, instances, events, etc.) -- there are no "defining characteristics". The dominance and subsumption relations of hierarchical structure tend to change across cases. Prototypes frequently tend to be misleading. In general, general principles are highly insufficient by themselves. Interactions of features in complex environments proliferate, introducing aspects of novelty and computational difficulty in the individual case. Which areas of knowledge have these properties? It turns out that all domains have a substantial component that is ill-structured, some more than others. (This is difficult to realize at first because of the widespread conspiracy of convenience that leads educators to artificially simplify the topics they teach. This avoidance of ill-structuredness makes it easier for teachers/trainers to teach, for textbook writers to write, for students to prepare for tests, and for teachers to construct and score tests. It is no wonder that students are frequently so unable to apply their school learning to the real world, which refuses to cooperate in this conspiracy.)

Consider the emphasis on case-based learning in most areas of professional education (e.g., medicine, business, political science). Why present so many individual cases (and still feel the need for students to acquire more experience after school) if you can much more simply provide students a set of general principles along with a handful of illustrative examples? Because the general principles won't work well enough by themselves. The world is more complicated than that. Aspects overlap. They combine into complex patterns. They depend on their application for an interpretation of the contexts in which they occur.

It is the ability to deal with these more ill-structured aspects of knowledge application that separates the well-schooled beginner from the experienced practitioner. An expert is not just someone who possesses more school learning and abstract knowledge. He is someone who can go beyond overly simplified prescriptions and appreciate an entire situation, with all of the complex patterns of interrelation that make it so frustrating for the novice practitioner (as well as the teacher). Then, from his weighing of the many facets of the complex situation, the expert arrives at an overall judgment of how to proceed that turns out more often than not to be correct. And yet he will frequently only be able to articulate some of his reasons. ("It was factors X and Y surely, but it was something more than that, something I can't quite put my finger on. . ."). The more difficult the decision, the more likely it is that a complete accounting of reasons will be impossible. The reason that the expert can do much more than he can tell you about is that he is doing a lot of things at the same time, each variably interrelated to the others. To convey it however, would require that all the factors being weighed simultaneously be split apart and sequenced, thus destroying their integrity and validity. We will return later to this issue of simultaneous consideration of multiple dimensions.

What enables the expert to make appropriate decisions under the conditions of uncertainty and indeterminateness found in ill-structured domains? What does he draw on? Experience. It is in the richly patterned detail of the numerous individual cases that an expert has been exposed to that the crucial information for correct performance based on intuitive judgment is to be found. Situations (cases, applications, examples, events) appear to us in various disguised forms; you need to see many of them to recognize the disguises. Situations involve numerous kinds of complex patterns; you need a lot of experience before you will have seen a high percentage of those patterns. Patterns tend to overlap and intertwine around each other in real situations; only after exposure to a large number of cases does it become possible to synoptically view these multiple interconnections. Thus, whereas in well-structured domains examples (cases, etc.) are helpful for purposes of illustrating general principles and then may be discarded as superfluous, in ill-structured domains examples are necessary and not just nice. It takes years to be exposed to enough cases to learn the myriad ways that patterns may relate to each other and to appreciate the practical significance of those relations.

PROBLEMS IN THE RAPID ACQUISITION OF CASE EXPERIENCE

Experience-Consolidated Systems are designed to shorten by many orders of magnitude the amount of time required to acquire large amounts of experience, without sacrificing the essential characteristics contained in experience. What are these essential characteristics that are retained by Experience-Consolidation Systems? Again, they are that the most important aspects of each case be presented in exhaustively rich detail (because of the importance of complex interactions and context-dependencies); that there be numerous cases; and that they be presented and arranged in a manner to facilitate the ability to recognize and appreciate pattern and context information. In the real world, the dilemma should be obvious: these essential characteristics are such as to work against any shortening of experience-acquisition time. First, real world cases unfold over durations long enough to prohibit any practical attempt to presenting a large enough set of cases within any training program. Second, cases come along in haphazard order, without any regard for instructionally efficacious arrangement. Third, and most important, even if lots of richly detailed case information could be presented in a short amount of time using some optimal arrangement scheme, it would quickly produce information overload. There would be too much to remember. The main technique for encoding large amounts of information, chunking similar bits in hierarchical fashion, cannot work in ill-structured domains by definition: if the information could be consistently chunked the domain would be well-structured. Experience-Consolidated Systems overcome each of these three problems.

<u>The Problem of Time</u>

This problem is addressed by assembling large numbers of cases (situations, examples, instances, events, etc.) and extracting from them the most significant multivariate information needed to fully characterize a case's environment, exhausting as many as possible of the perspectives that could be applied. (For technical reasons, the inevitable redundancy that goes with exhaustiveness is desirable to represent the entangled character of ill-structured domains.) Why are exhaustive representations

important? Because you don't know in an individual case what will and will
not be relevant. That's why you can't just hand someone rules or general
principles to go by, and instead have to rely on impressionistic judgment.
Also, the decision about the influence of any single factor will be highly
dependent on the context of what is going on with the other factors. Thus
you need to richly represent the context in which decision factors occur
in. A principle of Experience-Consolidation Systems is that in
ill-structured knowledge domains you teach contexts to teach concepts.

Note that each unit of multivariate information that is used represents
the result of some transformation of raw data; the unit is the output of a
"theory", of a cluster of considerations. By presenting a broad set of
theory outputs rather than individual features of situations, the goal of
exhaustively representing a situation from all points of view is attached.
For example, in the stock market timing application, information from a
theory of technical analysis produces just two or three values in the
complete situation's Experience-Consolidation System representation. These
values would be presented in the perceptually integrated context of outputs
from other global, comprehensive technical analysis theories, as well as
outputs from fundamental, monetary, and economic theories of stock market
behavior. All of the theories work sometimes and not others.
Experience-Consolidation Systems, by presenting the information from each
theory in the readily perceived context of each of the others, teach the
complex context characteristics in which the various theories work best
(with multiple entry points for future access also made possible.) The
whole point is to get people beyond relying on just the three or four
things that can be consciously monitored at one time. You want them to see
an ill-structured domain (like the stock market) as a complex, "living"
environment, in which different theoretical perspectives are interacting
parts. The perceptual displays of Experience-Consolidation Systems
(discussed below) allow you to see all the different perspectives in the
context of each other, as they interact, all at a glance.

Note as well that the multivariate information selected is everything
that readily available procedures, including advanced statistical modeling
techniques, do not address; the residuals, so to speak; the "apples and
oranges" for which current knowledge lacks a common metric of combination;
the complex, higher-order and nonlinear interactions that wouldn't be
discovered using regression procedures unless you knew to look for them.
In other words, the theory embodied in Experience-Consolidation Systems is
one in which approximate, impressionistic judgment takes over where
reason, explanation, and statistical prediction can go on further.

The Problem of Information Overload

This is the most difficult problem. How do you present lots of complex
case information for each of many cases in a short amount of time and still
get the user to take it all in. Experience-Consolidation Systems meet this
difficulty by presenting information using specially designed graphic aids
that are tailored to simultaneously convey complete sets of complexly
entangled patterns at a glance, tapping into everyone's finely developed
perceptual processing system. That is, Experience-Consolidation Systems
employ perceptual analogues of the conceptual situations that need to be
studied. As has been well established by experimental psychologists,
people have an extraordinary ability to remember large numbers of briefly
presented visual scenes. For example, in one study subjects were shown 600
pictures in approximately one hour. When later presented with the same
pictures or similar ones they had not seen, the subjects had an accuracy
rate of 98% in recognizing pictures from the original set. In another
study, 10,000 pictures where shown over a longer period of time, but again
with near 100% recognition accuracy.

One of the main types of visual aids used in Experience-Consolidation Systems is Chernoff Faces (a procedure for heuristic inspection of multivariate data developed by I. Chernoff). Think about all the information encoded in your memory of a friend's face: the size of the eyes, nose, mouth, etc.; the shapes of those features; how far apart the eyes are; how far the eyes are from the nose, and the nose from the mouth and ears; and so on -- one could list thousands of such relationships, all contained in a single image that may be stored in memory in a matter of seconds. In the Experience-Consolidation System training approach, each visual display corresponds to the features of a single situation (case, example, application, etc.). Thus, this powerful ability of human thought is now brought to bear to encode the manifold of features of ill-structured conceptual situations, situations which can be understood only by such a simultaneous appreciation of multiple, partially overlapping interrelationships.

The general procedures for Experience-Consolidation Systems (which differ slightly but not substantially across the various applications) involve rapidly presenting visual analogue displays (mainly faces) that each correspond to a single situation, case, example, or instance (what you would call it depends on the domain, but it all boils down to the same thing). Users go through a short acclamation period in which they learn a set of correspondences between facial features (when faces are the visual display mode used) built into the Experience-Consolidation System and a set of analysis categories appropriate to the training area. This procedure involves learning no more than 15-20 associations between output values for partly independent (i.e., incommensurable) analysis categories and the fixed facial features. It is a nontaxing time investment by the user that needs to be made just once, and then begins to pay increasing returns as the same analogues are used over and over for many different case presentations and representations.

Notice that this perceptual solution to the information overload and memory problem also provides the optimal kind of representation for conveying pattern and context information. The perceptual mode is par excellence that of simultaneous coordination of many dimensions multiply interrelated. A perceptual view comprehends many things juxtaposed, as coexistent parts of one field of vision. It does so in an instant. Consider again all the information that is taken in simultaneously in an image of a face, or of a landscape. Researchers in artificial intelligence have had little success in their attempts to get computers to model complex images and patterns. The best computer approaches are autocorrelational, in which each point in an image is correlated with every other point; it takes a powerful computer many hours to crank out these autocorrelations for complex scenes. People do it at a glance! And they store the image in memory very durably. And they operate easily on this stored perceptual information to readily detect patterns of resemblance and dissimilarity. In Experience-Consolidation Systems, the computer is a tool used to tap into a powerful processing system that people have and computers do not -- a system that is ideally suited to processing large amounts of complexly entangled case information in ill-structured knowledge domains.

The Problem of Arrangement

This problem is handled by sequencing the presentation of the special graphic aids that correspond to individual cases according to a unique system of criss-crossing arrangements that capitalizes on the power and flexibility of the computer. The arrangement system is designed to maximize retention of the rich case information, to highlight case information that might produce difficulties in application (e.g., superficially similar cases with different outcomes and different appearing cases with the same practical outcomes), and to effectively contrast cases so that a large number of complex resemblance patterns within the same outcome category can be learned. [See the discussion of the "family" and "gene pool" analogies below.] This highlighting of multiple connections and similarities between cases permits a deemphasis on the retrieval of precompiled schema in favor of enabling schema assembly to fit the needs of a given situation. This is an important consideration given the impossibility of having a prepackaged conceptual schema for every situation that might be encountered in an ill-structured domain. If training is to transfer in such domains, flexibility of knowledge representation is crucial.

It should be noted that the algorithm for instructionally efficacious sequencing of cases and sequence rearrangement in successive case presentations is a general one. Thus the case arrangement part of Experience-Consolidation Systems constitutes an automated authoring aide: the author instantiates the system's structural frame with contentive case information and sequencings (and perceptual adjuncts) are automatically generated.

A primary consideration affecting the arrangement of the displays is the classification of distinctions that need to be learned. These distinguished classes are called families. For example, an Experience-Consolidation System might help one learn to distinguish: Disease X from similar Diseases U, Y, and Z (or Treatment X vs. Treatment Y for Disease Z); general decision-making processes that are best fit to a given decision-making context; continuations vs. reversals of bull and bear market trends; whether to bet on Team A or Team B in a sporting event; which of a set of career choices one is best suited to; effective vs. ineffective military strategies given situational contingencies; Cause X from Cause Y or Z in some "presenting" context of motor vehicle failure symptoms. . . or electrical-system failures, or weapon-system failures. . . (in military recruit training for 1st-pass trouble-shooting in highly confusable repair problems: this is the "schema selection" problem); and so on.

RECOGNITION PROCESS IN DECISION-MAKING AND CLASSIFICATION

The Experience-Consolidation System principle underlying training to distinguish conceptual-family members is the same one that is involved in learning to recognize the members of real families based on their appearance: perceptual recognition of family resemblance. Just as different families have different gene pools that produce within-family resemblance of an ill-structured sort (e.g., no single feature need always be present to detect resemblance), so too will there be a "gene pool" for conceptual families. Not every case in which Disease X occurs will have the same presenting symptoms, but there will be a set of family resemblance patterns that will be different from that of Disease Y. Whenever events are not random and the past is a useful guide (however complex and inexact), then there will be a pool of features and configurations of features that emerge in new instances of the family (new cases) according to principles similar to biological gene pool inheritance. Gene pools partially govern the range of possible appearances of family members. Similarly, in Experience-Consolidation Systems, they govern the range of possible appearances a situation within a conceptual family may have.

Experience-Consolidation Systems arrange the integrated visual displays (say, faces) corresponding to individual cases in order to maximize the ability to distinguish the targeted families (rather than other distinctions that might be made, but which would be irrelevant). Faces are presented more than once in the context of a variety of surrounding faces; this domain "criss-crossing" treats the conceptual terrain like a physical object that can be held up and examined from many points of view, so that it can be recognized from all the points of view that it may later occur in. After seeing a large number of these systematically arranged face (case) contrasts, the user learns to recognize perceptual family resemblances in exactly the same way you would recognize that someone getting out of their car near your house was related to the neighbor on your left and not the one on your right, even though you had never seen the visitor before. This is a skill individuals possess in different degrees, but even those at the low end of the scale are very successful at it in everyday life. It is an important part of our evolutionary heritage. Again, the only assumption necessary is that the families to be distinguished really are distinct families with gene pools that don't perfectly coincide. That is, properties of cases cannot be randomly distributed among the family categories. If this assumption isn't met, then there obviously is not basis for greater than chance performance by even the most expert of practitioners. (Note that the best that can be hoped for in an ill-structured knowledge domain is rough accuracy of performance, something significantly greater than chance. If perfect performance were possible, the domain would by definition be well-structured and amenable to direct instruction in general principles or mathematical models. You wouldn't need Experience-Consolidation Systems. Unfortunately, there are no domains that are well-structured in all their aspects.)

CONCLUSIONS

   In summary, Experience-Consolidation Systems meet the requirements of conveying lots of case information about lots of cases while at the same time overcoming the problems of time, inefficacious arrangement, and memory overload. Thus experience is consolidated in a number of ways: 1) multivariate information is extracted from real situations (cases, examples, instances, events, etc.) and is presented in quickly processed visual displays so as to consolidate the amount of time required for exposure to large numbers of situations; 2) the mode of visual display is chosen so as to be able to represent at a glance all the partially overlapping relationships among the numerous variables that need to be tracked in any ill-structured situation, effecting a perceptual consolidation or integration of complexly interrelated information; and 3) the visual displays corresponding to individual situations are presented and represented in varying combinations with other situations using a computerized arrangement scheme designed to facilitate the noticing of different types of "family resemblance" across situations with similar and dissimilar outcomes, a consolidation of necessary "control" knowledge. In other words, lots of richly detailed case information is presented in a mnemonically convenient manner designed to foster the development of skill in perceptually recognizing family resemblances across past situations grouped according to their action recommendations and outcomes.

   Finally, it should now be clear how Experience-Consolidation Systems differ from the CAI approach they most closely resemble, simulations. Simulations facilitate learning by doing. They have the virtue of requiring active participation by the student. However, they are not directly concerned with the effective acquisition of the complexly patterned information in cases. They often do not convey all the multivariate features needed for future contextually based determination of appropriate classifications and courses of action. Even where they do, simulations cannot be presented rapidly enough to accumulate large numbers of cases in a short amount of time. They do not have special mechanisms for fostering the recognition of large numbers of partial similarities and dissimilarities in their patterns of irregular overlap across cases. They do not specifically address the mnemonic overload problems associated with exposure to large numbers of nonchunkable cases. Thus, Experience-Consolidation Systems complement the purposes of simulations.

THE USE OF INTELLIGENT AUTHORING TOOLS TO ENHANCE CBI IN TECHNICAL TRAINING

R. S. Perez and R. J. Seidel

U.S. Army Research Institute
Alexandria, Virginia, U.S.A.

INTRODUCTION

   The use of computer driven training systems for military training has increased over the last decade. This increase in the usage of computers as a delivery system for training can be partly attributed to the availability of relatively inexpensive and powerful micro-computers. Other factors that have contributed to the increased reliance on computer based training are the claim made by the mass media assertion of the importance of high technology and the hardware manufacturers' claims and advertisements that computer based training is motivating and enjoyable for trainees, that it can produce high quality, uniform and effective training. The use of computers as the delivery mechanism for instruction and training has been offered as a panacea to the much claimed decline in the educational quality of training and the United States public education system.

   Recent reviews of the effectiveness and use of computers in training and education have noted the effectiveness of computer-based training (Kearsley, 1983; Kearsley, Hunter & Seidel, 1983; Orlansky & String, 1980; Kulick, Kulick & Cohen, 1984; Kearsley & Seidel, 1985). The relative cost and quality of courseware developed for training, however, has not kept pace with hardware advances, aside from the perennial demonstrations that CBI can be effective given proper curriculum development.

CURRENT TECHNICAL TRAINING

   Currently the U.S. military, specifically the U.S. Army, is faced with the need to continually train a large number of soldiers possessing a wide range of abilities and needs in a broad spectrum of skills from the very basic to the highly complex skills necessary in rapidly changing technical systems. This training is required to be replicable across many, varied environmental conditions and scattered locations. Moreover, high quality training with maximum success rate is imperative, in spite of limited resources of time, money and human expertise. The U.S. Army, as well as the other military services, use a process of training development called the Systematic Approach to Training (SAT). The SAT procedures consist of five major steps in the SAT process. These steps are analysis, design, development, implementation and control.

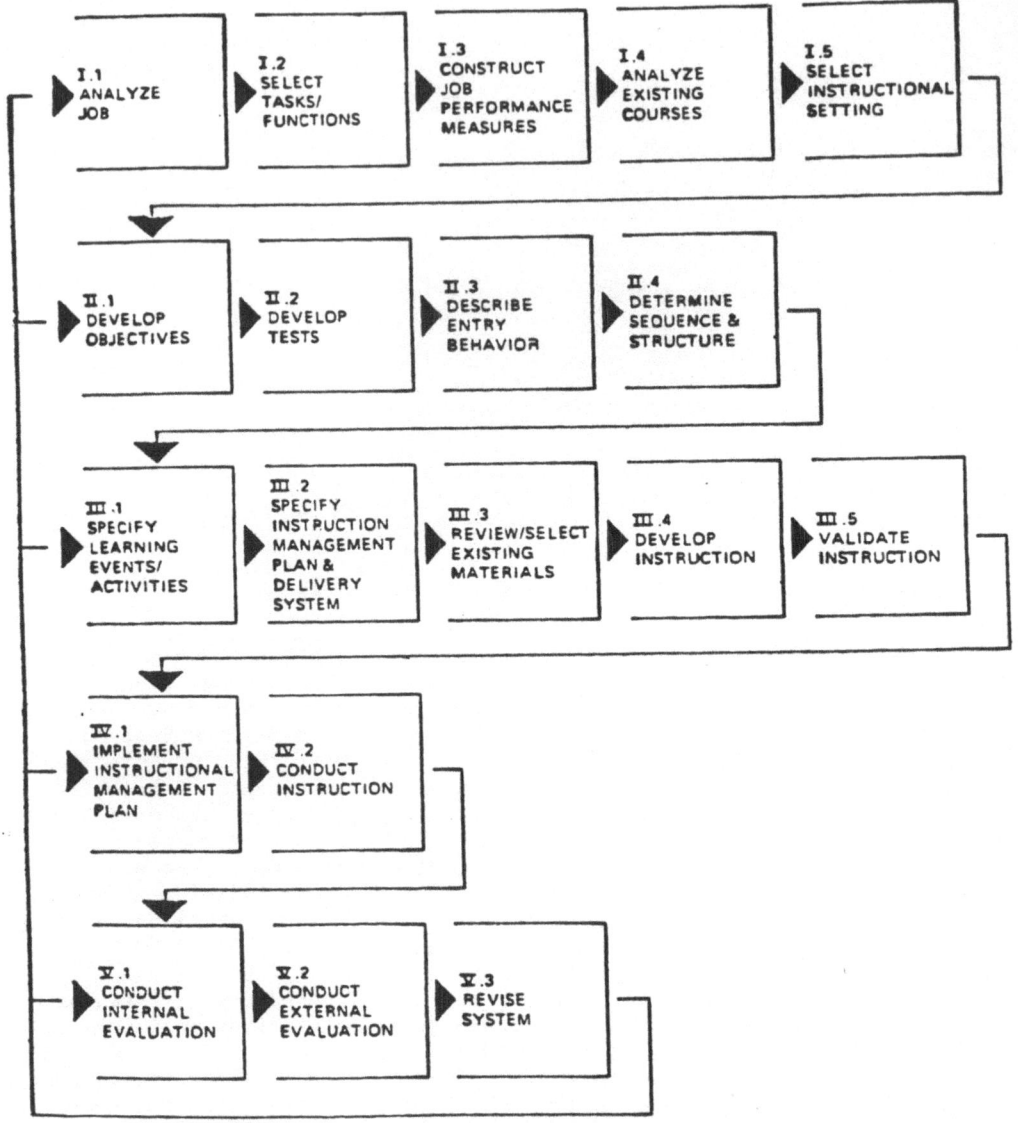

Figure 1. Systematic Approach to Training (SAT)

Andrews and Thompson (1982) have developed a model for estimating the costs of curriculum development using the SAT process. Their model considers the cost of resources (e.g., overhead plus direct labor) for development of instruction including the nature of the tasks to be developed, in terms of their complexity. The development of tasks requiring intellectual and cognitive strategies would be more labor intensive than those developing psychomotor skills and describing verbal information. A ratio of 30 hours of development time is required for each hour of instruction for tasks that have as their objective the development of intellectual skills and cognitive strategies. For tasks that require psychomotor skills and verbal information, the ratio is 15 hours to one hour of instruction. Using the Andrews & Beagles (1985) model, the developmental costs of a 300 hour-long course, designed to teach psychomotor skills and verbal information and delivered via platform instruction, would cost $186,000. This estimate does not include the operating costs associated with providing the course repeatedly, nor does it insure that the quality of the instructor used to deliver the training will be uniform. Thus, the associated cost of providing training for the U.S. Army is expensive using the SAT process and does not insure the quality of the instructor nor the instruction delivered via lectures (e.g., platform instruction).

Furthermore, platform instruction does not provide for individualized instruction. Benjamin Bloom (1983) and other researchers have suggested that the implementation of an instructional system that is sensitive, adaptive and personalized could enable over 90 percent of its students to learn at levels previously attained by only twenty percent of those students in conventional instruction. Bloom (1984) has presented evidence illustrating that student achievement varies depending upon which instructional condition they were taught under. He taught students under one of three conditions of learning: conventional, mastery learning and tutoring. It was found that about 90% of the tutored students and 70% of the mastery learning students attained the level achieved by only 20% of the students under conventional instructional conditions. In other words, students receiving tutoring performed at least two standard deviations better than students receiving group instruction.

In conventional instruction, students learn the subject matter in a class with about 30 students per teacher. Tests are administered periodically for the purpose of giving marks. In mastery learning, the same ratio of students to teachers exists except that the results of the formative tests are used to provide feedback to students and to determine corrective procedures. In the tutoring condition students are taught the subject matter with a tutor for each student (or two to three students). The instruction is followed by formative tests, feedback-corrective procedures and parallel formative tests. These results, of the effectiveness of tutoring or individualized instruction, are used to argue for the development of individualized training of highly technical, critical skills. The delivery mechanism for this individualized training has been CBI since the cost of providing human tutoring for two to three trainees would be prohibitive. Aside from the extensive savings that result from using CBI, research has found students are able to learn the material more quickly. Savings in student time using CBI has been found by several researchers who directly compared this method of delivery of instruction to traditional forms of instruction in private industry (Magidson, 1978; and Kearsley, Hillesohn, and Seidel, 1982). Orlansky and String (1979) have found that the greatest reason for time savings, demonstrated by students receiving computer-based instruction or computer-managed instruction, was their instruction was individualized. In sum, CBI has proven to be a more efficient teaching method in terms of both time and money, compared to traditional forms of instruction providing more uniform instruction and being tailored to the individual student.

The associated cost of developing CBI courseware is not trivial, nor is the expertise required of the authors. The cost of curriculum development ranges from 80 to 400 hours per each hour of instruction. McDonnel-Douglas has cited 130 hours per hour of instruction, using their Advanced Instructional System (AIS). Control Data Corporation suggests 200-225 hours of preparation time per hour of instruction. Boucher & Goldman (1983) found that the development of CBI in the military environment takes from 100 to 1,000 person-hours of effort by highly experienced personnel at costs of $5,000 to $50,000 to produce one hour of instruction, provided that the needed human expertise are available to produce it.

Thus, the production of computer-based training materials for essential technical skills consumes enormous amounts of human and financial resources. Wulfeck & Montague (1984) have found in their study of the effectiveness of training materials that present military personnel responsible for implementing the SAT process for training are untrained and inexperienced in teaching or training and lack fundamental knowledge required to design and develop appropriate instruction. Further, the SAT process itself has many methodological and implementation problems which provide stumbling blocks to the development of quality training materials. Although the costs of hardware used in the presentation and control of CBI have decreased over the decade, the costs of skilled human labor required to produce quality instructional materials, the most labor intensive aspect of the instructional development, have not. The instructional design process, although in part guided by scientifically derived principles of learning, in practice remains personal and highly artistic.

Therefore, the quality and quantity of CBI is highly dependent not only on such factors as instructional design principles but on the ability of the author to apply these learning principles to interpret and analyze the domain and/or task demands. Furthermore, a criticism often made of training materials developed using current ISD procedures is that the training is often proceduralized and superficial and is not designed to reach a "deep" understanding of the domain or task.

A solution to this problem of expensive, uneven and low quality CBI training materials is the development of intelligent authoring tools that aid the author in designing and developing CBI training programs.

In the remainder of this chapter we will argue that although the introduction of powerful affordable hardware and software are necessary components of an effective CBI system, they are not sufficient. The other components requisite for the development of high quality, inexpensive, portable and effective training materials are: 1) improved tools for aiding the authors in the development of instruction, such as intelligent authoring aids; 2) improved methodology and tools for deriving training requirements, knowledge engineering techniques; 3) the growing body of research knowledge on the representation of knowledge and procedures used in acquiring skills to perform a task; and 4) models of human information processing that form the bases of instructional theories. We also describe a set of intelligent authoring aids, a tool kit, that is intended to increase the quality of instruction and reduce the cost of producing computer-driven instruction.

USE OF COMPUTER-BASED INSTRUCTION IN THE MILITARY

Historically the introduction of computer-driven instructional systems in the U.S. military represents one solution to remedy the problem of the poor quality of available training materials. In the 1970's instructional technologists and engineering experts/computer scientists designed practical computer assisted instruction systems. These early forms of CBI were strongly influenced by Skinnerian behaviorism or neobehaviorism and are typified by a system developed around a static pedagogical model where learning is conceptualized as being linear and procedural in nature. However, later forms of CBI based on the programmed instruction paradigm have evolved to include other forms of instructional and learning principles. This conceptualization of learning as linear and procedural permitted the designers of the CBI systems to formulate a rather simplistic view of the CBI author. This view permitted the identification and specification of authoring functions. These specifications were used as guidelines to build a set of authoring tools that prompted the subject matter expert, who was the primary author in these systems, to author lesson material. The basic premise of this approach was that the subject

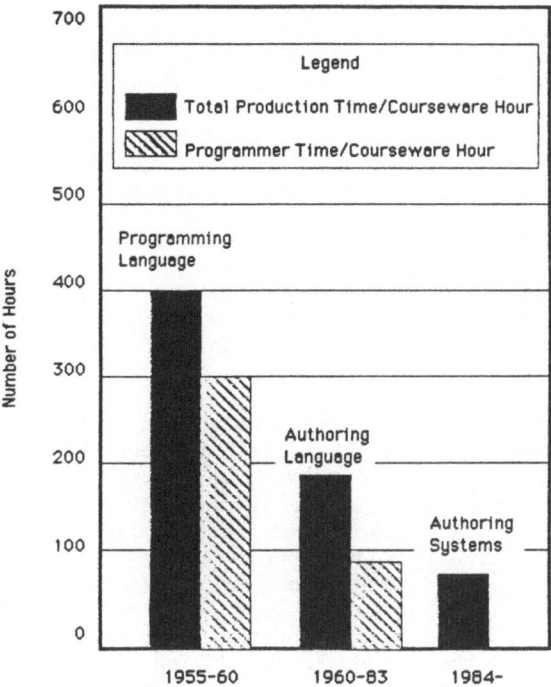

Figure 2. Courseware Production Time
(Hours per Courseware Hour)

matter expert could author training material without skill in, and knowledge of, computer programming or, more importantly, instructional theory or technology.

Because these early CBI systems were based on static pedagogical models they lacked instructional flexibility and restricted the creativity of the authors. These earlier systems were frame oriented. Instructional materials were organized beforehand into set presentations or frames. The "IBM Course-Writer" is an example of such a system. In an attempt to get around the static model limitation, many software and hardware developers like the Control Data Corporation, among others, developed authoring languages. "Tutor" is an example of a specialized language. This specialized computer language allows the author to use a variety of commands providing the author with the flexibility for input of information into several different instructional models. Authoring languages with the flexibility of Tutor are a powerful tool. However, authoring of training materials using these languages requires the authors to have expertise in three areas: the content domain, instructional technology and computer programming.

Present approaches to the development of instruction and training on computer driven systems rely heavily on authoring languages or systems that reduce the requirement of programming knowledge and skills. Szabo (1985) studied the impact of the use of authoring languages and systems on courseware development. The results of his study are presented in Figure 2. Figure 2 depicts the resultant reduction in courseware production time gained by the development and use of various authoring tools such as programming languages, authoring languages and, finally, authoring systems. The impact on courseware production is most notable when authoring systems requiring from 400 person hours to develop one hour of courseware are compared to the more recent authoring systems which require only 80 hours to create one hour of courseware. This reduction in production time of courseware does not, however, reduce the requirement that the author possess expertise in instructional design, nor do they reduce the amount of time and cost associated with the front-end-analysis and portions of the design. Seidel (1984), has estimated that 60 percent of the total development effort for the production of video-disk, a development process similar to CBI production, is in the front-end-analysis and portions of the design. Moreover, current authoring tools for CBI production have been focused on reducing the amount of time and skill the author spent in programming a CBI lesson. The development of these authoring tools has not affected the quality of current computer driven instructional systems. (See Kearsley's chapter for a further discussion of this point.)

In his review of current authoring tools such as authoring languages and authoring systems, David Merrill (1985) has concluded that none of the authoring systems he reviewed are true authoring systems. Rather, they are programming systems that have as their primary advantage special subroutines which facilitate educational programming, or they are menu driven editors which serve to reduce the amount of programming required. These systems fail to provide assistance to the author in the instructional design process. That is, they do not reduce the author's need to have knowledge of instructional design principles. Therefore, current authoring tools provide little to the author for producing quality CBI materials. In order for authoring aids to have a substantial impact on the quality and cost savings in the production of CBI, they must provide on-line helps and prompts in the design of instruction and aid the author in the knowledge acquisition process.

An example of current on-line helps for instructional design is contained in Control Data Corporation's PCD-3 authoring system in which an author can request help on-line in the form of information provided in menus advising them on how to format and write objectives, construct test items and conduct a task analysis. Authoring aids for FEA and knowledge acquisition have the greatest potential for reducing the cost of CBI (using the cost estimates provided by Boucher & Goldman [1983] one hour of instruction can cost anywhere from $5,000 to $50,000 to develop with current curriculum procedures). With the development and use of authoring tools, such a tool kit would make it possible to reduce the level of effort required to perform the front-end-analysis and the knowledge acquisition process. The resulting one hour of instruction costing from $3,000 to $30,000 would thereby reduce the estimated level of effort of the FEA from 60 percent (Seidel, 1984) to 30 percent, not to mention the expected increase in uniformity and quality of the training.

Further, present day computer driven training systems suffer from a number of deficiencies:

- They utilize deterministic algorithms limiting the flexibility of the system.

- They are task and content specific.

- They measure student results in terms of results instead of evaluating the deductive instructional process.

- Instructional models of the student or novice, are superficial.

- They do not distinguish between content and program domains.

- The creation of simulations are time consuming and complex.

- They are frame oriented and the presentations are static.

In later sections we provide suggestions of how these systems can be enhanced by technology from artificial intelligence, cognitive psychology and cognitive science.

APPLICATIONS OF AI TECHNOLOGY TO TRAINING

The quality of current computer based instructional systems and their developmental costs can be remedied by the application of Artificial Intelligence technology as aids, or "a tool kit", to the authoring process. Although current AI efforts can be characterized as examples of intelligent programming of well specified domains, these tools are domain dependent and are limited to those specific domains. However, these tools can be designed and developed to be generic and domain independent. Such tools are on-line tools for knowledge representation, tools for developing a student model and a set of tutoring rules or diagnostic rules that operate with and on the knowledge representation and on the student model. These tools would aid the author by providing intelligent functions within the instructional system. These intelligent functions could significantly improve the quality of instruction by providing instructional design aids. to the author and by reducing the complexity of the authoring task. Automation of portions of the process of FEA, design and development of instruction could reduce the amount of time required for the creation of instructional materials.

Authoring tools and procedures, which are currently available require of authors extensive development time and extensive knowledge of both the subject matter and of design principles to create instruction. Additionally, almost no CBI authoring tools exist for the design or creation of simulations. For example, it presently takes a subject matter expert with the assistance of a programmer up to three weeks to develop panel simulations using an authoring system like TICCIT, Freedman (1985). The development of intelligent authoring aids would enable authors to be more productive by automating some aspects of the authoring process, by reducing the need for subject matter experts and instructional designers, by increasing the quality and consistency of the instruction, by decreasing the time needed to develop instruction and by enabling training managers to reallocate scarce skilled labor. In order for the attainment of these goals to be realized, a prototype authoring system consisting of generic knowledge and skill acquisition tools for building behavioral and structural knowledge bases for a wide variety of tasks needs to be developed. This model authoring system must be a transparent, glass box and it must be made explicit to the author. The determination of what information should be presented in such a model, would be specified by explicit requests from the students or it could be driven by tutoring and diagnostic rules. One goal of this system is would be to reduce the gap between what the author knows, as represented by the model of the author, and the overall knowledge network. Present computer based training authoring aids attempt to aid the author by prompts, helps, menus and simulations. These authoring aids are not able to interpret what the user (author/student) wants to know and the basis for the mistakes he has made.

According to Merrill (1985), the design of intelligent authoring aids draws upon three areas of cognitive research according to Merrill (1985). These are first, the analysis of the instructional development process (authoring) as a cognitive task, acknowledging that some aspects of authoring is an art; second, the application of AI technology, techniques and methods such as intelligent tutors, expert systems and natural language interfaces; and third, the use of learning principles and analytic methods for task analysis from research in cognitive psychology and science.

ANALYSIS OF THE AUTHORING PROCESS

Second, we present our analysis of the instructional design process. We assume that this developmental process is logically structured with a series of proceduralized steps such as the Systematic Approach to Training (SAT) or a related model. In the authoring process the courseware designer must possess various types of skills which enable them to address the following questions: how to analyze the task to derive training requirements in terms of the prerequisite skills, knowledge, abilities and underlying cognitive processes; what and how to present information and in what sequence; how to structure and organize the content; how to measure and monitor student progress; how to diagnosis student errors; and finally, how, once student errors and misconceptions are identified, to remediate them. Second, that the authoring process although similar to teaching is different in important ways such as the dynamics and interactions between tutor and student may require a unique set of skills that include expert knowledge about the domain to be taught, the task, and knowledge of instructional design, development and evaluation. Present theories of instructional design that are used to guide the development of CBI are not adequate to specify the dynamic interactions between student and tutor nor do they address the micro architecture of tutorials.

MODEL FOR MACHINE TUTORING

A stated goal of researchers in the area of AI has been to emulate the functions of a human tutor and implement these in a computer tutor. The practical value of a computerized tutor to the military would be that of providing a "one to one" tutorial for the teaching of critical and highly complex technical skills. The successful implementation of such intelligent tutoring systems depends partly on evolving computer hardware and software. More importantly, it depends upon the development and expansion of a knowledge base in knowledge representation and human tutoring principles. To date, tutoring models that have been embodied in computer programs have, to a lesser degree, been based upon the research literature describing how expert humans teach. The exception to this observation is the work of Collins & Stevens (1983) which attempted to abstract a set of tutorial rules by observing expert teachers.

It is important to distinguish between traditional CBI and ICAI in that the latter has primarily focused on the tutorial as a strategy for instruction. CBI, on the other hand, has relied on several instructional strategies such as drill and practice, simulations, games and tutorials. Thus, the authoring process for ICAI programs may very well differ from the CBI authoring process given that ICAI programs emulate the dynamics between student and a tutor. Putnam (1985) has described a general model of tutoring which he based on his own empirical studies of expert tutors as well as previous models of teachers' thinking and decision making (Leinhardt, 1983; Shavelson & Stern, 1981) and on Collins & Stevens (1982) analysis of inquiry teaching. This generic model differs from other models of instructional design in that it includes knowledge from three domains: the mind of the teacher, the mind of the student and the behavior of the student. The key elements in this expert tutor model are: the agenda, the knowledge base and the student model. The agenda is the teacher's (author's) plans for a lesson – it is a dynamic plan that changes during the course of the lesson or tutorial session as the teacher acquires information about the students' ability and draws upon previous knowledge.

The agenda consists of the teacher's goals and subgoals of the agenda which determine the tutor's actions. The tutor's agenda is shaped by the knowledge base, the model of the student, and their performance (from which the tutor must infer what the student does or does not know).

The components of the tutor's knowledge base are Subject Matter Knowledge that is specific to the domain being taught and General Pedagogical Knowledge that consists of facts and theories about how students learn and general ways of presenting information and structuring lessons (instructional strategies) that are domain independent. The student diagnostic model is derived from an interaction between the knowledge base components of the tutor's previous experience with students, as well as their knowledge and understanding of the domain and pedagogical knowledge. Each of these components plays an important role in the tutoring process. Studies done by Rosenshine (1982), and Rosenshine & Stevens (1986) have from their empirical studies of teacher effectiveness in the classroom identified six teaching functions that are found in effective instruction. These functions are: (1) daily review and checking student(s) previous days' work with reteaching if necessary; (2) presenting new content, in small steps, but at a rapid pace; (3) providing instructional feedback and corrections to the student(s); (4) providing initial student practice with the tutor and monitoring student(s) understanding; (5) providing independent student(s) practice with a high rate of success (90-100%); and (6) weekly or monthly reviews. The last teaching function presumably serves not only to review previous materials, but also to integrate the material into a conceptual whole. Based on these researchers findings, in order that a machine tutor be successful it must contain, at the very least, these six functions to be effective.

The implementation of a tutorial system on a large scale is problematic for several reasons. First, the empirical knowledge necessary to verify the aforementioned model of tutoring is lacking. Second, the necessary skills required for the development of conventional CBI are not currently in the military environment. Thus, it is unlikely that individuals with all these skills are readily available (Kopstein & Seidel, 1967).

Therefore, ideally the development of CBI would be conducted by a team

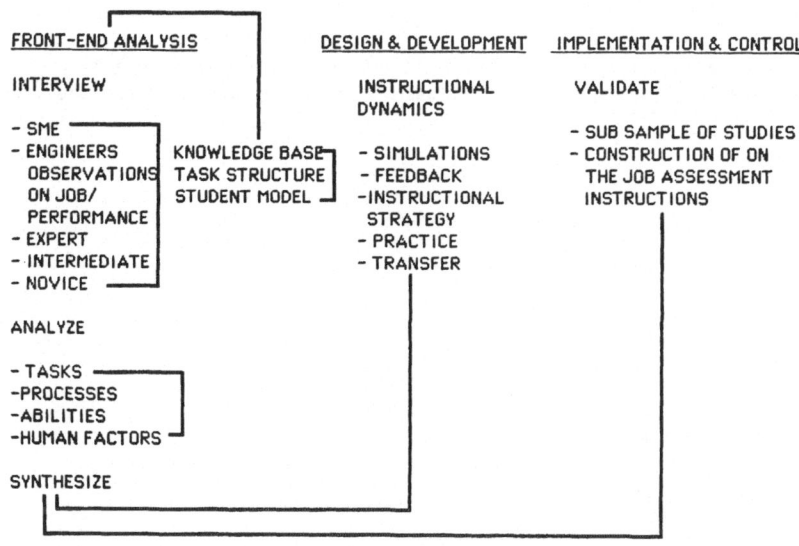

Figure 3. Authoring Process in Instructional Development

of individuals. This team would be comprised of an instructional designer, knowledge engineer, subject matter expert, task analyst, instructional developer, programmer and test specialist. Figure 3 summarizes our analysis of this process in terms of the specific skills, functions and knowledge required to perform the various tasks outlined in a representative instructional model. The next step is to identify and determine which of these skills, functions and knowledge can be automated by current state-of-the-art AI technology. These AI enhanced aids can serve to accomplish three general goals: first, they can provide tools which enable authors with a minimum of programming experience and skill and/or instructional design expertise to create effective instructional material; second, they can provide tools that allow authors, with considerable programming and/or instructional design skills, to create large amounts of instruction in a reduced period of time; and third, they can reduce the time and effort required to conduct a task/domain analysis for the design of instruction. Finally, they can provide, in an inexpensive way, methods for building simulation models that would lead to a deeper understanding on the part of the author of the behavioral and structural characteristics of the domain or task.

INTELLIGENT AUTHORING AID COMPONENTS

The conceptual model that this intelligent authoring system is based upon assumes that in order for it to be useful to an author it must contain three expert subsystems. These expert subsystems, illustrated in Figure 4, are: an Instructional Design Expert or tutor (IDE) that provides information to an author on the use of instructional strategies and principles; a Content Domain Expert (CDE) that models the knowledge of the content area (equipment) and advises the author on the domain (e.g., equipment characteristics); and a third expert, a front-end-analysis expert (FEA) or knowledge acquisition expert which advises and provides tools to build a knowledge base. In turn, each expert system would consist of two types of knowledge bases, structural and behavioral.

Each of these experts would interact with one another and would have the capability of modeling, displaying, demonstrating and explaining the system operation and the dynamics of their system. Monitoring of students' progress toward mastering the task would also be a capability of the system. For example, the instructional design expert would be capable of providing tutorials to the student (author) on any aspect of the instructional design and development process. The knowledge base in this expert system would consist of a student model, a set of tutoring rules and

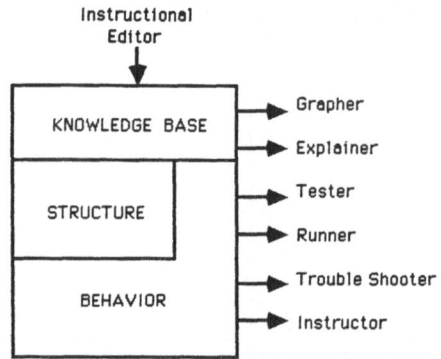

Figure 4. IDA System Diagram

diagnostic rules. Thus, in this system the user would be presented with
guidance in the form of "on-line helps" on how to present, organize and
structure information, when and what type of feedback should be included in
the instruction, how to provide explanations to students and how to
evaluate the student's performance. Each of the systems experts would be
comprised of four elements: a knowledge base, an intelligent tutor,
editor(s) and a glossary.

KNOWLEDGE BASES

   The description of Intelligent Authoring Aids is based on a proposal
for such aids developed by Wallace Feurzeig (1985) under contract to the
U.S. Army Research Institute. The knowledge bases that comprise each of
the expert systems are of two types, a structural knowledge and behavioral
knowledge base. The structural knowledge base of the instructional design
expert, for example, would provide a description of the overall structure
of the authoring systems, its organization and architecture (i.e.,
conceptual model of the authoring process) along with a description of the
purpose, role, functions of operation and how the authoring system
interconnects to the other subsystems of the system. In the
Front-End-Analysis (FEA) expert the training requirements are generated and
are then used as the content for the instructional design expert. On the
other side of the coin, the behavioral knowledge base provides descriptions
of the dynamic operations of a specific component or subsystem in terms of
how changes in one subsystem affects the behavior of the other components
in the system. Behavioral knowledge of the instructional design expert
would simulate the interactions between the FEA and Instructional Design
(ID) experts. This knowledge base would be illustrated by running
simulation models (engines) which could be either quantitative
(mathematical) or qualitative (functional). With respect to the ID expert,
the author could be presented with the overall structure of a lesson and
how its structure could be changed using different instructional design
models (theories). The dynamic quality of the running simulations of the
behavioral knowledge base can serve to illustrate to the author the
dynamics and interdependencies of various equipment subsystems within a
system. Forbus & Stevens (1981) demonstrated the value of such a
simulation program which generates and simulates the operation of a
hydraulic system. The interaction of these two knowledge bases, as
previously described, could be used to automate certain aspects of the
authoring process. Structural knowledge could be used to determine and
generate displays of schematic diagrams of the ID system depicting its
architecture and topology, physical and logical connections and paths,
narrative descriptions of the systems structure, its function and role and
mechanisms of any specific component. This would provide the author with
tests to access the users' knowledge of the system. Weld (1983) has
developed a comprehensive algorithm for generating explanations and
answering questions about the role, structure and functions for subsystems
of engineering devices. The behavioral knowledge could also be used by the
instructional designer (as opposed to the SME) to generate animated
displays of the schematic diagrams which would be created by the structural
knowledge base of the system to simulate the behavior of the subsystem.
These simulations could be used to provide the authors with a deeper
understanding of how the subsystem that they are developing training for
interacts, or to aid the author in programming frames. The creation of
these frames would enable the author to preview animate displays, such as
an on-line story board. These displays would also contain the explanations
of the running system, including specific events and their sequence, to
provide interactive environments for student explorations to be used in a
guided discovery instructional strategy approach, or in a mixed initiative
dialogue, to coach, in providing practice and aid in investigations by the

student of the system's systematic behavior, as in the introduction of specific faults and observing the subsequent behavior on the rest of the system. Steamer (Holland, Hotching, & Weitzman, 1984) is an example of this type of modeling applied to military training.

EDITORS

In addition to the knowledge bases, an instructional editor and a set of instructional specialists comprise this intelligent authoring system. The instructional editor is used by the instructional designer for developing and modifying the knowledge base and for setting parameters and conditions governing the operation of the instructional specialists. The instructional specialists are intelligent editors in the form of program modules designed to perform specific instructional tasks or functions. These modules are known as Grapher, Explainer, Runner, Tester, Trouble-shooter and Presenter. Each of these modules and their proposed function will be briefly described in the following section.

The Grapher is designed to generate schematic diagrams of the system using specialized iconic representations for drawing various system components. Its function is to generate animate displays that depict the system's behavior in conjunction with a runner module as it runs the qualitative simulation model that describes the system's operation. It may also be used to display state diagrams representing the progress of the model, as it runs through a sequence of states in an event chain. These state diagrams may be used as the graphics, in a lesson, describing the dynamic behavior of the system to the student.

The Explainer generates text explanations of a system's structure and behavior. Explanations of system structure can be generated recursively, covering the entire system, then its subsystems and components at all levels of the hierarchy. Explanations of the behavior of the system are generated as the qualitative simulation model is run in synchrony with animated graphic displays showing signal propagation, information flow and other dynamic effects. Alternatively, in the query mode, the student can request explanations about the structure or specific system components.

The Runner operates the qualitative simulation model. It uses the Grapher to demonstrate how the system behaves. It may allow the student to alter the states of the system components by designating their icons. It could also be used by the SME to verify the accuracy and completeness of the structural and behavioral knowledge bases. In this manner the student can introduce faults and see their effects on the behavior of the system. The Runner incorporates controls for single step operation and for operating the simulation until a specific condition is satisfied.

The Tester generates specific forms of questions and problems to assess the student's knowledge of the role, function and structure of the overall system and its components. Test presentations may involve displays as well as text items.

The Troubleshooter is a specialized module for use in applications involving maintenance of complex devices. There are two modes of operations in this module. First, in the demonstration mode it allows the student to enter a fault and then to study the troubleshooter's strategy as it displays its action and explains its reasoning using the other modules. The second mode of interaction is the practice mode. In this mode, the system enters a fault for the student to diagnose. It then monitors the student's actions in the course of his troubleshooting activity. The program may elicit the student's behavior and tentative hypotheses as the student attempts to isolate the fault and take remediative action. At the end of the session, the troubleshooter module reviews and critiques the student's performance.

The Presenter follows either the instructional strategy set designed by the instructional designer or selects a strategy for the SME. Then the presenter will control the selection and sequence of instructional tasks. The Presenter may perform these functions adaptively using differential models of student and expert task performance. Selection and sequencing may be controlled by the Program (tutorial model), entirely by the student (inquiry or exploration models) or shared (learner control or mixed initiative models).

The Instructional Editor, along with the other program modules and the intelligent editors, are designed to provide extensive capabilities for automating the development of instruction and aid the human instructional designer. A general knowledge representation language is available to the authors that enables them to "customize" the representation of knowledge to be taught to the student. Another feature of this module is that there are editors dedicated to the subject matter content. These modules would enable the author to develop a deeper understanding of the human expertise and the knowledge domain needed to teach students. The users of this system are seen as instructional designers and subject matter experts not AI systems programmers. Therefore, a natural language interface is a critical element of this editor. The goal of this editor is to provide the authors with knowledge aids to help him/her convey a concrete idea of the surface and deep structure of each domain to the student.

Another function of this editor is learning management. This facility enables the author to create and modify knowledge bases. The knowledge representation language incorporates current features of AI programming languages such as "Loops." It uses semantic nets, frames and production systems. The representation language will be used by the author to describe the conceptual structure and relationships among the knowledge bases and their elements. Similarly, to other AI programming systems, such as Loops (Stefik et.al., 1983), the intelligent authoring system provides an integrated environment designed for supporting multiple knowledge paradigms. Building domain-specific knowledge editors, presented in the language of the subject matter domain, will increase the likelihood of constructing complex structured knowledge bases that serve as the data base for authors to draw upon when designing high quality instruction without extensive cost or human resources.

COGNITIVE THEORY AND TECHNOLOGY

The introduction of intelligent authoring aids should contribute to reducing the cost of instructional development. However, improving the quality of instruction and training will depend upon continuing research in two areas: first, the development of conceptual and methodological tools for conducting a cognitive task analysis and second, the incorporation of research on knowledge representation and instructional theories from cognitive psychology and science must be incorporated. Feurzeig (1987), in a chapter in this book, has along with other researchers pointed out several limitations in current AI tutoring systems. In these systems, remediation of students' mistakes is often given at an incorrect level of detail. These systems either assume too little student knowledge or too much. Often it is not sufficient to tell a student he is wrong and indicate the correct solution method. An intelligent CAI system should be able to make hypotheses, based on a student's error history, as to where the real source of his difficulty lies (Barr & Feigenbaum, 1982). Current

AI tutorial systems assume a specific conceptual framework of the domain and thereby judge the students' responses on the basis of this critical framework (Sleeman & Brown, 1983). The tutoring and critiquing provided to the student by these tutorials are intuitively based rather than based on instructional or learning theory. The interactions afforded by these systems are restrictive to the students, limiting of students' responses and are unduly restraining of the diagnostic mechanisms. Almost all of these systems do not "learn" from their interactions with students. Although their content presentations are more dynamic than those of CBI systems, the tutoring mechanisms are static and not responsive to the individual differences of students. Feurzeig (1986) suggested several ways of building tutoring systems without these limitations. However, he has characterized this task as time consuming and difficult. He believes that the investigation of some instructional approaches may be productive in developing systems that do not have the aforementioned limitations. It appears that the integration of knowledge and technology from the fields of instructional design and theory (Park, Perez & Seidel, in preparation) and research on such cognitive science concepts as mental models (Genter & Stevens, 1985; Perez & Seidel, 1986) could serve as the building blocks for the development of more effective tutorial systems. Further, for the field to advance, empirical tests and research must be done to address several research questions. First, are the theoretical representation systems used by AI researchers adequate descriptions of the knowledge a person must have to perform a specific task? Second, what types of interactions between the tutor and student result in a successful communication of knowledge? Third, is a question raised by Bagget & Ehrenfeucht (1985) "What is the role of modalities of information (moving video, still photos, color graphs, verbalizations) with respect to their being able to execute concepts?" Fourth, are the cognitive structures of the student influenced and altered as a function of information presented by the tutor?

A major problem in the development of effective training materials and training programs for the operation and maintenance of highly sophisticated equipment has been the lack of appropriate methods for determining the necessary cognitive skills and processes that are required by the learners to take advantage of the leverage afforded by these complex systems. Current analytic approaches used in the design of training procedures and materials have been exclusively concerned with the training of "proceduralized" tasks (Nauta, 1983) or more aptly the "proceduralizing" of tasks and skills, rather than the development of training for such cognitive skills and tasks as generic troubleshooting, problem solving and decision making. These analytic approaches have resulted in the development of instructional materials and training that presents trainees with surface knowledge but does not provide the learner with a deeper understanding of the task. This limits the generality of the training and reduces the possibility of positive transfer. Further, this job-relevant and task oriented training has not taken into consideration human-machine interface factors such as the ease of equipment usage, its complexity in terms of the cognitive and attentional demands and the information processing requirements under varying environmental conditions. The solution to this problem is to develop analytic techniques for deriving training requirements that reflect the underlying psychological processes and knowledge structures needed by the trainee to competently perform a specific task. This analysis of training requirements, that specifies the psychological processes, knowledge structure and information needs of a domain or task, is a critical step in bringing the constructs of cognitive psychology to the instructional design process. Currently, analytic techniques that meet the needs of instructional designers and trainers do not exist. Furthermore, these analytic techniques must, if they are to be of use, must provide the instructional designer or knowledge engineer provide with guidance in identification of cognitive processes and knowledge structures that comprise the successful execution of a task and also explicitly describe procedures and techniques in such a way as to be learnable, functional and usable. Such an approach would combine AI technology (knowledge engineering techniques) with advances in cognitive psychology. An example of a cognitive task analysis approach is Kieras & Polson's (1982) application of GOM's model to technical training, proposed and developed by Card, Moran & Newell (1980). This approach allows the author of training materials to better specify the cognitive processes and knowledge structures needed to perform a task. This, along with powerful computing environments, could lead to the development of sophisticated simulations of physical systems. These analytical techniques could result in improved methods for the specification of how to present, structure and organize information to the student; enhanced analyses of cognitive processing requirements; planning; and enhanced use of the interactive characteristics of CBI -- of interactive teaching environments.

COGNITIVE INSTRUCTIONAL THEORY

Improved methods for the specification of cognitive processes and knowledge structures, required of a trainee to perform a task are important prerequisites for developing quality instruction, along with the formulation of an instructional theory. That would provide an instructional designer with guidance in selecting an instructional strategy to teach necessary cognitive processes and knowledge structures for competent task completion. In this section, we describe our view on what requirements are needed in an instructional theory such that it would enhance present computer driven training systems, smart or otherwise.

A Cognitive Instructional Theory should be capable of providing guidance to the instructional designer as to how to infer a student's initial stage of learning and at any point during training. Several researchers have demonstrated that differences exist in problem solving behavior between experts and novices (Reiff, Larkin & Brackett, 1976; Chi, Feltovich & Glaser, 1981). These differences go beyond the fact that one has knowledge and the other does not. The differences are of a qualitative nature. The expert differentially structures his approach to a problem solving task from that of a novice. To infer a student's stage of learning, however, requires additional research on experts and novices to include intermediate levels of expertise and more refined measures of the cognitive structures of experts and novices. Recent theory and research in cognitive science have provided a new framework in which to view instruction and training. This view suggests that an understanding of how people represent knowledge, think and solve problems are important and critical to how we train them. An important issue in the design of training programs for teaching these highly technically complex skills is not only a clear understanding of how experts represent knowledge and the ability to present these representations to trainees, but a prescriptive set of principles that describe how experts have acquired these knowledge structures. Considerable research has dealt with how people think and their use of mental representations in acquiring cognitive skills. It has been demonstrated how the structure of information in the learner's mind interacts with the structure of information learned (Anderson, 1977; Rumelhardt & Ortony, 1977; and Schank, 1980) have demonstrated how the structure of information in the learner's mind interacts with the structure of information to be learned. Other researchers (Greeno, 1977; Hayes & Simon, 1976; and Simon & Simon, 1978) have compared problem solving behaviors of novices to experts and demonstrated that the way the representation of the problem is defined influences the adequacy of the solution of the problem. These differences between experts and novices were studied further by Chi, Feltovich & Glaser (1981). They found that these observed differences were due to the use, by experts, of strategies to structure the knowledge. Research in this area of problem solving and cognitive structure can be applied to training. One application would be to design instructional materials that provide novices with guidance in solving problems such as troubleshooting.

The role of spatial representations and imagery in cognitive skill acquisition, memory and performance (Bower, 1970; Paivio, 1972; and Montague & Carter, 1974) has also been studied extensively. Visual imagery, including imaged information retrieved from memory, has also been studied in some detail by Kosslyn & Shwartz (1977) and Shepard (1977). It has been found that the spatial properties of images (e.g., their size and the relative distances among their parts) play significant roles in cognitive tasks, in that imagery can be a powerful tool for acquiring new skills in various domains, as Mayer (1979) demonstrated in his study of the use of mental models to teach computer programming. More recent research along this line is the work of Norman (1983) and Genter & Stevens (1984) on "mental models." A mental model is defined as an internal mental representation (model) of how things and people interact. This mental representation can be used by people much like a personnel metaphor in that it serves to predict and explain how a device or equipment work (Norman, 1983). According to de Kleer (1975 and 1979) mental models are a result of a "revisioning", i.e., forming a visual image of the system elements in order to assimilate the preparation of the elements of the system. Frederiksen (1986) suggests that the use of a mental model conceptualization has been demonstrated to capture the way in which experts reason in various domains. In electronics, for example, de Kleer (1985) has observed that "an engineer does not perform a qualitative analysis unless he first understands the circuit at a qualitative level." (p. 275)

The use of visual images to convey instructional information that would enable the student to develop a qualitative model would appear to be an effective instructional technique. However, a new type of grammar and a new set of prescriptive rules of how to use graphics in the design of instruction is needed. An attempt to find theoretical as well as practical principles for the use of different modalities is the work of Bagget & Ehrenfeucht (1983; 1985a; 1985b) in which they have developed a knowledge representation system that includes the use of different modalities in presenting a concept. A concept in their system can be represented as a graph with two kinds of associative links and modes corresponding to elements from different modalities. For example, a concept may be represented to a student with all or some of its elements in a number of different modes: the motoric or action, visual or pictorial and linguistic or abstract. It is their belief that the resultant memory is a single conceptual memory representation. This memory is connected to multiple processes which are used to process various types of input. This input may be either visual, auditory, or tactical information representing concepts. These processes function to convert input signals memory into form concepts. Therefore, a concept in this system can be composed of visual, auditory and motoric information. Presumably, an author who uses this system may be able to design instruction that includes concepts or the same concepts in multiple modalities.

QUALITATIVE MODELS AS AN INSTRUCTIONAL STRATEGY

The instructional or training goal of teaching students a "deeper" understanding of a domain and/or how a piece of equipment operates requires alternative conceptualizations of models of instructional strategies. These models or strategies must be able to simulate the exponent's qualitative reasoning processes and present their knowledge structures.

This qualitative model could then be used by the instructional designer to capture the reasoning process and knowledge structure of an expert. The value to an instructional designer of using a qualitative model is that it enables the designer to capitalize on the personal metaphor by which the learner models the subject matter domain. Further, using a qualitative model as an instructional strategy would equip the instructional designer with a powerful model on which to design instruction. Not only would the behavior of an expert, proficient at a task, be captured but underlying cognitive processes essential to the successful completion of similar tasks would be identified.

White & Frederiksen (1985) have demonstrated that a mental model can be used to reason qualitatively and casually about the effects of different faults on normal electric circuits. Frederiksen (1986) has argued further that mental models are central to expert performance on a number of logical grounds. These mental representations of how things and people interact improve the student's understanding of a specific domain. Additionally, they are memorable, adaptable, cognitively economical and extensive. For example, technicians trained using qualitative and mental models do not need to remember dozens of fixed procedures nor do they have to constantly refer to technical manuals in order to perform operation and maintenance tasks such as troubleshooting. In this conceptual framework of instruction, the student is provided with generalized, but complex, mental models from which they can derive specific procedures, insuring that performance based on the mental model can be adaptable to other unfamiliar systems. Since the reasoning process in problem solving tasks, like troubleshooting, in any system are similar, the mental model for this task is cognitively economic. Thus, specific procedures need not be learned and relearned for each new piece of equipment. The use of a mental model as a powerful instructional tool is demonstrated in the work of Kieras & Bovair (1984) in which they provide students with information about the structure and functioning of a technical system prior to providing them with instructions on how to use the system. The use of this instructional tool resulted in faster learning and less errors were made by the students. They also found that providing a mental model of how these "devices" functioned enhanced the ability of the students to localize faults.

As an instructional strategy for teaching highly sophisticated and complex cognitive skills, the use of mental models combined with AI technology to enhance the delivery of CBI in which the student is presented with simulations of the behavioral, structural and functional knowledge of a system will result in technicians that acquire operation and maintenance skills quicker and with less errors. Thus, it is our belief that the combination of AI technology, CBI and advances in cognitive psychology will lead to training systems that provide students with "deeper" understanding of a system or domain enhancing performance and increase the generality of the training.

REFERENCES

Anderson, J.R. (1985). "Skill acquisition: Compilation of weak-method problem solutions." Office of Naval Research, Technical Report 85-1. Arlington, VA.

Anderson, R.C. (1977). The notion of schemata and the educational enterprise, general discussion of the conference. In R.C. Anderson, R.J. Spiro & W.B. Montague (Eds.), "Schooling and the acquisition of knowledge" (pp 415-431). Hillsdale, NJ: Lawrence Erlbaum Associates.

Andrews, D.H. & Beagles, C.A. (1984). Estimating curriculum developmental costs: A model on the complexity of the learning tasks. "Proceedings of the 6th Interservice-Industry Training Equipment Center." Washington, DC

Bagget, P. & Ehrenfeucht, A. (1983). "Learning a procedure from multimedia instructions: The effects of film and practice" (Tech. Rep. No. 125). Office of Naval Research.

Bagget, P. & Ehrenfeucht, A. (1985). "Conceptualizing in assembly tasks" (Tech. Rep. No. 139). Office of Naval Research.

Bagget, P. & Ehrenfeucht, A. (1985). "A multimedia knowledge representation for an 'intelligent' computerized tutor" (Tech. Rep. No. 142). Office of Naval Research.

Barr, A. & Feigenbaum, E.A. (1982). "The handbook of artificial intelligence" (Vol II). William Kaufman.

Bloom, B.S. (1968). "Learning for mastery" (Evaluation Comment, No. 1 & 2). UCLA, CSEIF.

Bloom, B.S. (1984, June/July). The 2 sigma problem: The search for methods of group instruction as effective as one-to-one tutoring. "Educational Researcher," pp. 4-16.

Bower, G.H. (1970). Organizational factors in memory. "Cognitive Psychology," "1," 18-46.

Brown, J.S., Burton, R.R. & Bell, A.G. (1974). "Sophie: A sophisticated environment for teaching electronic troubleshooting" (BB&N Report No. 2790, March).

Card, S.K., Moran, T.P., & Newell, A. (1983). "The psychology of human-computer interaction." Hillsdale, NJ: Lawrence Erlbaum Associates.

Chi, M.T.H., Feltovich, P. & Glaser, R. (1981). Categorization and representation of physics problems by experts and novices. "Cognitive Science," "5," 121-152.

Collins, A., Stevens, A.L. (1982). Goals and strategies of inquiry teachers. In R. Glaser (Ed.), "Advances in instructional psychology" (pp. 65-119). Hillsdale, NJ: Lawrence Erlbaum Associates.

DeKleer, J. (1985). How circuits work. In D.C. Bobrow (Ed.), "Qualitative reasoning about physical systems." Cambridge, MA: MIT Press.

Feurzeig, W., (in press). Cognitive science, artificial intelligence, and complex training. In R.J. Seidel & P. Weddle (Eds.), "The use of CBI in military environments." The Hague, Netherlands: North Holland Press.

Feurzeig, W., Ash, W.L., & Ricard, G.L. Trio: An expert system for air intercept training. "Proceedings of the 6th Inservice Industry Training Conference" (pp. 45-48).

Freedman, R.S., (in preparation). OBIE-1: A knowledge-based software tool for simulation. "Proceedings of the 1985 New York Conference on Software Tools."

Forbus, K. & Stevens, A. (1981). "Using qualitative simulation to generate explanations" (BB&N Report No. 4490). Cambridge, MA.

Genter, D. & Stevens, A.S. (Eds.) (1983). "Mental models." Hillsdale, NJ: Lawrence Erlbaum Associates.

Greeno, J.G. (1977). Process of understanding in problem solving. In N.J. Castellan, D.B. Pison & G.R. Potts (Eds.), "Cognitive Theory," (Vol. 2). Hillsdale, NJ: Lawrence Erlbaum Associates.

Hayes, J.R. & Simon, H.A. (1976). The understanding process: Problem isomorphs. "Cognitive Psychology," "8," 165-190.

Holland, J.D., Hutchins, E.L. & Weitzman, L. (1984). Steamer: An interactive inspectable simulation-based training system. "The AI Magazine," "5(2)," 15-27.

Kearsley, G. (1983). "Computer-based training." Reading, MA: Addison-Wesley.

Kearsley, G., Hunter, B., Seidel, R.J. (1983). Two decades of computer-based instruction projects: What have we learned? "T.H.E. Journal."

Kearsley, G. & Seidel, R.J. (1985). Automation in training and education. "Human Factors," "27(2)," 67-74.

Kieras, D.E., & Polson, P. (1982). "An outline of a theory of the user complexity of devices and systems" (Working Paper No. 1). University of Arizona and University of Colorado.

Kieras, D.E., & Bovair, S. (1984). The role of a mental model in learning to operate a device. "Cognitive Science," "8," 255-274.

Kopstein, F. & Seidel, R.J. (1967). Computer assisted instruction versus traditional instruction. "Economic Adviser," "16," 147-175.

Kosslyn, S.M. & Shwartz, S.P. (1977). A simulation of visual imagery. "Cognitive Science," "1," 265-295.

Kulick, J.A., Kulick, C.C., & Cohen, P.A. (1984). Effectiveness of computer-based college teaching: Meta-analysis of findings. "Review of Educational Research," "50(4)," 528-544.

Magidson, E.M. (1978, August). Student assessment of plato: What the students like and dislike about CAI. "Educational Technology," pp. 15-19.

Merrill, M.D. & Wood, L.E. (1984). Computer guided instructional design. "Journal of Computer-Based Instruction," "11(2)," 60-63.

Merrill, M.D. (1985). Where is the authoring system? "Journal of Computer-Based Instruction," "12(4)," 90-96.

Montague, W.E. & Wulfeck II, W.H. (1983). Instructional quality inventory: A formative evaluation tool for instructional development. "Performance and Instructional Journal," "22," 11-14.

Norman, D.A. (1983). Some observations on mental models. In A.L. Stevens & D. Genter (Eds.), "Mental models." Hillsdale, NJ: Lawrence Erlbaum Associates.

Orlansky, J. & String, J. (1981). Computer-based instruction for military training. "Defense Management Journal," 46-54.

Paivio, A. (1972). "Imagery and verbal processes." New York: Holt, Rinehardt & Winston.

Park, O.K., Perez, R.S. & Seidel, R.J. (in preparation). ICAI: Old wine in a new bottle or is it a new vintage? In G. Kearsley (Ed.).

Rosenshine, B. (1983). Teaching functions in instructional programs. "Elementary School Journal," "83," 335-351.

Rosenshine, B. & Stevens, R. (1986). Teaching functions. In Wittrock (Ed.), "The Handbook of Research in Teaching" (3rd ed.). New York: MacMillian.

Rouse, W.B. & Morris, N.M. (1985). "On looking into the black box: Prospects and limits in the search for mental models" (Report No. 85-2). Atlanta: Georgia Institute of Technology, Center for Man-Machine Research.

Rumelhardt, D.E. & Ortony, A. (1977). The representation of knowledge in memory. In R.C. Anderson, R.J. Spiro & W.B. Montague (Eds.), "Schooling and the acquisition of knowledge." Hillsdale, NJ: Lawrence Erlbaum Associates.

Schank, R.C. (1980). Language and memory. "Cognitive Science," "4 (3)," 243-284.

Simon, D.P. & Simon, H.A. (1978). Individual differences in solving physics problems. In R. Stegler (Ed.), "Children's thinking: What develops?" Hillsdale, NJ: Lawrence Erlbaum Associates.

Sleeman, D. & Brown, J.S. (Eds.). "Intelligent Tutoring Systems." London: Academic Press.

Szabo, M. (1985). "Authoring aids." Paper presented at the 9th Annual Meeting of the Association for the Development of Computer-based Instruction Systems, Philadelphia, PA.

Vineberg, R. & Joynee, J.N. (1980). "Instructional system development: An analysis of needs and availability" (Special Report 82-37, August). San Diego, CA: Navy Personnel Research and Development Center.

Weld, D.S. (1983). "Explaining complex engineering devices" (BB&N Report No. 5489, November).

White, B.K. & Frederiksen, J.R., (1985). QUEST: Qualitative understanding of electrical system troubleshooting. "ACM SIGART Newsletter," "93," pp. 34-37.

Wulfeck, W. & Montague, W.B. (1984, Winter Quarter). Computer-based instruction: Will it improve instructional quality? "Training Technology Journal," "1(2)."

COGNITIVE SCIENCE, ARTIFICIAL INTELLIGENCE, AND COMPLEX TRAINING

W. Feurzeig

BBN Laboratories, Inc.
Cambridge, Massachusetts, U.S.A.

INTRODUCTION

During the past ten years there has been extensive work on the development of artificial intelligence methods for instruction. Interest in the instructional research community has shifted from traditional forms of computer-aided instruction (CAI) to new forms that employ "intelligent" methods, and are thus referred to as intelligent CAI (ICAI) systems or intelligent tutoring systems (ITS). Relative to the older CAI, the sheer technological power of ICAI methods is apparent and compelling. Systems such as SOPHIE, STEAMER and TRIO have demonstrated a variety of new and powerful computational capabilities in support of complex training tasks in areas such as electronic troubleshooting, naval steam propulsion plant operation, air intercepts and other important military application domains.

The complexity and sophistication of these systems is impressive. They incorporate a great deal of knowledge about their task domain, sometimes in the form of detailed dynamic simulations that are runnable, inspectable and semantically transparent. They are capable of making deep deductive inferences about the structure and behavior of the systems they model. For example, they can often simulate the behavior of a system under arbitrary hypothetical states and answer "what if" types of questions. Also, they can determine whether a student's actions or conclusions are logically warranted from the knowledge currently at hand and whether alternative actions or hypotheses are plausible.

ICAI systems often incorporate "experts" -- programs that are capable of performing the tasks to be taught in just the way the student is to learn to emulate. Some experts are "articulate", i.e., they describe and explain their own performance in carrying out a task as they perform it. Articulate expert programs are very sophisticated; nevertheless, it is a great deal easier to build the expert performance component of an ICAI system than it is to build the cognitive and instructional components -- those concerned with diagnosing the student's difficulties in performing the task, and deciding on appropriate instructional strategies to aid in overcoming them.

In an overview of recent work on intelligent tutoring systems, for example, the following are listed as some of their "acknowledged shortcomings" (Sleeman & Brown, 1983):

1. The instructional material produced in response to a student's query or mistake is often at the wrong level of detail, as the system assumes too much or too little student knowledge.

2. The system assumes a particular conceptualization of the domain, thereby coercing a student's performance into its own conceptual framework. None of these systems can discover, and work within, the student's own (idiosyncratic) conceptualization to diagnose his 'mind bugs' within that framework.

3. The tutoring and critiquing strategies used by these systems are excessively ad hoc reflecting unprincipled intuitions about how to control their behavior. Discovering consistent principles would be facilitated by constructing better theories of learning and mislearning -- a task requiring detailed psychological theories of knowledge representation and belief revision.

4. User interaction is still too restrictive, limiting the student's expressiveness and thereby limiting the ability of the tutor's diagnostic mechanisms."

The goal of building tutoring systems without these limitations is, indeed, very difficult; it is an ambitious long-term enterprise. Fortunately, however, there are other lines of development currently under investigation that address these issues differently and that have significance for military training. This note identifies some of the instructional approaches that appear productive and suggests directions for future work along such lines.

EXTENDED INSTRUCTIONAL PARADIGMS

A great deal of the advanced work in ICAI is focused on the development of powerful tutoring facilities, those where the initiative and control reside primarily in a sophisticated teaching program rather than with the student. Relatively little work has been done on the development of ICAI systems that integrate tutorial programs with complementary facilities for student exploration or practice. Yet these unprescriptive kinds of activities are essential to learning. However acquired, factual and procedural knowledge is assimilated and integrated through usage, by practice and by application.

A great deal of critical military training involves the acquisition of skill through practice in operation and maintenance of complex systems. Many current "trainers", though they incorporate powerful computers capable of supporting ICAI, do not in fact support any instructional programs. Their use in training requires an instructor. They are actually simulators that provide a training environment, rather than true training systems. The design of instructional capabilities to support such practice environments should be a primary area of military ICAI development.

The development of integrated training systems that support multiple modes of instruction, e.g., exploration, tutoring, and guided practice, is another important area for future work. The principles involved in the integration and use of ICAI systems employing multiple instructional paradigms are not yet established but the instructional benefits in military applications involving complex skill training appear to be considerable.

The technological issues involved in building environments for student exploration of concepts or processes are not as formidable as those typically encountered in building intelligent tutorial programs. What is often required instead is the imaginative design of task simulations that provide informative mental models of the objects of investigation or study. The development of facilities for student practice without guidance is straightforward. However, the development of intelligent facilities for guided practice is, in principle, even more difficult than the development of intelligent tutors because the program may have to understand the student's own conceptual framework to correctly diagnose his underlying difficulties.

Actually, however, it may be possible to provide instructionally effective guidance on the basis of a great deal less complete or deep understanding of the student's thinking. When a motivated student has difficulty in solving a problem it is often sufficient to tell him just two things -- where he went wrong and what he did wrong. This information may be all he needs to diagnose his own difficulty. Thus, in some cases, the direct approach of identifying and characterizing student errors obviates the need for deep diagnostic inferences. Even in instructional situations where this is not sufficient, however, there are other approaches to understanding the student's actions and intentions which do not depend entirely on AI inferencing methods. One of these is discussed in the next section.

DIAGNOSIS OF STUDENT PERFORMANCE

How can an ICAI system make plausible hypotheses concerning a student's knowledge state about a problem domain? The task of the diagnostic module of the system is to make intelligent inferences about the student's knowledge, knowledge gaps, surface bugs and, if possible, the associated underlying misconceptions. The essential starting point for such deep inferences is the observations of the student's task performance -- the sequence of actions taken by the student as he works on a problem. This constitutes the initial knowledge base of the student diagnostic module. This surface performance information is necessary for diagnosing and characterizing faulty behaviors, but it is not sufficient, even for diagnosing student difficulties in relatively simple intellectual tasks such as the performance of simple arithmetic computations using prescribed algorithmic procedures.

The diagnosis problem has been addressed by a number of ICAI systems, including WEST, DEBUGGY, SOPHIE, and QUEST. The concept of a differential student model was developed in WEST, a computer board game designed to teach computational skills through computation-based game playing strategy. The approach to diagnosis in WEST is to model the problem performance of an expert player and to contrast that with the observed performance of the student working on the same problem. This kind of performance analysis can identify weaknesses in the student's play but not the underlying difficulties responsible for them. For example, a poor move might be due to the student's failure to consider an alternative move or to an incorrect computation of a move, a distinctly different kind of difficulty calling for a qualitatively different instructional treatment.

DEBUGGY is the instructional form of the well-known BUGGY system for modeling the procedural bugs accounting for most student subtraction errors. In DEBUGGY, the diagnosis of a student's procedural bugs is done using a kind of pattern matching scheme. DEBUGGY incorporates a substantial data base of subtraction problem bugs -- faulty subtraction procedures obtained from empirical studies of subtraction problem work across large student populations. If a student's performance across a set of representative problems is identical to that of a buggy procedure in the data base, the system identifies the buggy procedure as the student's bug. This kind of approach is severely limited to those relatively simple types of problems for which there is a small enough set of distinct types of bugs to permit their explicit enumeration. It is not a feasible diagnostic methodology for the problems of typical interest in complex military tasks.

SOPHIE, an early ICAI system for electronics troubleshooting training, uses a general circuit simulation program as a dynamic knowledge base for evaluating the behavior of the circuit under working or faulted conditions. SOPHIE uses the simulator to make powerful deductive inferences about hypothetical, as well as real, circuit behavior. For example, it determines whether a student's troubleshooting inferences are warranted, i.e., whether the student has acquired information of the voltage and current states of relevant circuit components sufficient to unambiguously isolate the fault. However, though SOPHIE can infer such things as what the student should be able to conclude from his observations at any point, it does not try to determine what he has actually concluded or what strategic course he is taking. The system does not attempt to diagnose a student's specific misconceptions or difficulties in understanding circuit behavior or in troubleshooting faults.

The distinctive diagnostic feature of QUEST, (Qualitative Understanding of Electronic System Troubleshooting), which sets it apart from other current ICAI systems, is its facility for eliciting explicit information from the student about the intended purpose of his actions before they are performed and also about his conclusions afterwards (White & Frederiksen, 1984; Feurzeig, 1985). This interaction is carried out throughout the detailed course of the troubleshooting activity. A transcript from such a QUEST interaction with a student is shown in the Appendix. We believe that this fine-grained information about the student's intentions, expectations and conclusions can be uniquely valuable for understanding the student's performance and diagnosing his misconceptions and difficulties. Moreover, such information can only be elicited from the student: it is, at the very least, extremely difficult for an ICAI system based on present AI methods to infer the student's mental states from his surface behaviors. Thus, we believe that the QUEST work provides an effective starting point for development of a powerful student diagnostic module.

As the transcript shows, the present QUEST diagnostic module is invoked each time the student takes an action. This elicitation procedure is designed to be unintrusive and unforced. The student is not required or even requested to be deliberative about every single action he takes along the way. Nevertheless, a more sophisticated procedure, incorporating knowledge of the circuit and utilizing the information elicited from the student about his current plans, could be designed. This procedure would need to be invoked less frequently, at points corresponding to completion of a global operation sequence or to a shift in the student's current focus of attention. Further developments along these lines are planned so as to provide a rich and informative knowledge base for the student diagnostic module. The addition of information about what the student is actually doing is, we believe, essential to making informed and insightful diagnoses. This approach to diagnosis integrates common sense principles from cognitive science with powerful AI inferencing methods. It substantially enhances the power and reliability of ICAI inferencing capabilities. It has real importance for military training applications to complex systems maintenance and troubleshooting.

DIAGNOSIS OF PERFORMANCE IN REAL-TIME OPERATIONAL TASK DOMAINS

Virtually all AI systems development to date has concerned tasks which do not involve real-time decisions in time-critical situations. Medical diagnosis, electronic troubleshooting, geological exploration/prediction and computer systems configuration are representative of the kinds of task domains addressed in AI applications. In these kinds of tasks, the world within which the task is carried out (the task environment) does not significantly change while the user contemplates his next action. The user has essentially unlimited time between successive "moves". The AI system also benefits by having a great deal of time to process the user's inputs and make informed responses.

It is not surprising that considerably less AI development has been done in domains where interactions are complicated by the intrinsic need for real-time processing and response on the part of the system and its users. There is an important class of military tasks, those involving strategic or tactical decision-making in rapidly changing situations, in which real-time operations are essential, e.g., air traffic control or tactical decision making tasks such as radar intercepts, the task domain under development in the TRIO system (Trainer for Radar Intercept Operations) (Feurzeig, Ash & Ricard, 1984). AI systems for real-time operational tasks, e.g., the pilot's assistant, are only beginning to be developed. The AI methods and the instructional principles relevant to the design of the related ICAI systems for real-time training are beginning to emerge from work in progress on the TRIO system at BBN.

TRIO is an expert system for training F-14 radar intercept officers in the basic tactics of high speed air intercepts. The TRIO task environment supports simulations of airborne radars, interceptor and target aircraft operation, and weapons models. It provides dynamic displays of heading, bearing and displacement vectors, radar screens, flight instruments, intercept parameters, radar and missile envelopes, and interceptor/target aircraft ground tracks. It incorporates real-time speech recognition and synthesis subsystems including advanced capabilities for recognition of naturally articulated and extensive utterances.

TRIO supports three instructional modes: pre-flight demonstrations, in-flight monitoring and guided practice, and post-flight debriefing. Thus it is an example of the kind of ICAI system employing an extended instructional paradigm discussed above. TRIO is one of the first systems to introduce AI methods into real-time training. The real-time processing needed to support realistic simulation of high speed intercept engagements, together with the substantial processing demands of the AI articulate expert and daemon programs, pose computational requirements for TRIO considerably greater than those in previous expert instructional systems.

TRIO is an example of a distinctly different instructional domain from those (exemplified by STEAMER and QUEST) dealing with the operational and maintenance of complex systems. TRIO is essentially different in two fundamental ways. As discussed above, it is a real-time training system. Also, it is a man-in-the-loop system, a man-machine system in which the man is a part of the system he controls, and an integral component of that system, not an external agent. This contrasts with the role of the operator of the naval system power plant in STEAMER or the maintenance technicians troubleshooting the electronics systems in SOPHIE or QUEST, who are outside users of the systems they operate on.

TRIO is the subject of considerable interest in the military training research community precisely because it addresses the application of AI methods to the real-time tactical task domain, an enormously important part of the spectrum of critical military training tasks in which there has been little ICAI experience to date. In TRIO we are exploring the design and development of artificial intelligence methods for real-time monitoring and control of expert and student interactions.

The TRIO articulate expert is designed to provide the student with an exemplary model of intercept performance. The program performs the tactics to be taught in just the ways the student is to learn to emulate. The knowledge is represented using a special form of production rule system -- continuous running, interrupt-driven, goal-directed rules -- to operate an articulate expert program that runs within the simulation and that is capable of performing intercepts in real-time and explaining its actions and reasoning along the way. The expert has access to the identical information the student sees and drives the simulation through the same interface.

The expert system has to be efficient to work in this environment. The simulation has a lot of information to generate and display to provide real-time response from the interceptor, radar and target aircraft models. The high closing speeds of the two aircraft requires processing. The student is polled continuously for new intercept control instructions. The expert's performance must be attainable by the student, so the expert is only polled every few seconds. The correct and rapid performance of the expert is achieved through the shaping of the rules into a goal tree and the use of a clean control structure.

The expert's task is described as a series of high level goals together with associated actions for fulfilling each goal under any contingency. The goal hierarchy that guides the expert in running an intercept and that is taught to the student, is expressed as a set of rules. The top level rules expand to access the rule sets that are appropriate for the current situation. Each rule has several components including a test to check if this rule is to be fired now, an action to be taken (none for goals), a rule set to access next (none for actions), rules to remove from current consideration, and a rationale for why the current goal was established or the current action taken -- this becomes part of the explanation given to the student.

During practice mode, TRIO uses daemons to monitor a student's performance as he attempts to carry out an intercept. Each daemon monitor's the student's actions for a specific critical event such as imminent loss of missile threshold. If this occurs, the daemon can alert the student so that he can attempt to take corrective action.

Following a student run, the TRIO performance analysis system uses pattern matching methods to diagnose the student's actions relative to acceptable tactical performance behaviors as described in a solution space describing all allowable solution paths. The program structure is as follows. The student's intercept control actions are mapped into the solution space defined by the tactical doctrine. This enables the system to recognize student behaviors that are equivalent to those permitted. During the replay, correct actions are noted. Incorrect ones are pointed out on the TRIO visual displays. The student's errors are explained and the actions that should have been taken instead are described and justified in terms of the top level goals.

The problems of instructional design for ICAI applications to real-time tactical decision-making tasks are significantly different in important ways from those involved in complex systems maintenance and troubleshooting tasks. The knowledge acquisition problem is more complicated in the case of real-time tasks. Expert performers tend to "compile" their knowledge to enable efficient and rapid execution. They cannot explicitly or precisely describe how they do what they do. The development of indirect knowledge acquisition methods to characterize expert performance is essential here. Similarly, the problem of diagnosing student errors and performance behaviors is severely exacerbated by real-time constraints. It is not

possible to stop the world and interrupt the student's work to elicit the
reasons for his actions, in the way described for diagnosing the student's
troubleshooting behavior in QUEST.

Diagnostic methods and tools like those used in QUEST are very useful
in application to non-real-time tasks. However, real-time tasks call for
distinctly different methods, such as those investigated in TRIO
currently. The diagnosis of real-time performance, particularly in
rapidly changing tactical decision-making tasks, has to be carried out
after task completion. The performance analysis cannot be done in real
time. After the student run is over, however, the analysis can be quickly
performed and the ICAI system can replay the student's recorded run in a
debriefing session, critiquing the student's task performance along the way.

As noted above, the student diagnostic module currently used in TRIO
analyzes the student's performance so as to determine action sequences that
are deviant, i.e., those that could not be effective in realizing the
appropriate subgoals in the intercept solution space. This analysis
enables TRIO to generate explanations of what the student did wrong, where
it occurred, why it was wrong, and what he should have done instead. The
concept of a solution space as used in TRIO shows promise as a starting
point for the development of general AI methods for diagnosing student
performance in a large class of real-time tasks.

QUALITATIVE SIMULATION METHODS

Knowledge about the behavior of a system under a wide range of
conditions which cannot be anticipated in advance (i.e., for arbitrary
states of the system) is important for supporting the more powerful kinds
of instruction provided in ICAI applications. Such knowledge, even for
very complex systems, can often be represented by runnable simulation
models, either quantitative (mathematical) models or qualitative
(functional) models. A number of interpreters for implementing qualitative
models of electronic and digital circuits, adaptive control systems, and
various topics in physics, have been developed (deKleer, 1979; Forbus,
1981; Bobrow, 1985).

A substantial part of the understanding capabilities in the SOPHIE and
STEAMER ICAI systems is based on the use of mathematical simulation
models. SOPHIE used a general purpose circuit simulation package called
SPICE together with a Lisp-based functional simulator incorporating circuit
dependent knowledge (Brown, Burton, and Bell, 1974). These facilities were
essential for inferring complex circuit interaction sequences such as fault
propagation chains. SOPHIE'S capabilities for modeling and understanding
causal chains of events formed the basis for its powerful explanation and
question answering facilities.

The STEAMER system incorporates as a key part of its knowledge base, a
detailed mathematical simulation model of a steam propulsion plant, an
exceptionally complex dynamic physical system (Roberts and Forbus, 1981).
A major focus of the STEAMER work has been to provide interactive graphical
interfaces that are closely coupled to the simulation and that are designed
to provide highly informative displays of system operation. This kind of
environment is valuable in supporting instructional interactions designed
to foster the student's development of effective mental models for
understanding and reasoning about system behavior.

Humans think about the behavior of phenomena and systems in a
qualitatively different way from that used to describe such behavior in
mathematical simulation models. Experts in a domain (not only beginning

students) use qualitative models of thought and qualitative models to reason about system behavior. Thus, though it is necessary to employ mathematical simulations to obtain precise detailed descriptions of system behaviors, we generally want to teach conceptually sound qualitative reasoning. The use of qualitative simulation models for generating understandable explanations as well as animated displays of behavior, is valuable in supporting such instruction and in facilitating learning.

The principles and methods of qualitative simulation modeling are very much the subject of current research. A qualitative simulation model has recently been developed at BBN as part of the QUEST system. The model is used in the QUEST expert system for reasoning about, and troubleshooting simple electrical circuits including batteries, wires, resistors, coils, condensers, lamps, switches, and testlights (White & Frederiksen, 1984).

The model includes a representation of the circuit topology, a runnable functional model for each device in the circuit, rules for evaluating device states at each time increment, and circuit tracing procedures to aid in evaluating conditions for device states. The model can generate graphical representations of circuit operation. It will support a dynamic presentation environment within which an expert troubleshooting program can demonstrate troubleshooting concepts and strategy. It also supports a complementary instructional mode enabling student practice on troubleshooting problem work (Feurzeig, 1985). The model generates explanations of circuit operation in both working and faulted states, employing the same qualitative reasoning principles used in the execution of the troubleshooting strategy.

The use of qualitative models offers the promise of describing the behavior of complex systems and devices in a way that very closely mirrors the understanding we want students to acquire. This technology has the potential for wide applications throughout military training. There is need for further development of computer science methods to extend the scope and power of qualitative modeling. There is need to better understand the cognitive principles appropriate for guiding the effective instructional design and use of such models. This research together with the associated tool building, implementation and testing of qualitative simulation models, should be among the highest priority areas in ICAI development.

REFERENCES

Bobrow, D.G. (Ed.) (1985, December). "Qualitative reasoning about physical systems." Cambridge, MA: Massachusetts Institute of Technology Press.

Brown, J.S., Burton, R.R., & Bell, A.G. (1974, March). "SOPHIE: A sophisticated environment for teaching electronic troubleshooting" (BBN Report No. 2790). Cambridge, MA: Bolt Beranek and Newman, Inc.

deKleer, J. (1979). "Casual and teleological reasoning in circuit recognition" (AI-TR 529). Cambridge, MA: Massachusetts Institute of Technology, Artificial Intelligence Laboratory.

Feurzeig, W. (1985, January). "QUEST: A Computer System for Teaching Qualitative Understanding of Electrical System Troubleshooting--the Troubleshooting Practice Environment." Cambridge, MA: Bolt Beranek and Newman, Inc.

Feurzeig, W., Ash, W.L., & Ricard, G.L. (1984, October). TRIO: An Expert System for Air Intercept Training. "Proceedings of the Sixth Interservice Industry Training Conference" (pp. 45-48). Alexandria, VA: U.S. Army Research Institute.

Forbus, K. (1981). Qualitative Reasoning about Physical Processes. "Proceedings of the Seventh International Joint Conference on Artificial Intelligence" (326-330). Menlo Park, CA: American Association for Artificial Intelligence.

Forbus, K. & Stevens, A. (1981, March). "Using qualitative simulation to generate explanations" (BBN Report No. 4490). Cambridge, MA: Bolt, Beranek and Newman, Inc.

Hollan, J.D., Hutchins, E.L., & Weitzman, L. (1984, Summer). STEAMER: An Interactive Inspectable Simulation-based Training System. "The AI Magazine" (15-27).

Roberts, R. & Forbus, K. (1981, March). "The STEAMER mathematical simulation" (BBN Report No. 4625). Cambridge, MA: Bolt, Beranek and Newman, Inc.

Sleeman, D. & Brown, J. (Eds.). (1983). "Intelligent Tutoring Systems." New York: Academic Press.

Weld, D.S. (1983, November). "Explaining complex engineering devices" (BBN Report No. 5489). Cambridge, MA: Bolt, Beranek and Newman, Inc.

White, B.Y., & Frederiksen, J.R. (1984). "A qualitative simulation of simple electrical circuits" (BBN Technical Report). Cambridge, MA: Bolt, Beranek and Newman, Inc.

APPENDICES

OVERVIEW OF SCENARIO

In the following pages we describe a short scenario of a student troubleshooting a small circuit containing a battery, two resistors, a wire, and a bulb. This scene represents just a few minutes of such a session, which is itself only one of QUEST's (Qualitative Understanding for Electrical Systems Troubleshooting) modes of teaching.

The querying of the student proceeds effortlessly. The student is asked before each action (e.g., flipping a switch, inserting a test light) what he hopes to learn through this action. The action is carried out by the system, and he may repeat this several times. After the effects of the actions are seen by the student's calling for the simulation to be run, he is asked what he has learned.

Each question is answered with the mouse. To provide input to the system the student moves the mouse to position an arrow cursor on the screen so that it points to the object selected and presses a button on the mouse. This operation is called "clicking".

The student chooses from an appropriate range of responses. Some will take 2-3 clicks to indicate an intricate response, others are merely single clicks on a menu to indicate that he is exploring circuit behavior in a general way. The scenario shown provides examples across this spectrum, including the extremes.

This interface is easy and natural to use. After the session is over, a substantial knowledge base has been developed of the student's plans and goals with a minimum of interference.

APPENDIX 1

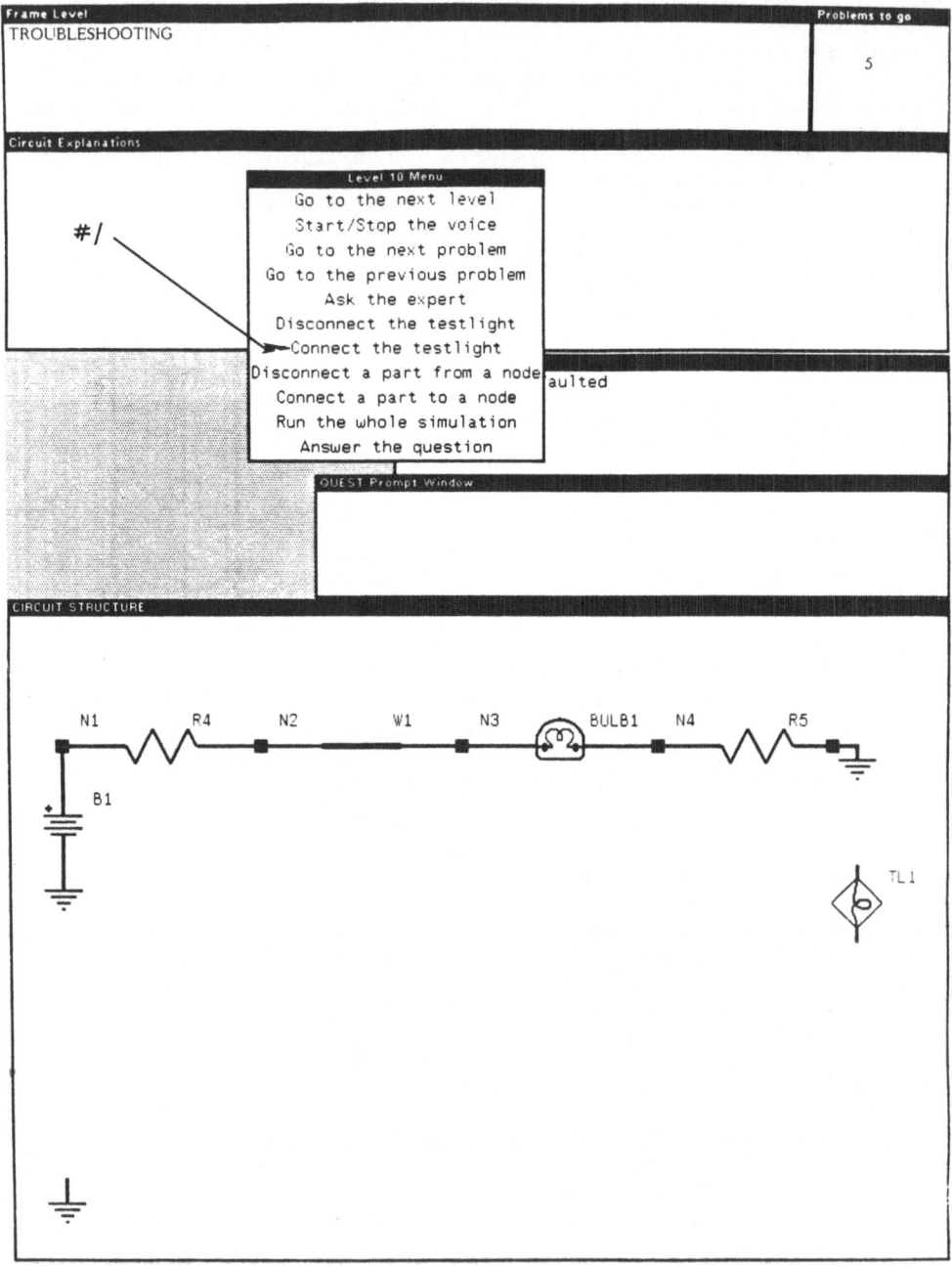

APPENDIX 2

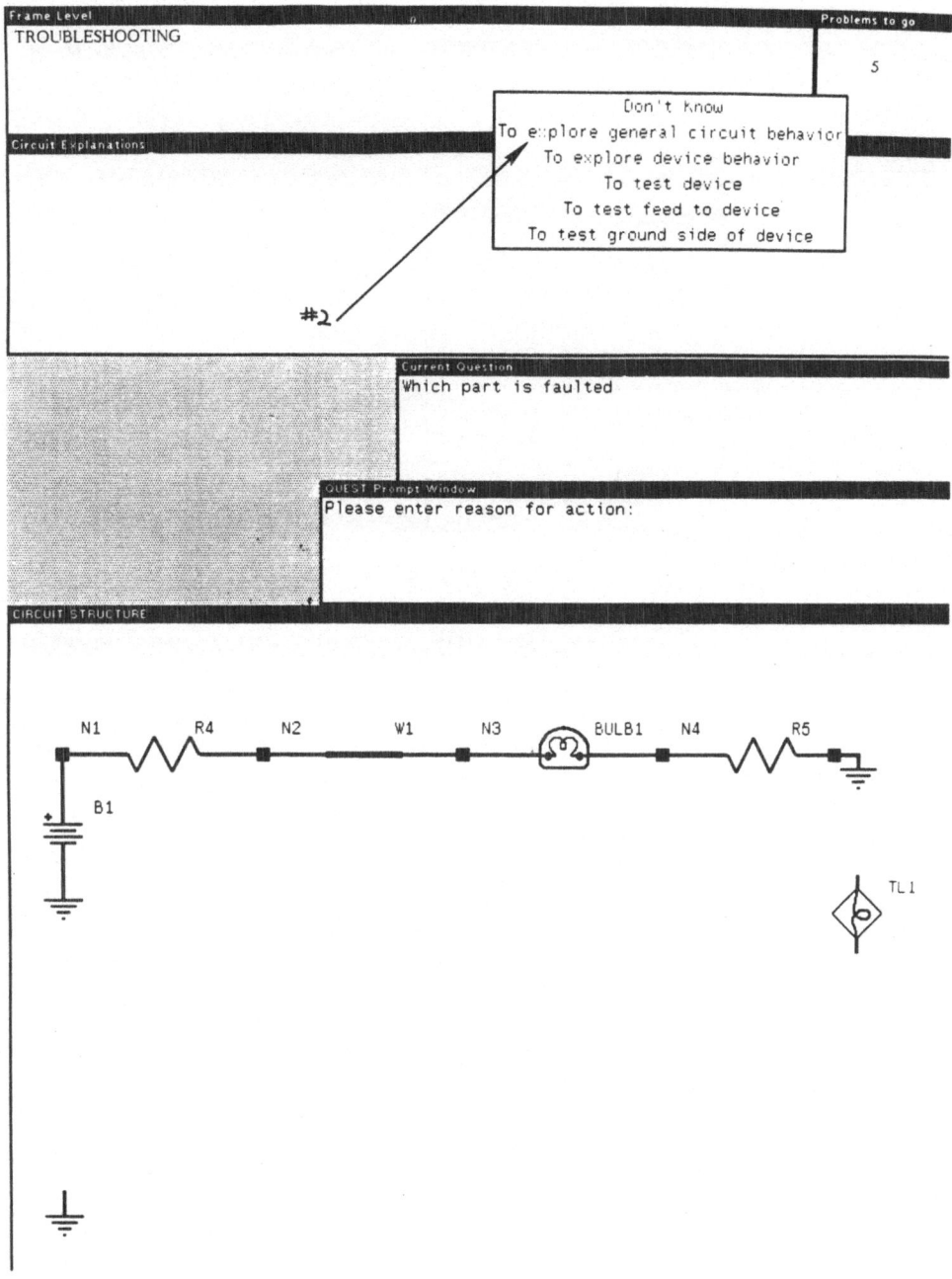

APPENDIX 3

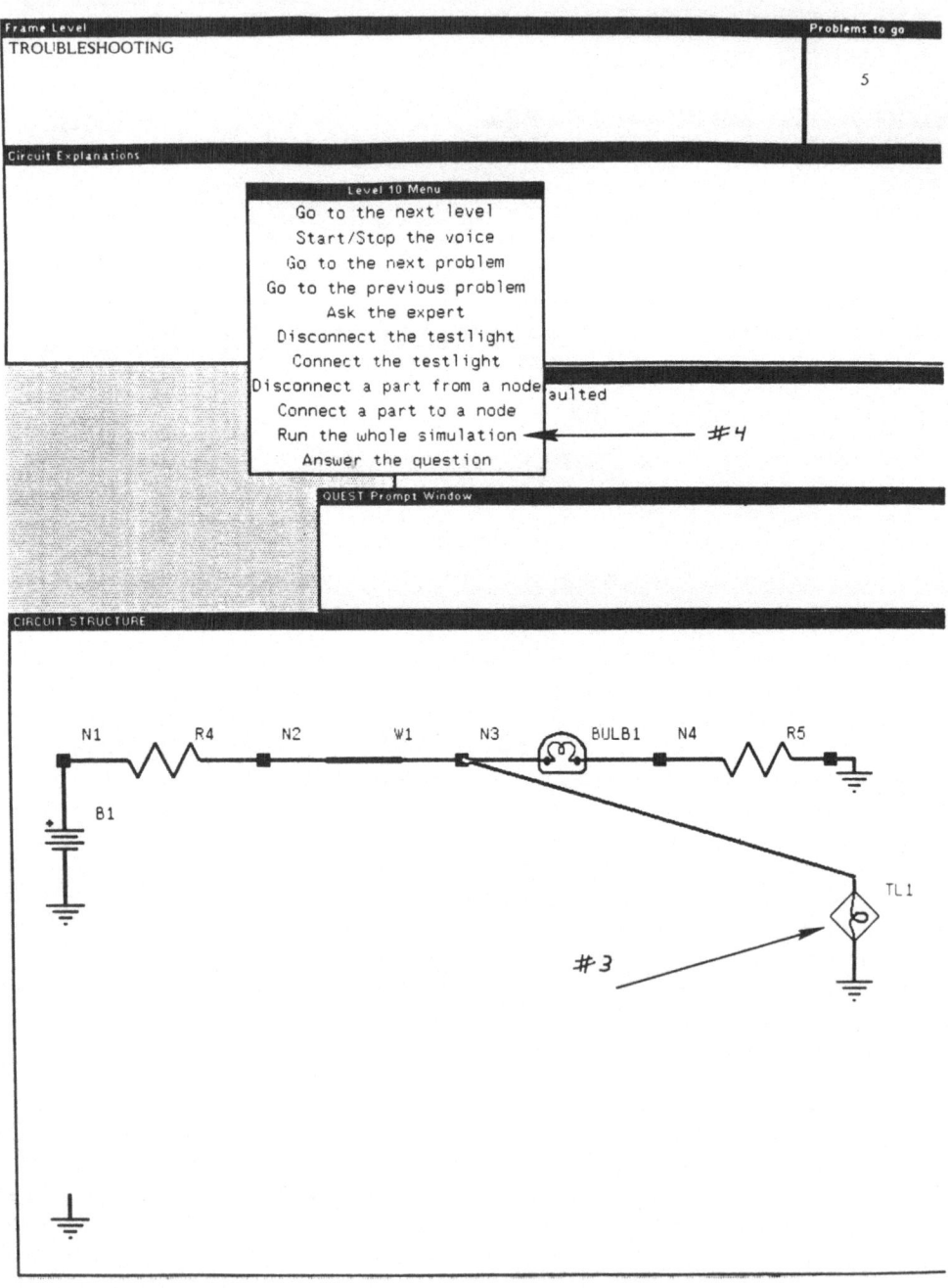

APPENDIX 4

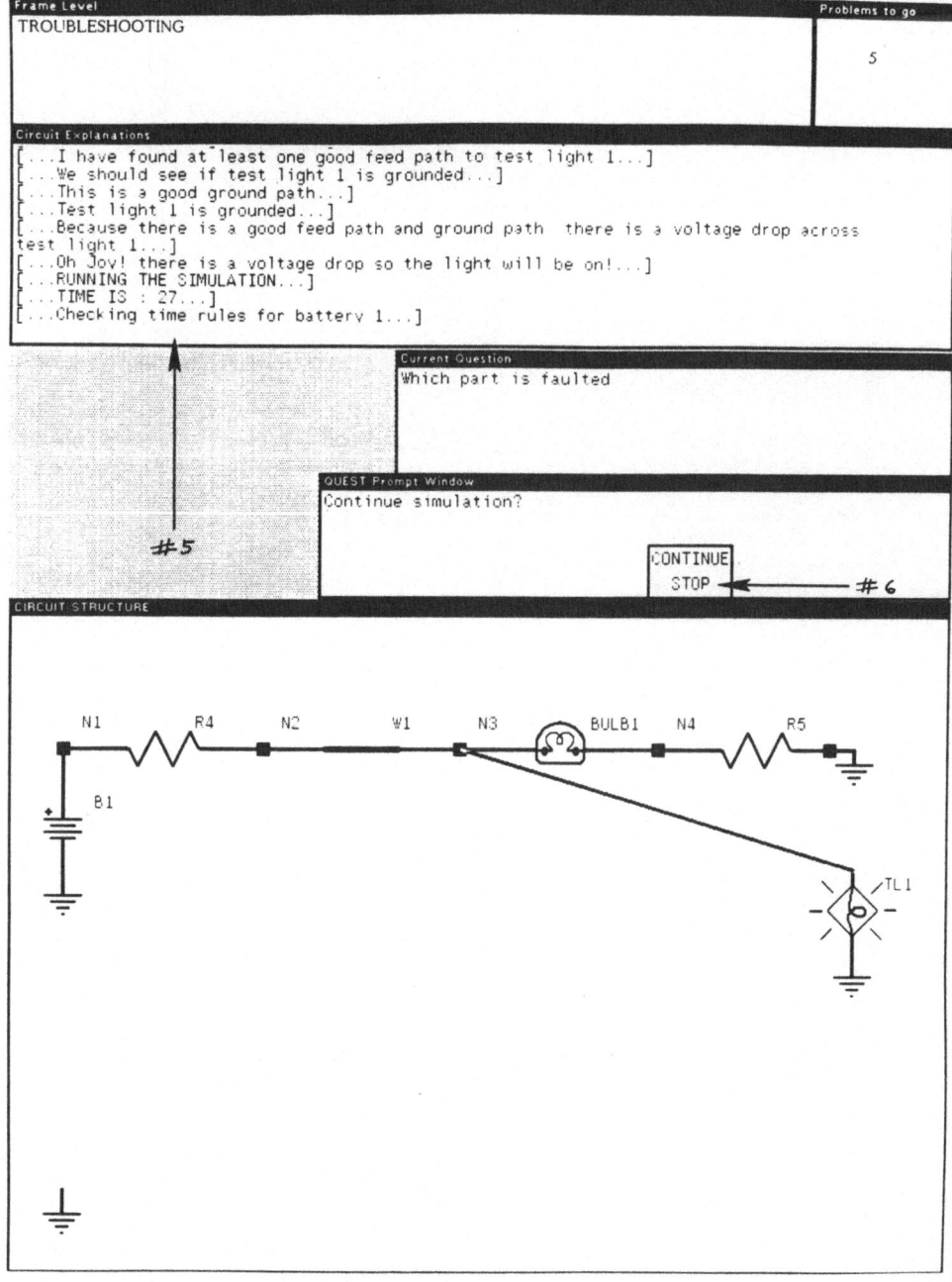

APPENDIX 5

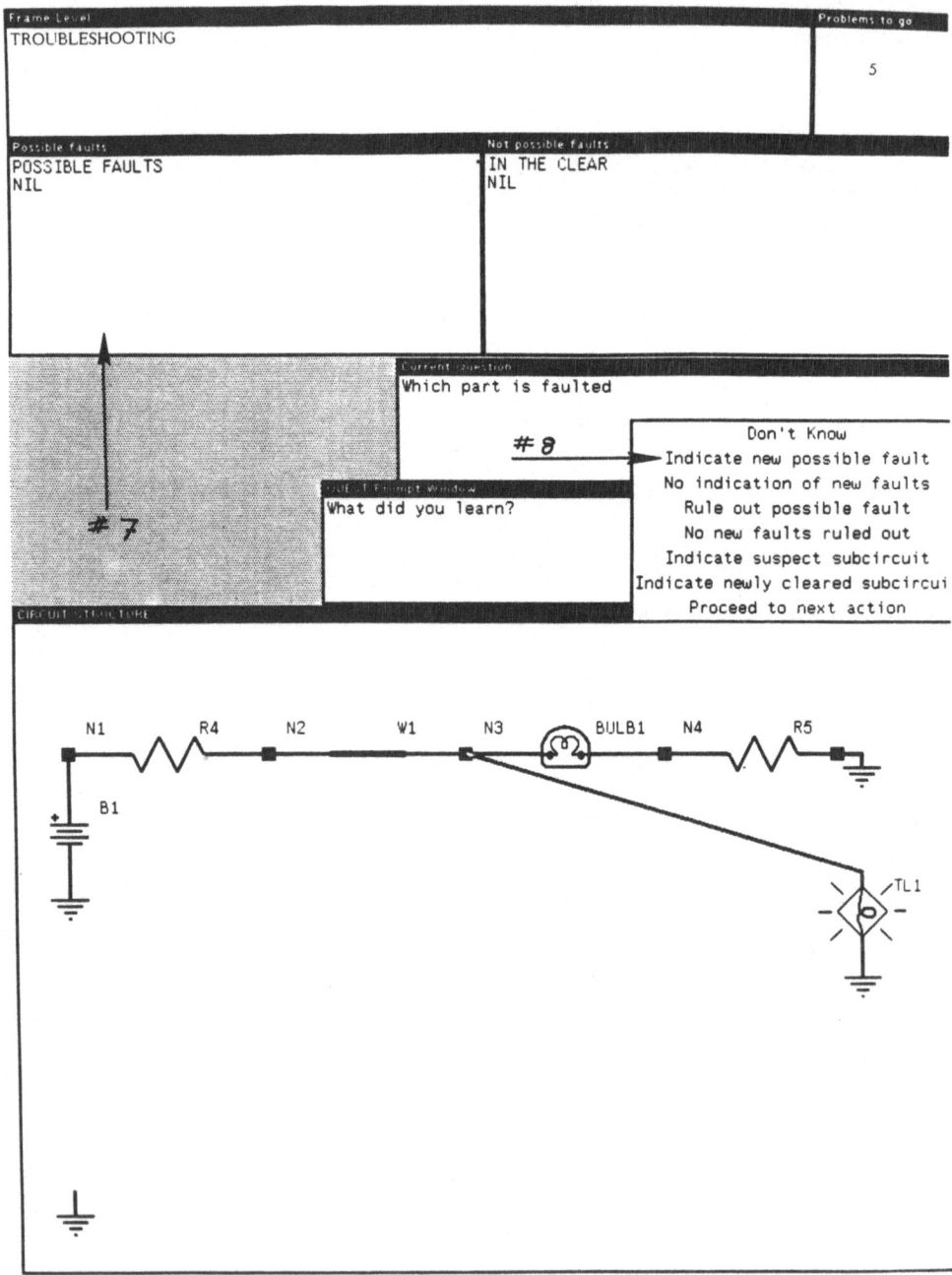

APPENDIX 6

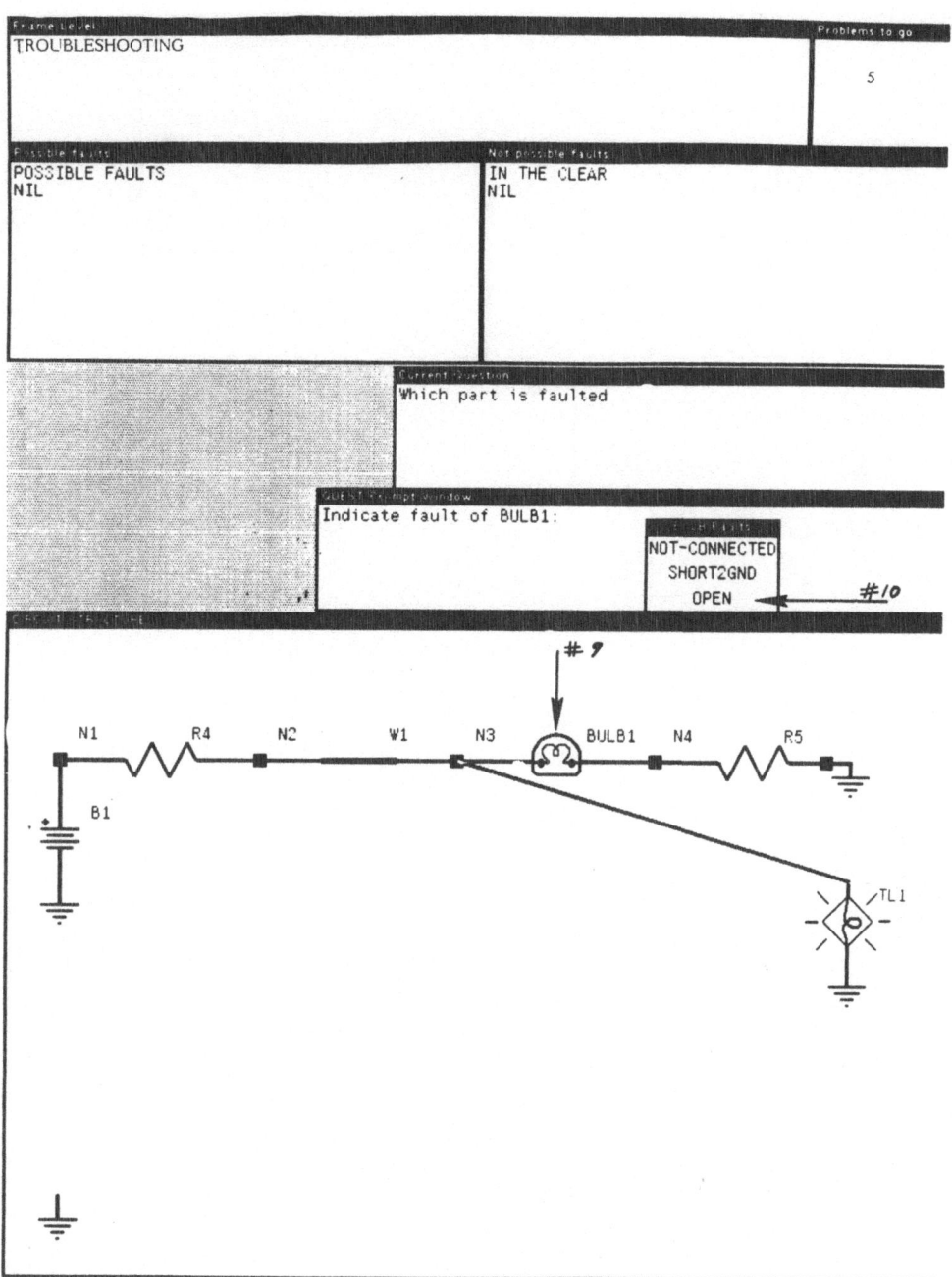

APPENDIX 7

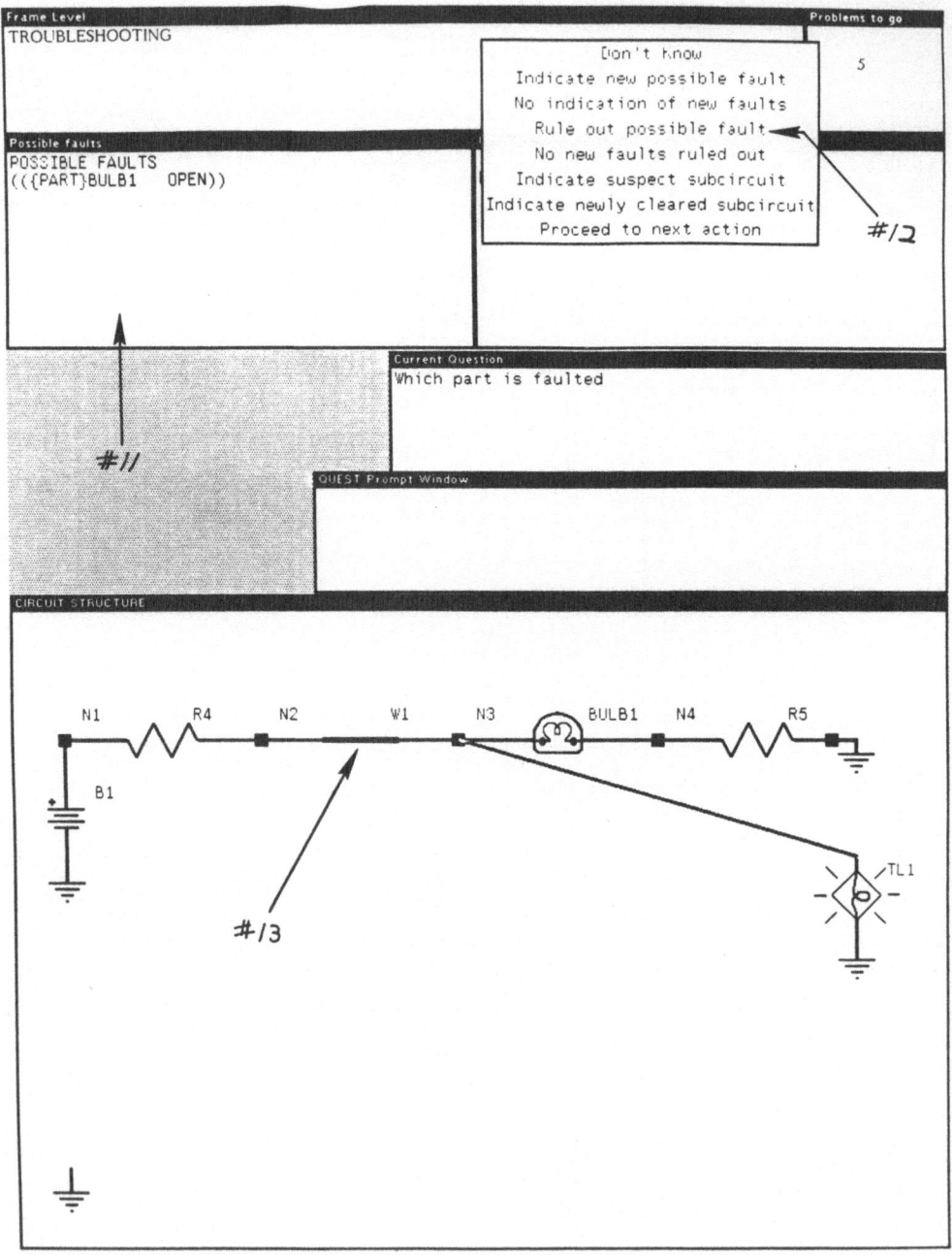

APPENDIX 8

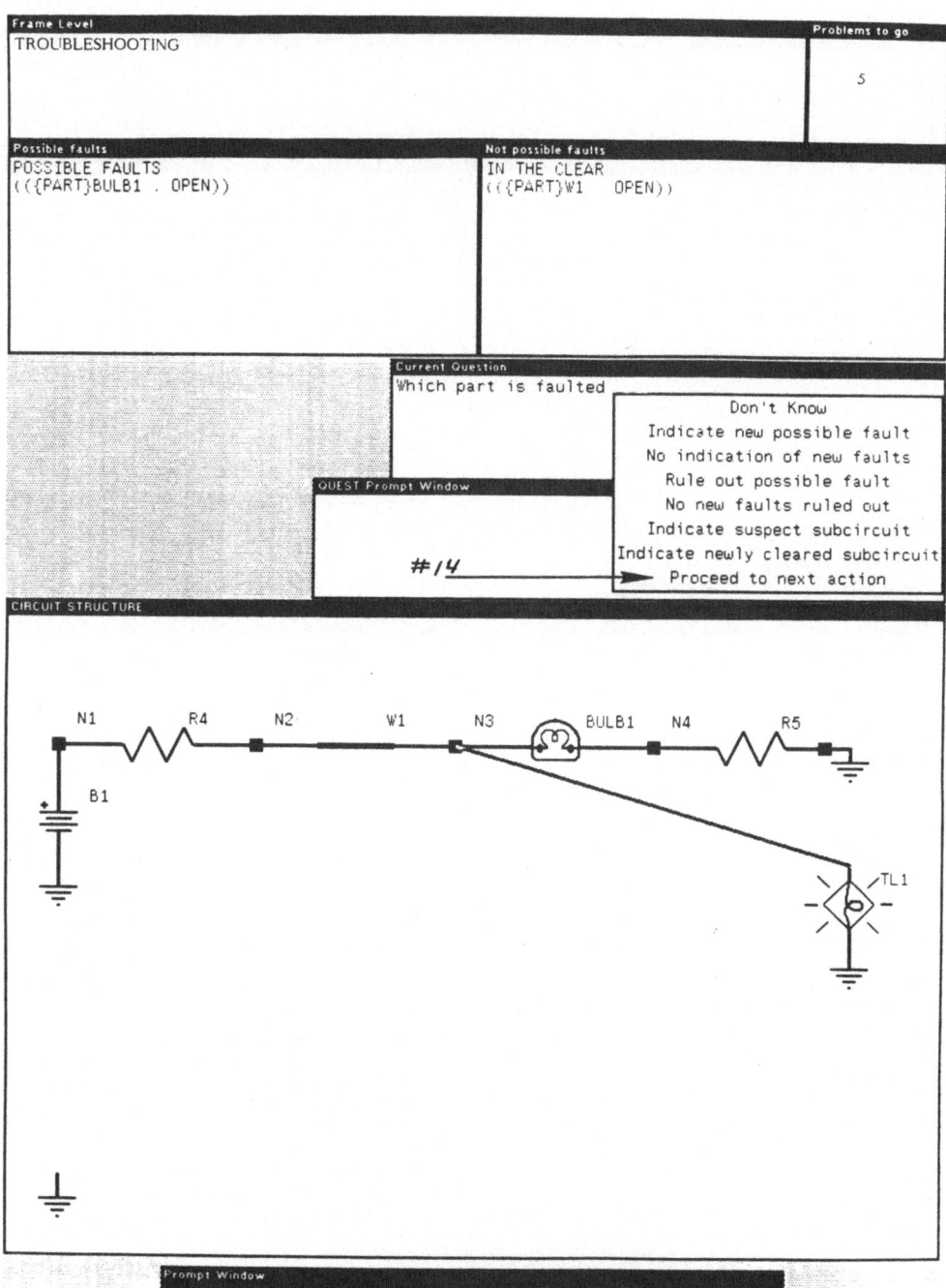

APPENDIX 9

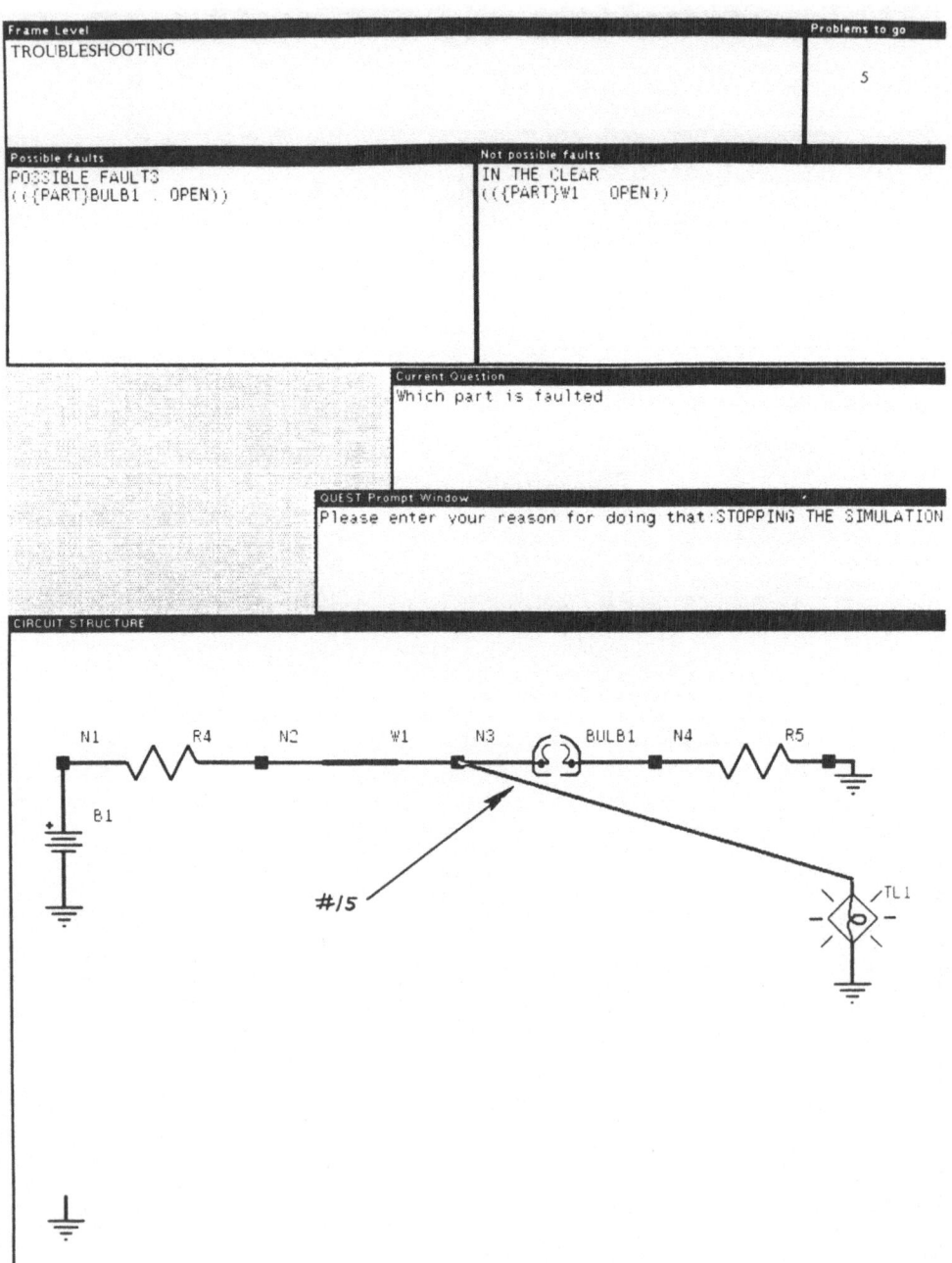

AUTHORING TOOLS: PAST, PRESENT AND FUTURE

G. Kearsley

Courseware Incorporated
San Diego, California, U.S.A.

INTRODUCTION

Authoring is the term used to describe the process of creating instructional software (courseware). Because this development process is complex and time consuming, the software tools used for authoring are of considerable practical importance. Furthermore, authoring tools play an important part in shaping the instructional strategies and pedagogy contained in the courseware. They determine what is easy, difficult and even possible to do in terms of learning or teaching via computers. So authoring tools are of considerable theoretical significance as well.

This article discusses the evolution of authoring software with primary emphasis on current and emerging research issues. This paper is not intended to be introductory or tutorial in nature; such treatments can be found in (Avner, 1979, 1984; Kearsley, 1982, 1985). Nor does it cover the practical aspects of authoring; these are also addressed elsewhere (e.g., [Kearsley, 1984, 1986; Gagne, Wagner & Rojas, 1981; Heines, 1983; Allessi, 1985; Bork, 1984]). After summarizing the past, present and future developments in authoring software, current research on intelligent authoring systems and automated instructional design being conducted by Courseware, Incorporated is described.

AUTHORING TOOLS: PAST

The earliest authoring of computer based instruction occurred in the early 1960s using the general purpose programming languages available at the time (e.g., FORTRAN, BASIC, Assembly). By the middle of the sixties the first author languages appeared such as Coursewriter (IBM) and Tutor for the PLATO system. With the development of new CBI systems, new author languages appeared. As additional hardware capabilities were added to the systems (e.g., color, sound, touch, graphics, fonts, etc.) more commands were added to the author languages.

There were also attempts to develop "generic" author languages that would run on a number of different machines and hence increase the transportability of courseware. Examples of such generic author languages are PILOT, PLANIT, and NATAL. However, despite a number of heroic attempts, generic author languages did not result in any significant sharing of courseware across different systems.

The next major development in authoring tools following author languages was the emergence of the first authoring system, APT for the TICCIT system. Actually, APT and TICCIT represented an important milestone in a number of respects. It was the first CBI system to be completely designed on the basis of instructional principles and research (component display theory). It also operationalized the concept of learner control in both the software and hardware of the system (Bunderson, 1974). Like all subsequent authoring systems, it provided a pedagogical framework which the author needed to conform to.

AUTHORING TOOLS: PRESENT

All three major forms of authoring tools (general purpose languages, author languages and authoring systems) are now used routinely for courseware development. There are system specific author languages available for each CBI system marketed. Examples include IIAS/PS (IBM mainframes), Producer (DEC Vax), Can-8 (Honeywell), USE (Regency) and many others. There are also hundreds of author languages or authoring systems available for popular microcomputers such as the Apple II or IBM PC. Recently, authoring tools have started to appear for machines which use the UNIX operating system. Specialized authoring tools exist just for the development of interactive video (tape or disc) materials.

No data is readily available which indicates the extent to which author languages or authoring systems are actually used relative to general purpose languages. The PILOT language (Starkweather, 1985) is available on most microcomputers and is popular for teaching how to design instructional software. In the case of dedicated CBT systems such as PLATO, TICCIT, or Wicat, the authoring software provided with that system must be used. However in the case of courseware which is developed for general purpose mainframes or microcomputers, languages such as C, Pascal, or LISP can be used. In fact, it appears that most organizations that produce educational software commercially use general purpose programming languages for authoring to maximize machine transportability and run-time efficiency.

Despite the plethora of authoring tools presently available, there are relatively few interesting developments from an instructional theory perspective. One exception is the authoring capability provided on the TeleLearning system designed to provide electronic lectures via computer conferencing. This capability provides authors with a large number of screen templates, each of which represents a particular microstrategy. For example, one such template might be two boxes with an arrow between them. This screen can be used to teach cause and effect relationships when the author fills in the appropriate text. Normally, this would be used as part of a questioning sequence; the author would expect the student to complete some part of the cause-effect sequence. To compose a lesson or course, the author uses whatever set of microstrategies seem appropriate.

Another interesting development in authoring systems from a theoretical perspective is the Authority system from Interactive Training systems of Cambridge, Massachusetts. The Authority system provides three different general formats that can be matched to a particular instructional application or student learning style. The three formats are inquiry (information presentation/acquisition), recognition (identification of concepts), and action (simulation of events/processes). Both the TeleLearning and Authority authoring systems are similar in that they provide the author with a choice of micro or macro teaching strategies. The provision of micro strategies would appear to be a new direction in authoring systems.

Even though authoring systems are capable of making the courseware development process more efficient, they have not been embraced very enthusiastically by major developers of courseware. Part of the reason is that the structure essential to making an authoring system work is often seen as too restrictive in terms of creative instructional design. Another problem is that most authoring systems do not facilitate the development of simulation or games which represent two of the most important ways of using computers for learning. There are also licensing and royalty complications associated with the use of authoring systems.

Probably the most fundamental dilemma with authoring systems is the common notion that they allow any instructor or subject matter expert to create their own courseware. In the strict sense this is true. But it misses the point that most individuals do not have the appropriate interest, background or ability to develop high quality courseware. We should no more expect most instructors or subject matter experts to create CBI lessons than to write textbooks or produce videotapes.

A much more promising idea than authoring systems that has emerged in the educational software world is the concept of customization. Teachers can customize programs to their own needs by adding, modifying or replacing data tables. This means that new vocabulary, problems, examples, etc., can be added to existing courseware as desired. However, there is no requirement that the program be created from scratch by the teacher. In essence, each program comes with its own self-contained authoring system.

AUTHORING TOOLS: FUTURE

Four major developments are likely to have major effects on the future evolution of authoring tools: window/icon oriented displays, embedded training, artificial intelligence and automation of instructional development. Each of these will be discussed in turn.

The emerging generation of microcomputers and workstations, as typified by the Apple® MacIntosh™ and LISP machines, feature high resolution bit-mapped graphics which allow multiple windows, iconic representation and control via mouse, trackball or joystick. This kind of interface makes it possible to develop authoring tools that make it easy to create and manipulate instructional materials. For example, Figure 1 illustrates an instructional strategy editor display which is part of an experimental authoring system under development by Control Development Corporation (Allen, 1984). It allows an author to change the instructional logic for a particular lesson by simply moving the icons on the screen.

There is an increasing tendency to building instruction directly into systems or products in the form of helps, tutorials, or advice systems (Kearsley, 1985). The major value of such embedded training is that it provides instruction as it is needed when learning to use the system or product. This kind of instruction is much more likely to be effective than more typical tutorials or simulations which are distinct activities from the use of a system in work tasks. Another advantage of embedded training is that it is also available to serve as an online job aid or refresher after initial training is completed.

The difficulty with embedded training is that it must be designed and implemented as an integrated part of the system or product. This means that training and human factors specialists must work with the system designers and engineers. Furthermore, it must be developed using the specific software and hardware available on the system. No real authoring tools exist to facilitate the creations of embedded training across such a

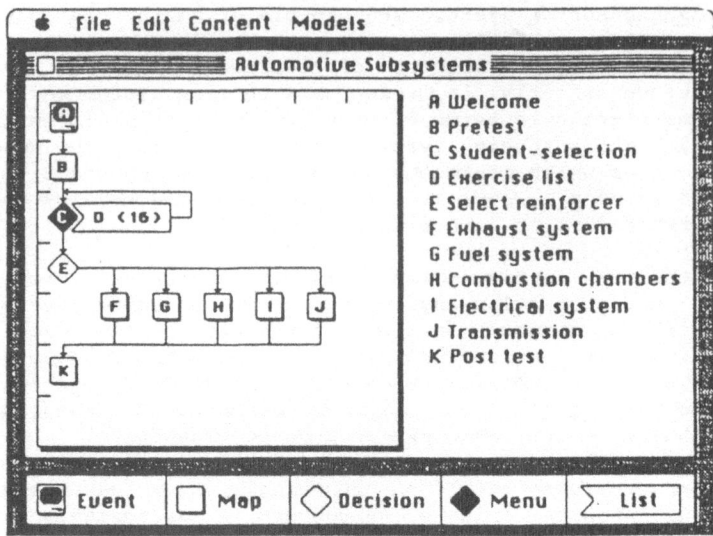

Figure 1. Instructional Strategy Editor Display from Experimental Authoring System under Development by Control Data Corporation

diversity of applications and systems nor is it obvious how to develop such general purpose tools.

The application of artificial intelligence to instruction has led to the creation of Intelligence CAI (ICAI) programs (see Sleeman & Brown, 1982; Brown, Burton & deKleer, 1982; Collins, 1977; Stevens & Roberts, 1983). ICAI programs differ significantly from traditional CBI. They usually provide a much more sophisticated diagnostic capability and allow the student to ask questions as well as answer them (so called "mixed initiative" capability). The main characteristic which distinguishes ICAI programs is that they understand what they teach in the same way that a human teacher understands the subject matter or task.

ICAI programs are normally programmed in an AI language such as LISP or Prolog and incorporate AIR programming techniques for knowledge representation and inferencing. Furthermore, a great deal of research is usually conducted about the subject or task to be taught in order to identify the teaching and learning processes to be programmed. ICAI programs are very time consuming to create, often taking years to complete. Clearly if ICAI is to be brought into the mainstream of education and training, new kinds of authoring tools are needed to expedite their development.

The fourth development that will affect the future form of authoring systems is the increasing automation of the entire instructional development process ranging from job/task analysis through to formative or cost/benefits evaluation. Current authoring tools only address the production step of creating programs. However, the majority of time spent developing courseware is involved in the analysis, design or evaluation steps. In order to really increase the efficiency of instructional development, all phases need to be automated. Past research has demonstrated the feasibility of automating different aspects of the instructional design process (e.g., Braby & Kincaid, 1981; O'Neil & O'Neil, 1979; Merrill & Wood, 1984).

These four areas of future development will result in new forms of

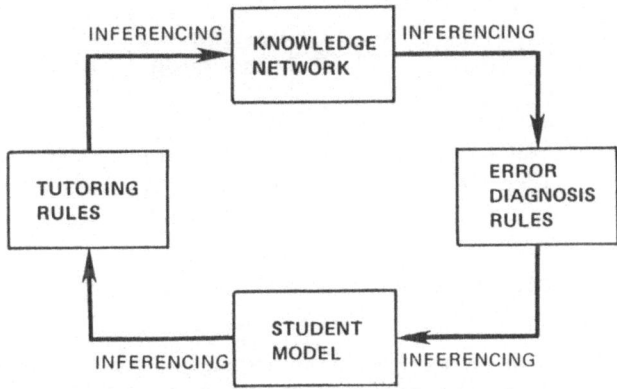

Figure 2. General Model of an Intelligent CAI Tutoring Program

computer based instruction and new kinds of authoring tools. The last two sections of this paper describe research projects being conducted by Courseware Incorporated in the areas of authoring systems for ICAI and automated instructional design.

INTELLIGENT AUTHORING SYSTEMS

Some of the general problems with authoring ICAI programs were introduced in the previous section. A major theoretical problem is that there has been very little attempt to synthesize the work of the past decade in ICAI. However, it is possible to taxonomize existing programs into broad categories such as coaches, mixed initiative tutors or microworlds and identify the characteristics of each category. This makes it feasible to develop authoring tools for different types of ICAI programs.

The oldest and best researched category of ICAI programs are mixed initiative tutors. Figure 2 depicts the basic components of such a tutor and how these programs work. The concepts and principles to be taught are represented in a knowledge network of some kind. The kinds of mistakes that students make in learning the subject matter are represented as diagnostic (error) rules. When a student responds to or asks a question, the diagnostic rules attempt to identify what aspects of the knowledge network the student understands or does not understand. This student model is updated to reflect this current representation of the student's understanding. Tutoring rules are matched against the student model to determine what concepts or questions are appropriate to present next. The teaching processing continues until the student matches the complete knowledge network (i.e., the student has mastered the subject completely).

To create this kind of ICAI program, the author must specify a knowledge network for the subject as well as diagnostic and teaching rules (the system builds the student model). Figure 3 depicts the structure of authoring system which helps an author build mixed initiative tutors. The discourse editor allows the user to identify dialogs (lessons) and the rules that govern branching from one dialog to another. It also allows that author to specify different discourse strategies to be used (e.g., generalize from examples, draw contrasts, etc.) The database editor assists the author in formulating knowledge of the subject into well structured knowledge items, diagnostic rules and teaching rules. The lesson assembler allows completeness and consistency checking of the database as well as creating the student model and helping the author

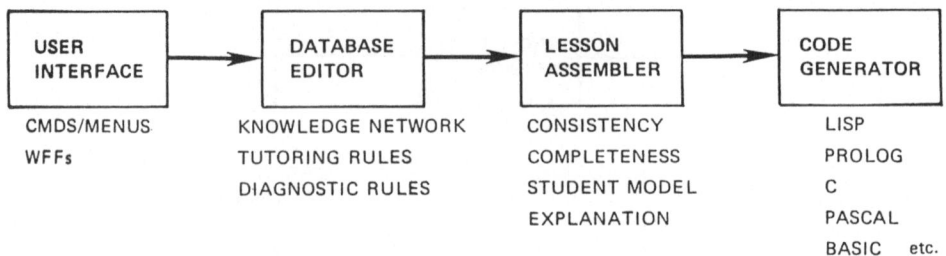

Figure 3. Structure of an Intelligent Authoring System

examine the inference sequences generated by the system. The fourth component of the system is the code generator which produces the actual ICAI program target language.

A prototype IAS as described has been implemented on a Burroughs ICON System. The System was written in C and generates Prolog programs. At the current time, existing ICAI programs are being used to evaluate the scope and robustness of the authoring system. It is envisioned that a family of such authoring tools would be needed to create the full range of ICAI programs which have been developed to date.

COURSEWARE INSTRUCTIONAL TOOLKIT

As already discussed, automation of the analysis and designs stages of instructional development is one of the current areas of research in authoring systems. The Instructional Toolkit is a prototype system implemented on an IBM/PC/XT that automates the functions indicated in Figure 4. The Toolkit is an open architecture system which uses off-the-shelf application software such as database, spreadsheet, graphics, word processing, and project management programs as well as any authoring software desired. The use of off-the-shelf programs allowed the system to be developed quickly and without programming support. The toolkit functions can be developed and maintained by instructional designers as needed.

The open architecture approach is made possible through the use of a system manager, a piece of software that acts as a pseudo-operating system and allows user-defined menus, helps and the transfer of data between different programs via windows. The system manager allows the particular applications software used to be hidden from the user. All the user has to learn to use are the actual instructional functions which are implemented in the applications software (see Figure 5). The system manager used in the current Toolkit is DESQ (Quarterdeck Systems) but other programs such as Topview (IBM), GEM (Digital Research) or Windows (Microsoft) are available.

Another important characteristic of the Toolkit is that it provides a user interface which accommodates variable experience in instructional design. In any organization or project, there will be very experienced designers as well as novices. If the system is to be useful to everyone, it needs to span this range. This one can be accomplished by providing a multilevel system of tutorials and helps for each instructional function. For example, for the task analysis function, there might be a general tutorial explaining what task analysis is, various examples of completed task analyses, a procedural job aid, and helps tied to the particular procedures implemented.

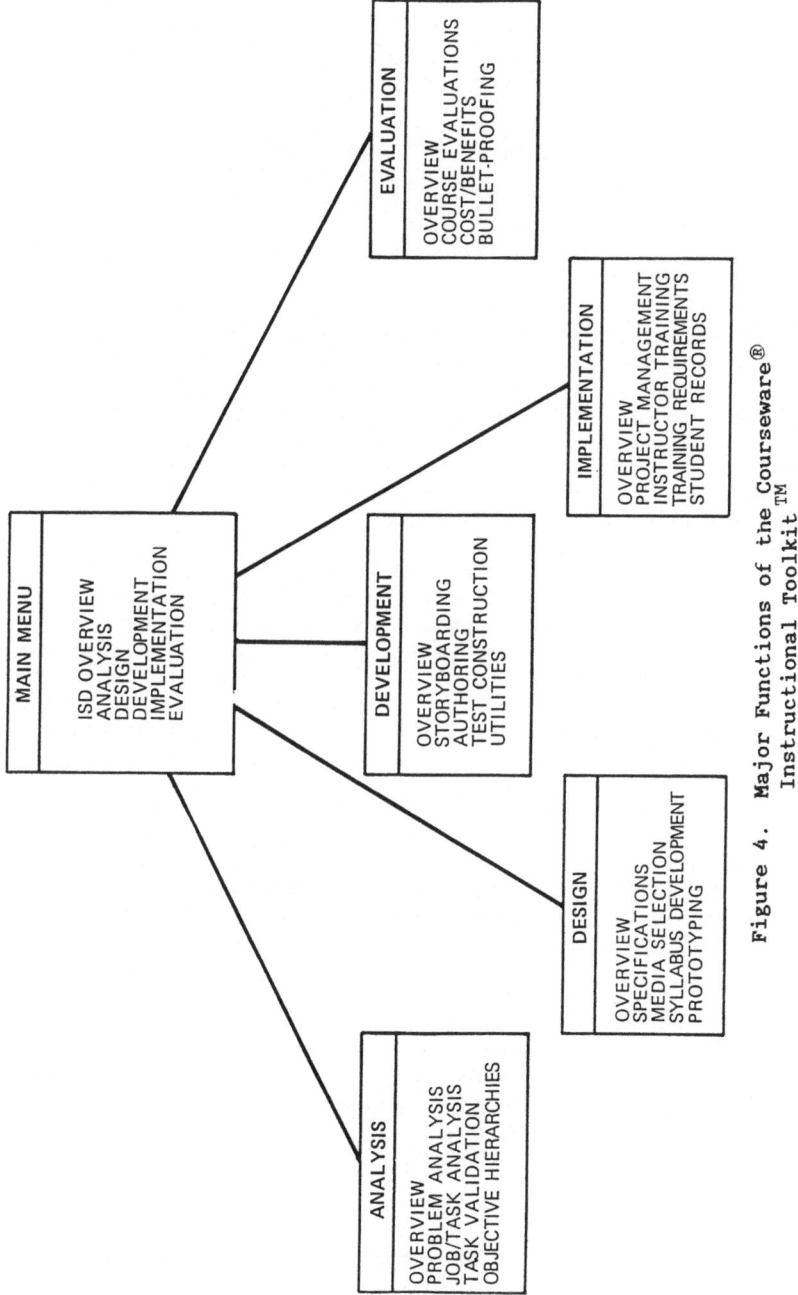

Figure 4. Major Functions of the Courseware® Instructional Toolkit™

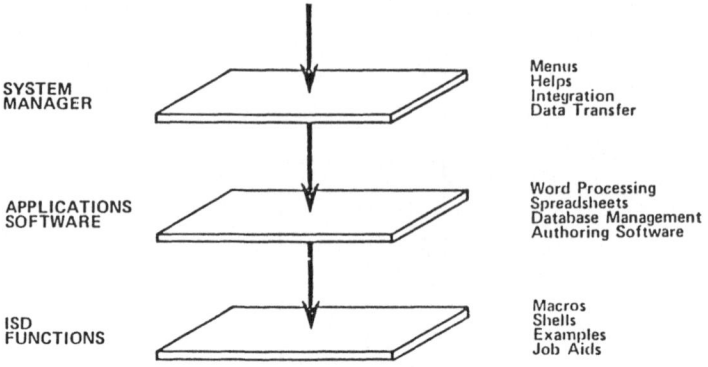

Figure 5. Functional Structure of the Courseware® Instructional Toolkit™

One of the practical benefits of the Toolkit is that it allows libraries of functions to be created and hence reduces the need to reinvent things. Most functions can be reused in subsequent projects producing considerable time savings. Furthermore, as multiple functions are developed for each aspect of instructional design, the designer is presented with a selection of options instead of just one approach. The Toolkit provides a means to introduce reliability into instructional design since each function works the same way each time it is used.

While the practical benefits of the Toolkit are numerous, it was really developed as a research vehicle to study the fundamental question of what could and could not be automated in instructional design. Our findings are that almost any instructional design task can be automated to some degree. However, almost every task has an intuitive or judgmental component that relies on the experience of the designer. Automation of this aspect of instructional design will likely require expert system approaches.

One of the most interesting research questions that the Toolkit allows to be examined is the interrelationships among different instructional tasks. Because it is possible to transfer data from one function to another, it is feasible to collect data on what kinds of transfers are most common. It is also possible to investigate the automation of such transfers, e.g., moving objectives to test construction, lesson specifications to scripts/storyboards, evaluation data to lesson content, etc.

It is not known how the effectiveness or quality of procedures conducted using the Toolkit compares to those done strictly manually. In order to make this kind of assessment, it will be necessary to measure the impact of instructional design methodology on training/learning outcomes, a nontrivial task.

CONCLUSION

This article has discussed the evolution of authoring tools from the earliest authoring languages to currently emerging developments such as intelligent authoring systems and automated instructional systems. This evolution is depicted in Figure 6. One of the important implications of this evolution as shown in the figure is that each authoring approach supplements the others in existence. In other words, as time goes on, an increasingly wider range of authoring alternatives is available. The

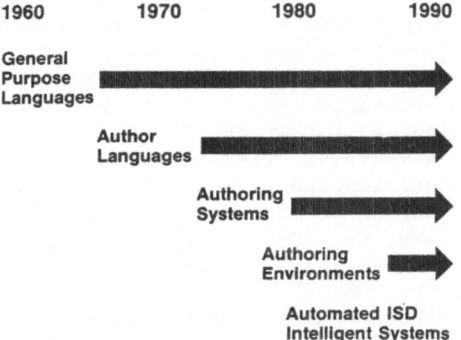

Figure 6. Increasing Variety of Authoring Tools Provides New Options for CBT

problem for an instructional designer or training manager is to choose what kind of tool (e.g., languages, system, environment) is best suited to the instruction to be developed. Little research has been conducted on this kind of authoring tool selection task, although there are some guidelines available (e.g., Locates & Carr, 1985).

One aspect of authoring system design that was not discussed in this paper was the incorporation of instructional theory into the workings of authoring software. Authoring tools present an opportunity to operationalize principles and procedures for good instructional design. For example, an authoring system could critique the design of screen displays in terms of cluttering, text spacing, color or font combinations, placing of graphics, reading level, etc. Similarly, authoring systems could identify missing examples, the need for more practice exercises, the lack of cohesion or flow among lessons, etc. Such efforts would allow us to put theory into practice in a much more effective fashion than at present. This should be an important aspect of future research and development in authoring software.

REFERENCES

Allen, M.W. (1984). A new approach to authoring CBE courseware. "Proceedings, Sixth Interservice/Industry Training Equipment Conference." Washington, D.C.
Allessi, S.M. & Trollip, S.R. (1985). "Computer-Based Instruction: Methods and Development." Englewood Cliffs, NJ: Prentice-Hall.
Avner, A. (1979). Production of computer based instructional materials. In H.F. O'Neil (Ed.), "Issues in Instructional Systems Development." New York: Academic Press.
Avner, A., Smith, S. & Tenczar, P. (1979). CBI authoring tools: Effects on productivity and quality. "Journal of Computer-Based Instruction," "11," 85-89.
Bork, A. (1984). Production systems for computer based learning. In D. Walker and R. Hess (Eds.), "Instructional Software." Belmont, CA: Wadsworth.
Braby, R. & Kincaid, J.P.(1981). Computer aided authoring and editing. "Journal of Educational Technology Systems," "10(2)," 109-124.
Brown, J.S., Burton, R.R. deKleer, J., (1982). Pedagogical, natural language and knowledge engineering techniques in SOPHIE I, II, and III. In D. Sleeman and J.S. Brown (Eds.), "Intelligent Tutoring Systems." New York: Academic Press.

Bunderson, C.V. (1974). The design and production of learner controlled courseware for the TICCIT system: A progress report. "Journal of Man-Machine Studies," "6," 479-491.

Collins, A. (1977). Processes in acquiring knowledge. In R.C. Anderson, R.J. Spiro and W.F. Montague (Eds.), "Schooling and Acquisition of Knowledge." Hillside, NJ: Lawrence Erlbaum Associates.

Gagne, R.M., Wager, W. & Rojas, A. (1981). Planning and authoring computer assisted instructional lessons. "Educational Technology," "21," 17-26.

Heines, J.M. (1983). "Screen Design Strategies for Computer Aided Instruction." Bedford, MA: Digital Press.

Kearsley, G. (1982). Authoring systems in computer based education. "Communications of the ACM," "25," 429-437.

Kearsley, G. (1984). Microcomputer software: Design and development principles. "Journal of Educational Computing Research," "1(2)," 215-226.

Kearsley, G. (1985). Helps, simulations and intelligent tutors. "Data Training."

Kearsley, G. (1985). Instructional design and authoring software. "Journal of Instructional Development," "7(3)," 11-16.

Kearsley, G. (1986). "Authoring: A Guide to the Design of Instructional Software." Reading, MA: Addison-Wesley.

Locates, C. & Carr, V. (1985). Selecting authoring systems. "Journal of Computer-Based Instruction," "12(2)," 28-33.

Merrill, M.D. & Wood, L.E. (1984). Computer guided instructional design. "Journal of Computer-Based Instruction," "11(2)," 60-63.

O'Neil, A.F., O'Neil, H.L., Author Management Systems. In H.F. O'Neil (Ed.), "Issues in Instructional Systems Design." New York: Academic Press, 1979.

Sleeman, D. and Brown, J.S. (1982). "Intelligent Tutoring Systems." New York: Academic Press.

Starkweather, T. (1985). A User's Guide to PILOT. Englewood Cliffs, NJ: Prentice-Hall.

Stevens, A. & Roberts, B. (1983). Quantitative and qualitative simulation in computer based training. "Journal of Computer-Based Instruction," "10(1&2)," 16-19.

INDEX

Advanced Instructional
  System (AIS), 145-148,
  150-154, 295
Artificial Intelligence,
  6, 9, 12, 14, 18,
  28, 42, 56-57,
  153, 175-177,
  231, 242-243,
  246-247, 286,
  289-299, 310,
  313, 317, 320-321,
  333-334
Audio-visual systems, 216
Authoring, 4-6, 59, 62-63,
  65, 74, 111, 151-153,
  163-166, 169-170,
  175, 197, 201, 203-204,
  206-207, 265,
  267-268, 290,
  296-305, 311,
  331-336, 338-340
  intelligent authoring
    aids, 296, 299,
    302-303, 305
  languages, 5-6, 102,
    164, 170, 173,
    212, 223, 226-227,
    297-298, 338
  tools, 164, 293, 296-299,
    331-336, 338-339

Basic Acoustic Trainer (BAT),
  95, 98, 101, 103-104
Basic Radar Skills Trainer
  (BRST), 95, 97-98
Battlefield Engagement
  Simulator and
  Trainer (BEST),
  278, 280, 281

CAI, see Computer-assisted
  instruction, 5, 10,
  57-58, 91, 98,
  103-104, 146, 152,
  154, 175, 198, 200,
  238, 255, 305, 311,
  313, 334-335
CAITER, 59, 63-68
CBI, see Computer-based
  instruction, 1-10,
  30-32, 40-43, 46,
  53, 55, 59-67, 74,
  145, 152-153, 163-
  164, 181, 197-202,
  293, 295-301, 306-
  307, 309-310, 331-
  334, 339
CHIP, see Computerized Hand-
  Held Instruction
  Prototype, 237-238
Classroom instruction, 97-
  98, 146, 151
Cognitive psychology, 105,
  251, 283, 286, 299-
  300, 305-307,
  309-310
Cognitive science, 7, 9, 56,
  171, 299-300,
  305-307, 310-311, 313,
  316
Computer adaptive testing,
  10, 108-109,
  113-114
Computer-assisted instruction,
  (see, also Computer-
  based instruction,
  2, 6, 10-12, 20,
  57, 101-146, 181,
  197, 255, 296, 311

341

Computer-Assisted/Managed
    Instructional
    Language (CAMIL),
    145-146
Computer-Assisted Management
    of Learning (CAMOL),
    69
Computer-based instruction,
    1, 10, 29-30, 41,
    45, 57, 59-60,
    62-63, 66-68, 74,
    145, 153-154, 163-
    164, 175-176, 197,
    202, 283, 285, 295-
    296, 310-312, 331,
    335
  courseware, 59, 60, 66
  hardware, 59, 215
  software, 59, 68, 215
Computer-based testing
    and assessment,
    105
Computer-based training,
    5, 45, 56, 74,
    95, 145, 203,
    207, 215, 228,
    231, 293, 295,
    299, 310, 340
Computer-managed instruction,
    2, 146, 197,
    255, 295
  reports, 146
  software, 255
Computerized Hand-Held
    Instructional
    Prototype, 237
Cost effectiveness of
    CBI systems, 176
Courseware, 3-6, 8, 43,
    59-63, 65-67, 74,
    96, 181, 197, 199,
    202, 204-213,
    256-257, 293,
    295, 297-298,
    300, 331-336,
    338-340

Curriculum, 14, 17, 23-24,
    116, 153, 204-207,
    209, 211, 220,
    225, 293-295,
    298, 309

DES, see Domain Expert
    System, 22-23,
    26-27

Diagnostic, 11-14, 45,
    57, 105, 109, 117,
    119-120, 136-138,
    142-144, 259, 299,
    301, 303, 306,
    314-316, 319,
    334-335
  decision aid, 6
  feedback, 43-44, 54
  job aids, 11, 16
  maintenance, 13
  testing, 109, 117-118,
    120
Domain Expert Systems
    (DES), 22-23,
    25, 27

Educational psychology,
    20, 57, 259
Embedded training, see
    Training, 8, 333
Environment, 2, 5-6,
    12-14, 17-18,
    31-32, 40, 51,
    62-63, 65,
    67-68, 74-75
    92, 94, 146,
    151-153, 156,
    159, 170, 173,
    181, 198, 209,
    215, 235, 243,
    268-269, 272,
    275-278, 281,
    286-288, 303,
    305, 307, 310,
    314, 317-320,
    339
  military, 1-4, 10,
    163, 179, 181,
    215, 232, 269,
    295, 301, 310
  nontraditional, 4, 6, 7
  traditional classroom,
    2
Experience-Consolidation
    systems, 285,
    287-292
Expert, 4, 12-14, 17-18,
    21, 27, 29, 31-33,
    36, 40, 42, 44-
    46, 51-52, 55,
    159-160, 164-
    165, 168-169,
    174-176, 179,
    200, 203, 206,
    244, 249, 257,

Expert (continued)
263, 265, 296–297, 299–300, 302–303, 305, 307–310, 315, 317–320
  model, 29–31, 168–169
  systems, 2, 12–13, 20–26, 28, 42–43, 75–76, 153, 177, 242–243, 246–247, 300, 302–303, 310, 317–318, 320, 338
  tutor, 12, 300

Flight simulators, 2, 10, 43, 272, 279, 281

Generator, 3, 18, 22–25, 64–65, 91, 221, 224, 255, 336
  support generator, 29–30, 34–35, 38
  teaching generator, 22–25
Graphics, 3, 4, 6, 8, 18, 44–45, 55–56, 60–64, 110–111, 119, 152, 179, 206, 212, 216, 222–224, 226–227, 232, 265–268, 272, 278,–280 283

Hand-held computer, also Hand-held tutor, 7, 107, 231–233, 238
Hunter Killer Simulation (HUNKS), 29–32, 35–38, 40

ICAI, see Intelligent computer-assisted instruction, 4, 6, 7, 9, 11–14, 17–19, 21–24, 28, 153, 156, 158, 161, 300, 311, 313–320
Individualized instruction, 6, 8, 145, 150–151, 295

Information processing, 175–177, 188, 282, 296, 306
Instructional, 2, 5–10, 12–13, 17–19, 28–30, 32, 43, 55, 57, 66, 68, 71, 81, 95–97, 102–103, 106, 109, 116–119, 145–148, 151–156, 158–160, 162–166, 169–171, 176, 179, 181, 198, 100, 203, 209, 232–238, 276, 282–283, 295–299, 301–315, 317, 319–320, 331–334, 336, 338–340
  design, 150–151, 162, 164, 166, 169, 171, 176, 202–204, 207, 232, 238, 296, 298–300, 302–303, 306, 311, 318, 320
  interface, 19
  management functions, 200
  strategies, 14, 18–19, 109, 160, 164, 169, 209, 300–303, 306, 311, 313, 331, 333
  systems development, 10, 153, 311, 339
Intelligent computer-assisted Instruction, 4, 6, 11–12, 20, 153, 155–156, 197
Intelligent Teaching System (ITS), 6, 29–33, 38, 40
Intelligent Teaching System for Self-Organised Learning (ITSSOL), 32–34, 36–37, 40

Interactive, 1, 5, 7,
    11, 44, 66,
    90, 109, 118,
    145-146, 153,
    163, 166, 168-
    170, 173, 175-
    176, 182, 188,
    203, 206, 255-256,
    303, 307, 310
  systems, 177
  videodisk, 332
Item Response theory, 108,
    111, 120-121

Job aids, 7, 12, 262-263,
    267, 333, 336
  diagnostic, 11, 16
  job performance aids,
    11, 160, 261, 269

Knowledge base, 13, 21-27,
    176, 299-305, 310,
    315-316, 319, 321
Knowledge engineers/
    engineering, 17,
    27-28, 56, 296,
    302, 306-307
Knowledge representation,
    56, 290, 299-300,
    305, 308, 310,
    314, 334

Learner model, 29-30, 33,
    36, 309
Learning strategies, 238

Maintenance training, see
    Training, 8, 11-12,
    14, 283
Mental model, 9, 15, 18,
    171, 306, 308-
    311, 315, 319
Microprocessor Controlled
    Video Simulators
    (MCVS), 271, 274-
    277, 283
MicroTICCIT, 204, 206-207, 212

Natural Language
    Interface (NLI),
    22, 24-25, 27, 300, 305

On-line help, 5, 163-164,
    168, 170, 175-177,
    298, 303

Part-task training, see
    Training, (also
    Part-task simulation)
    8, 104, 277, 279
Performance aids, 11, 160
Personal Electronic Aid
    for Maintenance
    (PEAM), 7, 262,-269
Portable Aircrew Trainer
    (PAT), 6, 46, 48-56
Programmed cases, 249, 252-
    259
Programmed learning method,
    216, 219
Programmed languages,
    10, 204, 226,
    297, 305, 331-332

Savings, 5, 12, 71-75,
    81-83, 89, 113,
    148, 150-151, 187,
    198, 295
  cost, 73-75, 181, 198,
    298
  student time, 147-148
  training time, 147, 150, 152
Self-organised learning,
    6, 29-34, 38-40
Simulation, 2, 4, 6-7,
    10, 13-19, 29,
    41-46, 50-51,
    54-55, 69, 72-
    73, 75-76, 89-
    90, 92, 94-95,
    111, 243, 275,
    277, 279-280,
    282-283, 285,
    291-292, 313,
    215-321, 332-
    333, 340
Student model, see Learner
    model, 6, 22-25,
    27, 160, 315, 335
Subject domain, see
    Domain, 22, 24-26
Subject matter expert, 8,
    17, 164-165,
    169, 265, 296-
    297, 299, 302,
    305, 333

Test, 15, 19, 25, 30, 36,
    52, 98, 103, 106-
    123, 125, 136-
    138, 142-144,
    146-150, 153,

Test (continued)
    159, 174-182,
    208,-210, 218,
    220, 228-229,
    231-233, 235-
    238, 242, 251,
    257-258, 265-
    266, 268-269,
    271, 286, 295,
    298, 302-304,
    306, 318, 321
  administration, 106
  analysis, 70, 81-82,
    106, 146
  computer adaptive
    testing, 107-109,
    113-114
  diagnostic testing,
    109,117-118,
    120
  diagnostic adaptive
    testing, 117
Time Shared Interactive
    Computer-Controlled
    Information Television (TICCIT) 4,
    57, 60-62, 65,
    68, 163, 209,
    299, 332, 340
Trainer for Radio
    Intercept Operation
    (TRIO), 46, 56,
    313, 317-320
Training, 1-3, 5-10, 11-12,
    14, 16-17, 19-20,
    22, 31, 40-44,
    46, 52, 55-57,
    69-76, 81-85,
    89-96, 98-104,
    111, 118, 120,
    176, 179-182,
    185-188, 200,
    202,-209, 212,
    215-221, 224,
    227-229, 231-
    233, 235-240, 249,
    252, 256-257, 259,
    261, 263-264, 269,
    271, 274-282, 285,
    287, 289-290, 290,
    293-300, 303, 305,
    310, 312-314, 317,
    320-321, 332-334,
    338-340, 349

Training (continued)
  combat training, 92
  decision making,
  devices, 10, 18, 43,
    56, 73, 95-96,
    199, 220, 231-
    232, 271, 276-
    277, 282, 285
  electronics training,
    76
  embedded, 8, 333
  flight, 45-46
  gunnery training, 277
  introductory training,
  in military, 1-4, 7,
    10, 41, 43,
    57, 89, 95,
    118, 154,
    176, 197-199,
    202, 215, 271,
    293, 304, 311
  maintenance, 8, 11-12,
    14, 283
  part-task training,
    104, 277, 279
  perceptual skills
    training, 99
  procedural skills
    training, 99
  sonar training, 98, 100
  technical, 6, 14, 91,
    145, 153-154,
    283, 293, 307
  tactical, 73
  transfer of, 43, 100
  troubleshooting
    training, 316
  weapon training, 89,
    91, 93-94

Tutor, 2, 13, 21-29, 45,
    61, 159-160, 170,
    173-174, 177,
    232-238, 295,
    297, 300-303,
    306, 310, 314-315

User, 3, 5, 7-9, 13,
    17, 24, 62, 67-
    68, 70, 106,
    110, 114, 152,
    163-177, 179-187,
    197, 199-204, 234,
    238, 248, 262, 264-
    269, 275, 277-278,
    285, 288-289, 291,

User (continued)
 299, 303, 305, 311
 friendly, 181, 183, 203
 interface, 24, 65, 75-177

Videodiscs (<u>also</u> Video disk),
 4, 18, 65, 91, 119,
 216, 220, 222-224,
 226-227, 229, 298
Video Game, 271-178, 280,
 282-283